Mosby's Fundame

ANIMAL HEALTH T.

PRINCIPLES
OF
PHARMACOLOGY

Mosby's Fundamentals of
ANIMAL HEALTH TECHNOLOGY

Series editor

Roger G. Warren, V.M.D.

SMALL ANIMAL ANESTHESIA
Roger G. Warren

SMALL ANIMAL SURGICAL NURSING
Diane L. Tracy, *Editor*

SMALL ANIMAL RADIOGRAPHY
Lawrence J. Kleine

PRINCIPLES OF PHARMACOLOGY
Richard Giovanoni

Mosby's Fundamentals of
ANIMAL HEALTH TECHNOLOGY

PRINCIPLES
OF
PHARMACOLOGY

Richard Giovanoni, B.S.Pharm., M.S.Pharm., M.Ed.

Director of Pharmacy,
Massachusetts Eye and Ear Infirmary,
Boston, Massachusetts

Roger G. Warren, V.M.D., Series editor

The University of Florida, School of Veterinary Medicine,
Gainesville, Florida

with 57 illustrations

The C. V. Mosby Company

ST. LOUIS • TORONTO • LONDON   1983

MOSBY

A TRADITION OF PUBLISHING EXCELLENCE

Editor: Eugenia A. Klein
Assistant editor: Jean F. Carey
Manuscript editor: Stephen C. Hetager
Book design: Jeanne Bush
Cover design: Diane Beasley
Production: Susan Trail

Printed in the United States of America

The C.V. Mosby Company
11830 Westline Industrial Drive, St. Louis, Missouri 63141

Library of Congress Cataloging in Publication Data

Giovanoni, Richard.
    Principles of pharmacology.

    (Mosby's fundamentals of animal health technology)
    Bibliography: p.
    Includes index.
    1. Veterinary pharmacology.   I. Title.
II. Series.   [DNLM: 1. Drug therapy—Veterinary.
2. Pharmacology.   SF915 G512p]
SF915.G56   1983   636.089'57   82-14534

ISBN 0-8016-5402-5

C/VH/VH   9   8   7   6   5   4   01/B/078

To

my family

whose respect for all life forms provided me
with sympathetic insight

to the

authors

of the other volumes in this series
for sharing their medical expertise with me

and to all

future students of veterinary technology

who will provide a fresh approach to its study

Mosby's Fundamentals of
ANIMAL HEALTH TECHNOLOGY

Since the inception of the first formal college-level training program for animal health technicians (AHTs) in 1961, the demand for skilled veterinary paraprofessionals has grown appreciably. In 1975, the American Veterinary Medical Association (AVMA) assumed the responsibility for the accreditation of AHT programs and established the Committee on Animal Technician Activities and Training (CATAT). In the same year, the Association of Animal Technician Educators (AATE) was formed for the purpose of assuring quality instruction for students, providing guidance to graduate AHTs, and assisting educators and practitioners. Since then, many state veterinary licensing boards and practice acts have instituted examinations and certification requirements for AHTs.

In spite of a well-established and well-organized educational foundation, there has been no compilation of text material written expressly for the AHT. The Mosby series addresses this need by providing comprehensive information that will enable educators and practitioners to blend this material with both formal and in-service training programs. The text material is liberally illustrated and presented in a way that facilitates student and curriculum evaluation. Specific performance objectives are provided at the beginning of each chapter to aid the instructor in developing a curriculum or training program and to help the student in comprehending the focus of the material.

It is our hope that this series will expand and improve in concert with the burgeoning field of animal health technology.

Roger G. Warren

Preface

This volume is an introductory guide to the study of drug composition, mechanisms by which drugs interact with biological systems to produce beneficial or detrimental effects, and drug administration as a therapeutic tool. These considerations constitute the field of study known as pharmacology.

An introduction to a medical discipline such as pharmacology is most effective when it presents overviews of and generalization about current principles. This volume is intended to provide coherent, rational, and scientific explanations of currently accepted principles underlying the clinical use of medications. When these principles are complex, I have taken liberties to present simplified explanations in the hope that they will create a climate for further investigation by the reader. Individual chapters may be supplemented by books, articles, and lectures that more thoroughly discuss the areas of pharmacology introduced in this volume. The aim of this volume is to systematically expose, rather than elaborate on, certain pharmacological principles.

This book is concerned with the mechanics of drug actions and with the discussion of drug classes. It is hoped that an understanding of the concepts behind drug classes will prompt further research by the reader.

Although dose-related responses are discussed, this book is not a primer for the exclusive study of dosimetry. It will be emphasized on many occasions that dosage should be a function of a practitioner's judgment and an animal's overall condition; it does not depend solely on the published literature about a drug. Wide fluctuations in dosage are inevitable and necessary, since a practitioner must deal with many pathological conditions and many species.

This volume is broad in scope, reflecting the myriad considerations that constitute current pharmacological rationale. The first and second chapters deal with principles, observations, and theories associated with drug bioavailability and elimination. It is intended that the reader will apply this information to subsequent chapters, which discuss diuretics, central nervous system drugs, selected anti-infectives, anti-inflammatory drugs, and cardiovascular drugs.

It is my hope that this book will provide a worthwhile introduction to pharmacology. I welcome comments about the volume and would appreciate suggestions for future editions.

Richard Giovanoni

Contents

1 Drug absorption, 1

2 Drug distribution and elimination, 22

3 Diuretic drugs, 46

4 Drugs affecting the central nervous system, 58

5 Anti-infective drugs and immunologicals, 104

6 Anti-inflammatory drugs, 164

7 Cardiovascular drugs, 203

Appendix A Guide for intravenous administration of drugs, 226

B Federal classification of and regulations for addictive drugs, 228

1

Drug absorption

PERFORMANCE OBJECTIVES

After completion of this chapter the student will:

- Explain the difference between acid-stable and acid-labile drugs
- List two methods suggested to administer drugs that are irritating to the gastrointestinal tract
- Explain the relationship between undissociated drug molecules, pH, and degree of drug absorption
- Compare the relative importances of pH, partition coefficient, and enzyme transport systems with respect to drug absorption
- Calculate the partition coefficient of a drug when given its lipid and water solubilities
- List two advantages and two limitations of each of the following: intromuscular drug administration, intravenous drug administration
- List four general guidelines to be observed when drugs are being mixed in a solution intended for intravenous administration
- Differentiate between "intravenous bolus" and "intravenous infusion" of a drug
- Categorize epidermic, diadermic, and endodermic ointment bases in terms of relative skin-penetrating ability
- List three factors that influence the absorption rate of inhaled drugs

Chemicals that are used to prevent, diagnose, or treat disease are called drugs. Some drugs are discovered accidentally; others are intentionally designed for use against certain disorders. It is vital to remember that drugs are not mystical entities that ignore principles of chemical reactions, but are substances that act in a predictable quantitative and qualitive fashion within the environment they are placed. For the purposes of this book, this environment consists of the biological systems of various animals. The reaction of a biological system to a drug is a function of the peculiarities of the drug. These peculiarities range from simple considerations, such as how fast the drug in a certain dosage form dissolves (dissolution rate), to presumptions about complicated, only partially understood tissue receptor reactions with drug molecules. In vitro studies of a drug's characteristics are equally as important as in vivo observations of its clinical activity. The amount of a drug that is ultimately released into a particular biological system is measurable; it is expressed as the degree of drug bioavailability.

ORAL ADMINISTRATION

The route of administration of a drug has a marked impact on the degree of bioavailability and therefore is a consideration when manufacturers formulate a drug product. The oral route is a popular and convenient means of drug administration for most animals, with the exception of cats and cows. Tablets, capsules, and liquids are examples of oral dosage forms.

The vast majority of oral tablets and capsules are not exclusively composed of active ingredients. Generally, solid oral dosage forms contain nonactive ingredients, which may include the following:

1. Binders, such as lactose—added to avoid breakage of tablets during manufacture, transportation, and administration
2. Lubricants, such as magnesium stearate—to prevent adhesion of the ingredients to the production machinery parts, especially the dye molds that compress the powdered formulation under great pressure to produce a tablet
3. Dissolution aids, such as sodium bicarbonate—to decrease a tablet's disintegration time once it comes into contact with an aqueous medium
4. Desiccants, including silica gel—to avoid premature degradation of the active ingredient(s) by humidity
5. Diluents (bulk-producing agents), the most common being lactose (milk sugar)—to make a tablet or capsule large enough so that administration can be facilitated. It is generally accepted that a tablet approximately the size of an aspirin is the most convenient to administer to either animals or humans. Smaller tablets can become misplaced in the mouth and begin to dissolve, imparting an undesirable taste and making further administrations more difficult. Large tablets or capsules also cause problems of acceptance, especially in smaller animals.

Manufacturers' package inserts usually list both the nonactive and the active ingredients present in drug products.

For purposes of uniformity and technical correctness, in this book the term "drug" will refer only to the medicinal or active ingredient(s) present in a dosage form. Consequently, terms describing dosage forms (such as tablet or capsule) will include the drug(s) as well as other ingredients in the formulations.

For reasons to be considered shortly, the oral route is not always optimal from the standpoint of drug stability and/or patient acceptability, especially when drugs are administered to veterinary patients.

Acid stability and lability

The stomach is the first major organ to significantly degrade foodstuffs and other agents entering the gastrointestinal tract via the oral cavity. The degradation process relies largely on the presence of hydrochloric acid, which is secreted by the gastric glands located in the mucosal portion of an animal's stomach. As a result, the normal physiological environment of the stomach is usually about pH 1. This acidic environment is beneficial for activation of certain digestive enzymes found in the stomachs of some species. These enzymes also participate in the initial process of food biodegradation. Some drugs, most notably epinephrine and insulin, are significantly destroyed by the stomach environment and thus are termed *acid-labile* drugs.

Acid lability is not absolute; that is, drugs are degraded in varying degrees, with some not being measurably affected. If a drug is degraded to the extent that the anticipated clinical activity is marginal or absent, the drug is considered *clinically acid labile* and should not be administered by the oral route. For most species, benzylpenicillin (pencillin G), for example, is clinically acid labile. However, it can be orally administered to dogs and display clinically significant anti-infective activity. As will be noted throughout this book, general observations about drug activity must be qualified according to the particular species in question. The practice of veterinary medicine encompasses a wide variety of biological systems.

The amount of drug degradation resulting from the stomach environment can be lessened by adjusting the dosage schedule. If a drug is sensitive to gastric secretions, it may be administered with anticipated results when the stomach is *empty*, since less acid is present and the pH is slightly higher. A clinically practical time for administering a drug when the stomach is empty is *1 hour before a meal or 2 hours after a meal*, providing the animal is not a ruminant. Although individual drugs within a therapeutic drug class can be either acid stable or acid labile, it is prudent to administer all drugs in a class by the same dosage schedule.

An advantage of administering a drug on an empty stomach is that *drug absorption is hastened*. The drug passes through the stomach quicker in the absence of food because it is not delayed in the digestive process. This reduction in contact time with the stomach can lessen the amount of biodegradation a somewhat acid-labile drug undergoes.

In some instances acid-labile drugs can be either chemically or physically altered to make oral administration feasible. Chemical alteration involves changing the drug molecule to render it less acid labile. It was mentioned earlier that penicillin G is acid labile in most species. However, the addition of a phenoxymethyl group and potassium to penicillin G changes the molecule to potassium phenoxymenthyl penicillin, which is markedly less acid-labile in most animals:

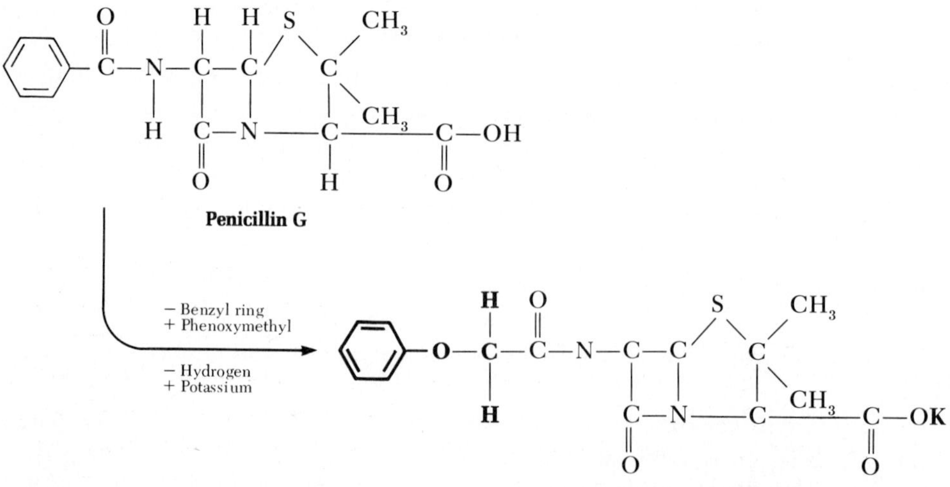

Penicillin G

− Benzyl ring
+ Phenoxymethyl

− Hydrogen
+ Potassium

**Potassium phenoxymethyl penicillin
(penicillin VK)**

After removal of its benzyl group, penicillin G serves as the core structure to which organic molecules, such as phenoxymethyl, are attached. Commercially all semi-synthetic penicillins are manufactured by first removing the benzyl group through fermentation processes and then chemically substituting various organic side chains in its place.

Physically coating a drug with a material, such as synthetic waxes or polymers, that is impermeable to gastric juices can protect an acid-labile drug from stomach acidity. Once the drug passes the stomach, the different pH range of the duodenum and small intestine (approximately 7 for many animals) can serve to dissolve the coating, causing the drug to be released into a more favorable environment. Although technically possible, this alternative is not generally chosen by manufacturers, because of the additional expense that would have to be passed on to the client. Usually, acid-labile drugs are prepared in other dosage forms (such as injections).

Drugs that are not affected by gastric secretions are termed *acid stable*. Like acid lability, acid stability exists in varying degrees. Consequently, a drug that is clinically affected by biologically synthesized hydrochloric acid can be referred to as acid labile even though not all of it is destroyed, and a drug that is not clinically affected by stomach acid can be called acid stable even though a percentage of the drug may be degraded by stomach acid. The following drugs, all of which are antibiotics, are considered acid stable; however, their therapeutic effectiveness is best ensured if they are administered in the absence of food.

Amoxicillin	Dicloxacillin	Penicillin G‡
Ampicillin	Griseofulvin*	Penicillin V
Cephalexin	Hetacillin	Phenethicillin
Cephaloglycin	Oxacillin	Penicillin V
Cloxacillin	Oxytetracycline†	Tetracycline†

Drug irritability

The discussion of acid lability or stability centered around the harmful effects biological systems can have on some drugs. The following discussion deals with the undersirable effects a drug can have on biological systems.

Gastrointestinal secretions are of two types. The first type includes hydrochloric acid and digestive enzymes, both of which are responsible for biodegradation of foodstuffs. The second type, an example of which is mucus, is secreted in all areas of the gastrointestinal tract and is primarily responsible for protection of the tract lining from the digestive secretions. Mucus is a high-molecular-weight substance that is classified as a mucoprotein; it is resistant to almost all biological digestive secretions. Consequently it prevents the penetration of gastric digestive secretions into deeper layers of the stomach mucosal lining. Since the stomach secretions are hostile to unprotected stomach tissue, the entire surface of the stomach is covered by mucus-containing cells. If the integrity of mucous cells is interrrupted, the deeper lining of the stomach becomes vulnerable to destruction by gastric secretions, especially hydrochloric acid. The innate chemical nature of some drugs may irritate mucous cells, and repeated exposure to these drugs can destroy these protective cells.

Since an orally administered drug is most often given in a solid form (such as a tablet or capsule), it settles in a very small area of the stomach and can concentrate its irritant effects in a confined area. The ultimate result of repeated doses is the destruction of mucosal cells and the formation of ulcers because of acid-mediated destruction of stomach lining. The use of proper dosage schedules for irritating drugs can reduce the impact on mucous cells. If a drug is mixed with food, the

---

*If food is given, it should be very low in fat content to avoid drug binding to fatty food.
†If food is given, it should not consist of dairy products (for example, milk, cheese) or be high in iron content.
‡Considered acid stable only in dogs.

physical presence of food in the stomach and intestinal tract dilutes the amount of drug available for contact with the gastrointestinal lining, while peristaltic action keeps the drug particles in motion, thereby further lowering the possibility of prolonged contact.

If a drug is to be administered with food, it must be acid stable, since it will be exposed to prolonged contact with large amounts of gastric secretions. Traditionally, practitioners have suggested concurrent administration of an antacid when an irritant drug is administered. The purpose of antacids is to neutralize stomach acid. Theoretically this may be of benefit, since it would diminish the amount of acid available to attack the stomach lining (providing the animal could be administered the antacid.) Care should be taken, however, not to give excessive amounts of antacid, which could elicit an acid rebound phenomenon. Acid rebound results in an excessive secretion of hydrochloric acid into the stomach to compensate for the unphysiologically high pH brought about by too much antacid. (Commonly used antacids, such as Maalox or Mylanta, are usually combinations of metallic salts such as aluminum and magnesium hydroxides.) An alternative is to administer the drug with large amounts of a bland fluid that exhibits negligible buffering capacity. Milk is acceptable for most animals; however, certain drugs, such as the tetracyclines, are inactivated in its presence.

The concept of coating a drug with an acid-resistant agent that delays drug release, which was mentioned in the dicussion of acid-labile drugs, can sometimes be applied to protect the stomach lining from the drug. Experience with enteric-coated, *delayed-release* potassium chloride tablets, however, has shown that this is not always a desirable alternative, since drug-induced ulcerations can be formed in the small intestine rather than the stomach. Enteric coatings are designed to dissolve in the small intestine, thus releasing the drug there rather than in the stomach. With delayed-release forms all of the drug is made available for absorption in a very short time at one location. Enteric *sustained-release* dosage forms differ from enteric delayed-release forms in that the former releases a drug over a long period of time (up to 12 hours) as it travels along the intestinal tract, thereby avoiding drug concentration in a small area. Intestinal irritation is more likely to occur with delayed-release forms, since all of the drug is liberated within a relatively small area of the small intestine.

In early sustained-release dosage forms, a drug was implanted within an insoluble, nonabsorbable matrix composed of synthetic polymers and/or waxes. As a tablet traveled along the intestinal tract, intestinal fluids eventually invaded the matrix, dissolving the drug and leaching it from the core. Newer methods have employed the same concept of gradual erosion of the coating, but in place of a single drug receptacle, hundreds of small receptacles, usually spheroidal, contain the drugs(s). These spheroids are usually enclosed in a gelatin capsule, which dissolves in the stomach. The spheroids, however, do not dissolve until they reach the intestines. Different spheroidal coating thicknesses and/or different coating compositions are responsible for releasing medication over extended time periods as the spheroids travel through the intestinal tract.

Several factors, such as drug solubility, pore size of the matrix, and resistance of the coating to erosion, have been demonstrated in vitro to affect sustained drug release. Biological factors, such as peristaltic activity, can also affect drug bioavailability, by altering the rate of drug population along the intestines. If intestinal contents move too rapidly, some of the drug could be eliminated in the feces, resulting in therapeutically inadequate blood levels. On the other hand, since more than one dose of the drug is incorporated into the sustained-release dosage form, the possibility exists that high, toxic blood levels could result if the actual rate of drug release is quicker than anticipated.[1]

Although sustained-release preparations offer a mechanism to administer acid-labile or irritant drugs, their main advantage is that they make possible the attainment of continuous therapeutic blood levels through infrequent dosing, as shown in Fig. 1-1.

Sustained-release pharmaceuticals are generally more expensive than common dosage forms. Therefore their use should be justified by a demonstrable need.

Certain drugs, such as aspirin, incorporated into a delayed-release dosage form have had good success in reducing the potential for gastric disturbances. It seems only prudent, however, that animals receiving chronic drug therapy with enteric

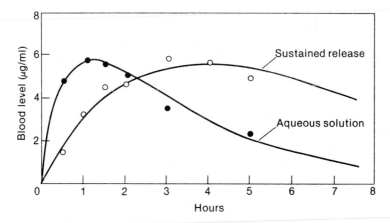

Fig. 1-1. Drug blood levels after administration of a sustained-release drug in dogs. An anthelmintic drug formulated as a sustained-release product and the same drug in a "regular" aqueous solution were given to six dogs. The sustained-release dosage form required more time to reach maximum blood concentration but persisted longer than the aqueous dosage form. (Modified from Wiegand, R.G., and Taylor, J.D.: Kinetics of plasma drug levels after sustained-release dosage, Biochem. Pharmacol. 3:256, 1960.)

TABLE 1-1

Drugs that irritate the gastrointestinal tract in many animals

Drug	Therapeutic cateogry	Enteric form available
Aspirin	Analgesic	Yes
Aminophylline	Bronchodilator	Yes
Dexamethasone	Anti-inflammatory	No
Erythromycin	Anti-infective	Yes
Flumethasone	Anti-inflammatory	No
Fluprednisolone	Anti-inflammatory	No
Hydrocortisone	Anti-inflammatory	No
Meclofenamic acid	Anti-inflammatory, analgesic	No
Medroxyprogesterone	Anti-inflammatory	No
Methylprednisolone	Anti-inflammatory	No
Phenylbutazone	Anti-inflammatory, analgesic	No
Prednisone	Anti-inflammatory	No

dosage forms be intermittently screened for occult blood in feces. Table 1-1 lists drugs generally considered irritating to the gastrointestinal tract and indicates whether enteric dosage forms are available.

Occasionally a practitioner must prescribe an irritating, acid-labile drug. In such a situation, experience with the drug, the animal's overall condition, and the nature of the pathological condition must all be considered in the final determination of the dose schedule.

pH

Consideration of a drug's pH and the pH of its environment is essential to understanding the drug's absorption profile with respect to rate and location. A substance's pH is an expression of the degree of acidity or alkalinity the substance exhibits. Any substance dissociates (dissolves) to some extent in an aqueous medium, forming electrically charged particles called ions. Positively charged ions are termed *cations,* and negatively charged ions are called *anions*. The interaction of these cations and anions in the aqueous medium results, in a measurable effect that can be classified as a basic, acidic, or neutral response. No chemical is absolutely soluble (dissociates 100%), and likewise no chemical is absolutely insoluble. When placed in an aqueous vehicle, all substances dissociate into ions to some extent, but never entirely. Consequently three forms of a pure chemical can exist simultaneously in an aqueous environment: anions and cations (the dissociated components) and the undissociated, *non-charged* component, consisting of electrostatically bonded atoms (which become ions upon dissociation). The degree of dissociation dictates the concentration of a chemical in each phase. Very soluble chemicals, including drugs, have most of their weight in the dissocated phase; the opposite is true for relatively insoluble chemicals. These concepts can be summarized as follows:

"Insoluble" compounds
[Anions]$^-$ + [Cations]$^+$ $\rightleftarrows$ **[Anion and cation combined]**

"Soluble" compounds
[Anions]$^-$ + [Cations]$^+$ $\leftrightarrows$ [Anion and cation combined]

The extent of a compound's solubility is proportional to the number of ions in solution. As solubility increases, the number of distinct anions and cations increases while the nonionized (undissociated) portion diminishes.

Drugs adhere to the same dissociation principles as nontherapeutic chemicals. All drugs, on the basis of their degree of dissociation and interaction of ions, can be classified as acidic, basic, or neutral chemicals. Therefore when the three forms (anions, cations, and undissociated molecules) concurrently exist in an aqueous medium, the drug exhibits an inherent pH value determined by the interaction of its three forms. For example, the pH of tetracycline is approximately 2 (strong acid), while aminophylline is usually pH 11 (strong base). The high pH of aminophylline is primarily responsible for its irritating action on the gastrointestinal tract.

It is fundamental to remember that *drugs are more undissociated (nonionized) at their inherent pH and become more dissociated (ionized) the farther they move away from that pH*. Tetracycline exists primarily in the undissociated form at pH 2 and primarily in its ionized form (as anions and cations) at pH 11. This principle is a major consideration, since different compartments of the body have markedly different pH values. Thus as a drug moves from one area of the body to another, the relative amounts of drug in each form will shift significantly, thereby altering its absorption rate.

A companion fundamental principle to remember is that *drugs are absorbed from the gastrointestinal tract only in the undissociated (nonionized) form*. Since the pH environment of a biological system affects the dissociated/undissociated equilibrium, it can enhance or discourage drug absorption. If the undissociated form is favored, absorption is promoted; conversely, if ionization is promoted, absorption is discouraged. Fig. 1-2 illustrates this principle by comparing relative amounts of ionization for some common drugs in various body compartments.

During normal situations relatively few drugs are absorbed from the stomach. This is primarily due to the low pH environment of the stomach, which favors ionization of most oral drugs, and the lack of substantial enzymatic activity. The small intestine is the primary focus for absorption of orally administered drugs, since its pH environment is markedly higher than that of the stomach, thereby

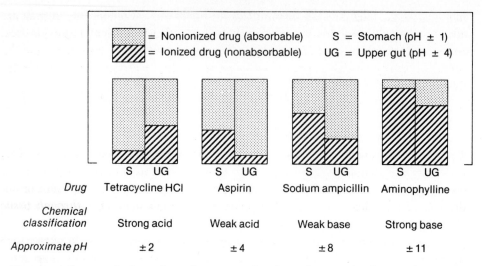

Fig. 1-2. Influence of pH on drug absorption. The closer the pH of a drug to the pH of its biological compartment (such as the stomach or intestine), the more nonionized the drug will be. The amount of drug represented by the dotted area is potentially available for absorption. As the pH of a drug's environment moves farther away from the drug's own pH, the more ionized the drug becomes and the smaller the amount that will be available for absorption (striped area).

promoting the nonionized form of many drugs. The amiable environment for drug absorption in the small intestine can be illustrated by the fate of orally administered aspirin in most nonruminant animals. If 600 mg of aspirin is given, in most species approximately 390 mg is ionized in the stomach and 210 mg is nonionized and available for absorption. Most animals exhibit minimal absorption of aspirin from the stomach; thus somewhat less than 600 mg moves into the small intestine. In the small intestine (pH about 7) approximately 540 mg is nonionized and absorbable into the bloodstream while less than 60 mg is in the ionized form.

Partition coefficient

Although the degree of nonionization is a major factor is determining a drug's rate of passage through tissue barriers (for example, from gastrointestinal tract to bloodstream), a measure of the drug's relative lipid solubility is of equal importance. Lipid solubility is a measure of how much drug dissolves in a nonaqueous medium. Most often, in vitro tests to determine a drug's partition coefficient use nonaqueous organic solvents, such as n-heptane, benzene, or cottonseed oil, adjusted to physiologic pH ranges. Unfortunately there is no way to determine which organic solvent(s) is most similar to cell membranes. The more soluble a drug is in a lipid solvent, the less soluble it is in an aqueous solvent. To measure how much more soluble a drug is in one solvent than in the other, equal amounts of drug are added to equal amounts of water and an organic (lipid) solvent under identical conditions. The amount of drug that dissolves in each solvent is measured, and the relative solubilities of the drug in each solvent are then compared by means of the following formula:

$$\text{Partition coefficient} = \frac{\text{Lipid solubility (grams)}}{\text{Water solubility (grams)}}$$

The higher the numerical value, the more lipid soluble the drug. *Lipid solubility is directly proportional to the degree of drug nonionization in vivo.* A high partition coefficient value indicates low water solubility and therefore a large amount of undissociated particles, a situation that *enhances a drug's movement through tissue barriers.*

It may seem contradictory that some drugs that are very soluble in water, such as the short-acting barbiturate sodium secobarbital, attain therapeutic blood levels shortly after oral dosing, indicating absorption from the stomach. The pH of sodium secobarbitual is around 10, and therefore this drug is almost exclusively ionized in the stomach, where the pH is 1. However, like many drugs, sodium secobarbitual exists simultaneously in the ionized and nonionized forms while in the stomach. Its nonionized form has a very high partition coefficient, which favors immediate diffusion through the stomach wall into the bloodstream, thereby removing it from the stomach and upsetting the equilibrium between the two phases (ionized and nonionized). In order to preserve the equilibrium, drug in the ionized form is converted to the nonionized form, thereby reducing the amount of nonabsorbable (ionized) drug in the stomach. In turn, the nonionized drug passes through the stomach wall into the bloodstream, causing more ionized drug to be converted to the nonionized form, and so on. Consequently a therapeutic blood level is quickly attained, as a result of the concept illustrated in Fig. 1-3.

Enzymatic activity and membrane transport

Enzymes, which are usually high-molecular-weight chemicals containing nitrogen, can be produced by living cells regardless of whether the cells constitute only a portion of the total organism (as in higher species) or are themselves entire living organisms (for example, bacteria). The evolutionary need for intestinal enzymes came about largely for reasons of food absorption. In higher organisms, specific bacteria found in the intestinal tract manufacture enzymes necessary for the movement of food molecules from the intestinal tract to the bloodstream. Since foodstuffs contain the same elemental atoms, molecules, groups of molecules, and chemical bonds that many drugs contain, these enzymes are likewise instrumental in drug absorption. Some enzymes are unique to a particular species, owing to their evolutionary synthesis and particular function, while others are relatively commonplace, being found in most species.

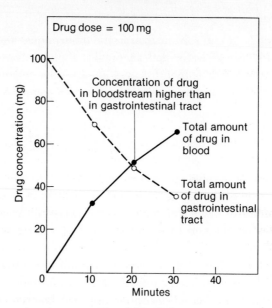

Fig. 1-3. Comparison of gastrointestinal and blood drug concentrations. As drug molecules leave the gastrointestinal tract (dotted line) and enter the bloodstream, their concentration in the bloodstream increases (solid line). The higher the partition coefficient of the drug, the quicker it will pass from the gastrointestinal tract into the bloodstream. Depending upon the rate at which the drug is removed from the blood, eventually a condition can occur in which more drug is in the blood than in the gastrointestinal tract. The excretion rate also determines whether this condition will persist for a long time or be brief.

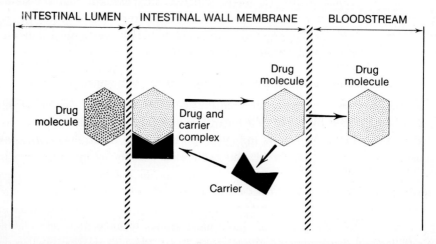

Fig. 1-4. Carrier concept. Movement of drug molecules from the intestinal tract to the bloodstream sometimes requires the attachment of a carrier, which may be an enzyme or another agent used to facilitate the passage of the drug. Occasionally the drug's composition can be altered by the carrier's attachment; thus the drug delivered to the bloodstream is chemically different from what was in the gastrointestinal tract.

With the exception of pepsin, which is found in the stomachs of many animals, enzymes are complex molecules having many *reactive centers* that can combine with substances called substrates to hasten chemical reactions within a biological system. Some reactions are responsible for biodegradation, which involves the breaking down of foodstuffs to smaller, more absorbable moieties, while others are anabolic in character, contributing to the synthesis of new tissue. Some enzymes are found only in certain species because these enzymes function only within narrow pH and temperature ranges. Although enzymes are primarily catalysts for chemical reactions associated with synthesis and elimination of waste from the body, they are also indispensable for rapid assimilation of foodstuffs from the gut.

As was mentioned earlier, two requirements for rapid drug absorption are non-ionization and high lipid solubility. These prerequisites ensure that the drug molecule will be soluble in the cell membrane separating the intestinal lumen from the bloodstream. Such solubility is necessary for the drug's diffusion and/or transport across the membrane to the bloodstream. Some drug molecules, or portions of drug molecules, that are otherwise insoluble in the cell membrane can form complexes with cellular enzymes and possibly with enzymes in the intestine, thereby allowing their passage through the membrane by either passive or active enzyme-mediated transport mechanisms.

The formation of an enzyme "complex" depends on one or more of an enzyme's reactive centers spacially fitting the molecular configuration of part or all of a drug molecule (substrate). The degree of enzyme specificity to the substrate depends on how well the enzyme "fits" the drug's molecular configuration. The traditional description of how enzymes and substrates interact is the "lock and key" theory. According to this theory, the substrate (lock) is any molecule that the enzyme (key) can chemically interact with to form a new molecule. The enzyme (or carrier) is separated from the substrate-enzyme complex and then recycled to perform the same function innumerable times. This active transport requires energy expenditure by the carrier enzyme, while passive diffusion does not. Oftentimes the substrate-enzyme complex results in a chemical change in the substrate (drug) molecule, and it is the newly created molecule deposited in the bloodstream that exerts the clinical effect. The carrier concept, expressed schematically in Fig. 1-4, is helpful in explaining why some insoluble drugs can be transported from gastrointestinal tract to bloodstream and why only portions of other drugs are found in the bloodstream immediately after their movement from the intestinal tract.

Differences in digestive systems among species

Milleniums of selective species evolution has resulted in a host of different physiochemical and anatomical mechanisms for absorptive, metabolic, and excretory functions. Chemical mediators such as enzymes and anatomical differences associated with absorption developed in response to the different foodstuffs available to different species. Other features, such as detoxification and elimination mechanisms, developed partly in response to the particular biological substances each species was exposed to during its evolutionary development.

Thus anatomical variations associated with the digestive function have an impact on drug therapy. The fate of orally administered drugs in animals with single-chambered stomachs is more predictable than it is in ruminants. When administered with food, drugs can remain in the rumen for up to 3 days, being constantly exposed to ruminal secretions and endemic microbes. Consequently some medications, such as digitalis, that are acid stable in species with single-chambered stomachs are not clinically effective in ruminants, presumably because of biodegradation in the rumen.[4] Some antibiotics administered orally to animals with single-chambered stomachs demonstrate minimal intestine-related side effects, such as diarrhea, because of their efficient transport from the gut. Since antibiotic absorption from the rumen is delayed, contact time is extended. This can result in overt destruction of beneficial endemic microbes, thereby upsetting the normal microbial flora of the rumen and causing diarrhea and possibly dehydration.

The greater the complexity of the digestive tract, the greater the period of time required to produce therapeutic blood levels of an orally administered drug. If a situation requires that therapeutic blood levels be attained quickly, routes other than those employing the digestive (enteral) system should be used, especially in ruminants.

RECTAL ADMINISTRATION

Partly because of the restraining measures that are usually necessary, rectal administration of a drug is limited to situations in which the oral route is not suitable. If an animal is vomiting, the oral route is not recommended, even for antiemetics. Oftentimes, nauseated animals resist oral medications, and the consequent struggling can trigger vomiting episodes. Some gastrointestinal diseases preclude the use of oral medications. If the gastrointestinal tract is decompensated (as in ulcerative colitis), the administration of drugs that ordinarily are not associated with gastrointestinal problems in healthy animals can serve to aggravate the condition. The physical presence of a solid dosage form such as a capsule or tablet can exacerbate already decompensated digestive tract tissue, possibly causing spasms. Increased or otherwise erratic peristaltic gut activity lessens the chance of predictable drug absorption and can result in subtherapeutic blood levels.

Traditionally, enema feeding, (the instillation of nutrients in a liquid form directly into the colonic area) has been used as an alternative to oral feeding. However, with the advent of sophisticated protein hydrolysate and free amino acid solutions, which can be administered by the intravenous route, rectal feeding can no longer be considered the optimal alternative to oral feeding.

Rectal administration can sometimes be used to promote specific response (such as rapid catharsis) or to treat localized inflammation (for example, treating regional enteritis with steroidal enemas). In these situations a drug can be applied directly to the affected area, thereby lessening the potential for systemic side effects.

Drug vehicle considerations

Usually drugs are administered rectally by aqueous lavage or by means of suppositories. Suppository vehicles, the inert material in which drugs are dissolved or suspended, are either lipoidal (fat soluble) or aqueous. Lipoidal suppositories are usually made of cocoa butter, with the drug being suspended uniformly throughout the suppository. Upon insertion the cocoa butter melts because of the ambient colonic temperature, thereby releasing the drug. Water-soluble suppository bases are usually made of polyethylene glycol (PEG) combinations. Unlike cocoa butter suppositories, PEG suppositories are miscible with aqueous media and dissolve in the colon, thereby releasing the drug. Medication release from PEG-base suppositories is independent of temperature but requires an aqueous environment.

Once medication has been released from the suppository vehicle, its degree and rate of absorption are governed by the same principles (pH, partition coefficient, and enzymatic activity) that govern the absorption of orally administered drugs.

It is difficult to generalize about the differences in time required to obtain therapeutic blood levels between the oral and rectal routes. The physiology and anatomy of the entire digestive tract, as well as the characteristics of drug and vehicle, play important roles. Although the colonic area is highly vascular and the route of administration is direct, absorption is often unpredictable.[3]

PARENTERAL ADMINISTRATION

The term "parenteral" is derived from the Greek *para,* meaning "alongside of," and *enteron,* meaning "intestine." Clinically the term has come to mean administration of medications, diagnostics, and nutrients by way of veins, muscles, and subcutaneous tissue. The two most common routes of parenteral administration are intravenous (IV) and intramuscular (IM). Many parenteral medications should not be administered by both routes; a practitioner must read manufacturers' labels to be sure about proper dosage routes. It is not advisable to administer parenteral suspensions or injectables designed for prolonged activity by the intravenous route, because of the potential for emboli formation. Likewise, some intravenous medications, such as potassium chloride and diazepam, can cause pain and skin necrosis at the injection site when administered by the intramuscular route. Parenteral routes are employed most often if rapid blood levels are needed or if a medication would be clinically degraded by the gastrointestinal environment.

Intradermal (ID) injection—the injection of a drug into the dermis —is usually used for diagnostic procedures, such as allergy testing or tuberculosis screening. Subcutaneous (SC) injection involves the placement of drug directly below the dermis, into the alveolar connective tissue. A prompt response generally occurs, and the dose is normally about half the oral requirement. Insulin is routinely given by this route, for the treatment of diabetes mellitus.

Intramuscular injection

When the intramuscular route is used, the drug is injected through the layers of skin deep into skeletal muscle. If aqueous solutions rather than suspensions are injected, absorption is quicker than with the subcutaneous route, because of the higher vascularity of muscle tissue.[3] A unique advantage of intramuscular administration is that prolonged drug levels can be obtained with a minimum number of injections. Extended blood levels are achieved by incorporating the medication into a solid matirx composed of inert ingredients similar to those used for oral sustained-release drugs. These injectable dosage forms, usually called "pellets," are implanted into deep muscle tissue, where the drug is very slowly leached from the matrix. Medications, such as steroids that enhance anabolic reactions associated with weight gain in mammals are given by this route.

Intramuscular injections (other than those involving pellet implantations) create a fluid depot in the tissue. How long this depot remains is a function of the drug state (dissolved or suspended), the vehicle (aqueous or lipid [oleaginous]), and fluid supply to the area.[3] The depot is created by compressing tissue cells at the injection site. If the volume of fluid injected is inordinately large, the cells are compressed to a degree that results in pain. Usually, not more than 2 ml is recommended for small animals and not more than 10 ml for large animals in any one site. If a medication or its vehicle is irritating to tissue, this situation increases any discomfort and causes it to persist until the fluid is dispersed from the injection area. Often times procaine, a local anesthetic, is combined with a medication to lessen discomfort.

When a medication is injected as suspended particles rather than in solution, movement of the drug out of the depot depends on (1) how quickly in vivo processes can dissolve the drug and (2) blood supply to the injection area. The dissolution processes require time; consequently movement of the medication from the injection site is delayed, resulting in a gradual, prolonged entry of the drug into the bloodstream. As is true of orally administered drugs, the movement of a drug from extravascular tissue to the bloodstream is facilitated by a high partition coefficient, nonionization of drug molecules, and enzymatic transport activity. In order to obtain therapeutic drug levels, medications intended for prolonged release are more concentrated than their aqueous counterparts, which are intended for rapid blood levels. Another method used to attain prolonged drug action is to mix a medication in lipid (oleaginous) vehicle, if the solubility characteristics of the drug allow. Introduction of an oleaginous depot into muscle tissue delays leaching into surrounding aqueous tissue and blood vessels. A drug's release rate from an oleaginous vehicle is governed by the drug's partition coefficient, the surface area of the oil globule (or depot), and the blood supply to the injection site.[3]

Intravenous injection

Intravenously administered drugs are most often injected into a peripheral vein. Intravenous administration is the most rapid means of getting drugs into the bloodstream, since a blood level is attained immediately. Irritating drugs and drugs administered in high concentrations are given by this route, since they will be immediately diluted by the blood. However, care should be exercised when irritating or highly concentrated drugs are infused, so that localized inflammation of the inside of the vein (phlebitis) does not occur. Such inflammation disrupts the normally smooth inner surface of vein (intima), causing it to become uneven and rough. As blood cells collide with the intima, they lyse and their remains tend to clump together. These masses of debris may become entrapped on the rough vein surface, causing thrombi to be carried through the circulatory system as emboli. This situation is potentially crippling or even lethal. Likewise, if medications are not properly diluted their contact with blood elements can cause lysis and clot formation. Such side effects are best protected against by proper dilution of drugs and use of appropriate rates of administration.

The phenomenon of emboli formation resulting from blood cell destruction can also occur in response to the presence of an indwelling needle or catheter. As blood cells collide with the needle, they are lysed by its sharp edges and tend to clump. To avoid this situation, heparin, an anticoagulant, is routinely administered through indwelling needles or catheters.

Particulates (foreign matter) entering the bloodstream likewise collide with blood cells, promoting emboli formation. This problem is more complex if these particulates are microbial, since sepsis must be anticipated. Careful examination of all intravenous solutions and their containers must be an integral part of intravenous administration procedure. Glass bottles should be checked for cracks, which most often occur at the base below or along the metal band used to hang them. A bottle should be checked for the presence of particulates by holding the bottle upright and rotating the wrist so as to create a whirlpool effect in the fluid. As the vortex disappears, any visible particles settling to the bottom of the container should be considered particulates and the solution should not be administered. Plastic containers should be inverted before they are checked for particles that settle. Since plastic containers are not as clear as glass ones, it is more difficult to detect particulates in them.

Particulates can also be created in a solution as a result of mixing drugs that react chemically with each other to form a precipitate. Such drugs are said to be "incompatible" with each other. Although no hard and fast rules govern which drugs are incompatible with each other, a few general guidelines exist:

1. Drugs having acid (below 7) pH values should not be mixed with drugs having basic (above 7) pH values.
2. Generally, vitamins should not be mixed with antibiotics, especially those of the penicillin type.
3. Antibiotics belonging to different categories should not be mixed.
4. Antifungal drugs (for example, amphotericin) should not be mixed with any other drugs.
5. Steroidal drugs (for example, hydrocortisone) should not be mixed with antibiotics.

See Appendix A for more specific information about which drugs should not be mixed together for intravenous administration.

Plastic containers holding intravenous solutions should be firmly squeezed before hanging to ensure that no pinhole puncture are present, which would allow microbial contamination. Since an intravenous administration line allows the outside environment direct access to the bloodstream, aseptic technique should be strictly followed when an infusion is started and the cleanliness of the injection site should be strictly maintained.

Different categories of medication lend themselves to different intravenous administration techniques. In addition, the nature of the pathological condition being treated affects the choice of techniques. Generally, three techniques are used. *Intermittent intravenous therapy* (also known as "piggy-back'" administration) involves diluting a drug dose in a small volume of fluid and administering it during a period of 30 to 60 minutes by means of an administration set. This is repeated a number of times during each 24-hour period. Blood levels of antibiotics are best maintained by this method. *Infusion* of fluid may be clinically defined as the administration of large volumes of fluid continuously over extended periods of time. This method is appropriate for the administration of irritant drugs such as electrolytes (for example, potassium chloride and sodium chloride), which also could have harmful effects on cardiac function if they were infused too rapidly. Nutritional agents such as amino acids should also be administered by prolonged intravenous infusion. (The term "infusion" can be misleading, since the intravenous administration of any drug over any time period can technically be called "infusing" the drug. For example, a drug can be "infused" by means of the intermittent therapy technique). *Bolus intravenous administration* involves injecting a drug in a very small volume of fluid, with only a syringe and needle rather than a standard large-volume container and administration set. Usually, bolus administration is employed in life-threatening situations, when immediate high concentrations of drugs are needed and concern about phlebitis is secondary to concern about patient survival. While offering the advantage of immediate high blood levels, bolus intravenous administration does not allow for prophylactic measures to combat side effects such as anaphylactic drug reaction (for example, injecting a small amount of the drug and observing for reactions to it). Complications such as this must be met by symptomatic treatment.

TOPICAL ADMINISTRATION

Drug absorption through unbroken skin (percutaneous absorption) depends on a drug's ability to penetrate layers of skin cells, hair follicles, sweat glands, and sebaceous glands. All skin cells and glands are at least partially lipoidal, and, like passage through gastrointestinal membrane, drug penetration through skin is thus proportional to partition coefficient. Drug penetration into deeper skin layers is enhanced if (1) the ointment base or the drug can remove or disrupt the outermost layer of skin, (2) the drug dissolves or mixes with the protective serum (oily phase) of skin, (3) the drug is rubbed in vigorously, thereby disrupting the outer skin barrier, and (4) the drug concentration is increased. The absorptive ability of skin varies with illnesses. Generally, a systemic illness promotes absorption through the skin, as does lack of skin integrity (for example, wounds or debrided skin). The site of application and the length of time an ointment remains in contact with the skin are important factors relating to drug penetration. Ointments are semisolid preparations of such consistency and composition that they soften, but do not necessarily melt, when they are rubbed on the skin. Penetration is most efficient when the outer layer of skin is thin and contact time is prolonged. Thick, highly keratinized areas of skin, such as paw pads, retard penetration.

Ointment bases vary in terms of degree of penetration, in accordance with the considerations just mentioned. Use of the proper ointment base for the type of drug activity desired is a critical aspect of product formulation, since the base can play a key role in determining the rate and amount of drug penetration. Ointment bases can be classified into three types according to their penetration ability:

1. Epidermic ointment bases. These demonstrate no or very slight skin penetration. Generally they are used as emollients (agents that promote skin softness) or protective agents. These ointment bases have a very greasy, tenacious consistency, and it is therefore best to clip the hair at the application site before they are applied, to promote cleanliness. Bases that contain waxes and petrolatum are found in this group.

2. Endodermic ointment bases. These penetrate into deeper skin layers; however, systemic absorption of drugs mixed with them is not to be expected. Usually these bases are composed of lanolin and/or wool fat.[3]

3. Diadermic ointment bases. Ointment bases in this category penetrate skin layers, thereby offering a better chance for systemic absorption of the medication. Ointment bases containing water or those that are water soluble are included in this group.

Ointment bases can also be classified as either *hydrophobic* or *hydrophilic*. This classification does not consider penetrability but rather is a measure of how much water a base can absorb before losing its consistency. Hydrophobic ointments do not absorb water and should not be applied over weeping lesions because the ointment could be lifted off by the aqueous discharge. It is also possible that the ointment could block desired drainage, leading to disruption of the healing process and possibly promoting infection.[4] Hydrophilic bases can absorb up to twice their weight in water and as a result can be applied to draining wounds without washing away or losing their consistency, if applications are frequent enough.

Certain drugs, such as salicylic acid and lactic acid, disrupt epidermal integrity and can be added to ointment formulations to enhance their penetrability. However, their use is not advised if the skin is already broken.[3]

In general, topical administration of drugs is used only for local treatment. In some cases, even though it is not desired, percutaneous drug absorption occurs, causing systemic side effects that are attributable to the applied drug. Although various ointment bases facilitate drug absorption into the bloodstream, if a drug is intended for systemic effect the percutaneous route should not be the route of choice, since absorption is not consistent from one application to the next.

INHALATION

The expansive alveolar surface of the lungs is excellent for absorbing gaseous, volatile, and microcrystalline medications. The speed of onset of systemic effects from inhaled medications is second only to that from intravenous therapy.

The rate at which an inhaled drug is absorbed through the alveoli is a function of (1) the thinness of the absorbing membrane, (2) the available surface area, (3) the concentration of the drug in the airway, and (4) the degree of vascularity in the area. Pathological conditions such as emphysema or bronchitis, which restrict airflow to the alveoli and cause secretions to form within the bronchi, significantly reduce the effectiveness of nebulized drugs (drugs administered as a fine spray intended for inhalation). The anatomy of an animal's pulmonary system is also a major factor in determining the effectiveness of inhalation therapy. The longer, more winding the airway is, the less probable it is that deep penetration of a drug into the lungs will occur. Upon nebulization, droplets containing the drug can collide, forming larger droplets, which tend to precipitate rather than travel along the airway. The purpose of inhalation therapy therefore dictates the intial particle size. If inhalation is required for treatment of a local condition in the bronchi, the particle size should range from 1 to 10 μ in diameter. If systemic effects are desired, the particles should be less than 1 μ in diameter preferably 0.5 μ. Particles smaller than 0.5 μ are generally not retained in the lungs of most animals, since air currents keep them from settling.[3]

Inhaled drugs used commonly for local conditions include bronchodilators, electrolytes, mucolytic enzymes, antibiotics, and, rarely, steroids. Bronchodilators increase the airway lumen and can be used as ancillary, prophylactic medication when other drugs are nebulized, since inhalation of most nonbronchodilators can cause pulmonary spasms.[2] Prolonged inhalation of electrolyte solutions, most often saline, is especially indicated to offset electrolyte loss and to liquefy secretions in the treatment of chronic bronchial inflammation when secretions are abundant. Drugs containing mucolytic enzymes liquify thick mucous secretions, thereby making their removal from the lungs easier. However, these drugs can cause mucosal irritation, leading to bronchospasms; therefore a bronchodilator, such as isoproterenol, is usually given prior to their inhalation, to ensure maximum penetration and to prevent spastic bronchoconstriction. The parenteral route is preferred for the administration of antibiotics to combat most lung infections. Unfortunately some antibiotics, such as polymyxin, neomycin, and bacitracin, are not absorbed well. However, when inhaled they are effective in the treatment of topical lung infections. Generally, the dose of antibiotics used for inhalation drug therapy is the same as for parenteral therapy. Systemic effects resulting from steroid nebulization occur readily, and therefore steroids are not commonly administered in a nebulized form.[2]

REFERENCES

1. Goldstein, A., Aronow, L., and Kalman, S.M.: Principles of drug action, New York, 1968, Harper & Row, Publishers, Inc.
2. Lambert, Ivan: The chief pharmacist as the director of inhalation drug therapy, a research report for master of science degree in hospital pharmacy, Boston, 1968, Northeastern University.
3. Martin E.W., and others: Remington's pharmaceutical sciences, ed. 13, Easton, Pa., 1965, Mack Publishing Co.
4. Spinelli, J.S., and Enos, L.R.: Drugs in veterinary practice, St. Louis, 1978, The C. V. Mosby Co.

2

Drug distribution and elimination

PERFORMANCE OBJECTIVES

After completion of this chapter the student will:

- Describe the relationship between a "target organ" and "drug bioavailability"
- Plot a blood level curve, identify its axes, and indicate (1) the peak serum concentration point and (2) the area representing total amount of drug absorbed
- Differentiate between "drug bioavailability" and "drug bioequivalence"
- Explain how the concentration gradient phenomenon affects in vivo drug distribution
- Differentiate between "bound" and "unbound" drug with respect to (1) transport sites in the bloodstream, (2) comparative rates of detoxification, and (3) comparative lengths of biological half-lives
- List and define the four major enzyme-mediated chemical reactions responsible for drug detoxificaton
- Discuss the effect of "enzyme induction" on the rate of drug detoxification
- List similarities and differences between the blood-brain barrier and the placenta with respect to drug passage through each
- Discuss the relationship between a drug's rate of hepatic detoxification and its rate of renal excretion
- Differentiate between "drug clearance" and "drug excretion"
- Complete the drug kinetics study outline (Fig. 2-3)

Ic can be recalled from the first chapter that a drug can enter the circulatory system by intravenous injection or by absorption from depots where it has been placed. In the latter case the drug must generally pass through at least one semi-permeable membrane in order to reach the bloodstream. Most commonly the depot is the gastrointestinal tract, the drug having been taken by mouth or administered by rectum. Other depot areas result from intramuscular, subcutaneous, or other parenteral drug administration routes. Usually the blood is not the drug's site of action but rather is used to transport the drug to its target organ(s). Natural in vivo reactions assure that the drug molecules are rendered soluble when they reach the bloodstream since undissolved particulates offer potential for clotting. Likewise it is necessary to ensure that only sterile solutions are administered parenterally in order to prevent the introduction of pathogens into the body.

DOSAGE CONSIDERATIONS

Only a small fraction of a drug's molecules react with target organs. Most of the drug remains dissolved in interstitial fluid, plasma, storage sites such as fatty tissue, and nontarget organ. It has been postulated that, in order to exert an effect, drug molecules must react with specific target organ *receptors*. A receptor is a specific area on a tissue cell upon which compatible drugs can fit and interact with cellular components to exert their biological effect. Most animal cells are 80% fluid, and receptors constitute only a very small fraction of the remaining dry cell weight. Consequently, even if every receptor of a target organ were in contact with a compatible drug molecule, only a small portion of the administered dose would be involved.[4] Since the entire dose of a drug cannot react with suitable receptors at one time, the amount of drug in each dosage form (tablet, capsule, and so on) takes into account that most of the drug will be distributed into areas where it is not active or desired. Placing an excess amount of drug in each dose ensures that after the drug has been distributed throughout the animal's body, enough will contact target receptors to elicit a desired response.

DRUG BIOAVAILABILITY

The amount of drug that reaches the bloodstream can be correlated with the drug's clinical efficacy. For example, if clinical studies indicate that a drug is effective at a dose of 250 mg administered four times daily, we can assme the effect is a result of (1) the maximum concentration of the drug in the bloodstream (peak serum concentration), (2) the speed at which the drug was absorbed after administration, and (3) the total amount of drug absorbed.[2] The amount of a drug that an animal is able to biologically absorb is the amount that becomes biologically available, or "bioavailable." It is not essential that a drug be bioavailable to be effective. Laxatives such as dioctyl sodium sulfosuccinate and anthelmintics such as piperazine salts do not enter the bloodstream but exert their effects totally within the intes-

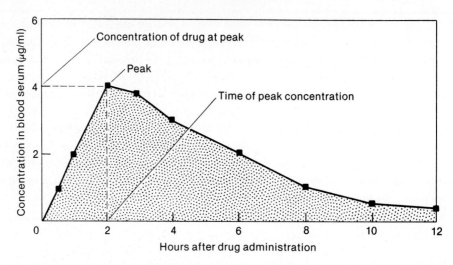

Fig. 2-1. Measurement of drug bioavailability. After administration of a drug, blood samples are taken at specific intervals and the amount of drug found is plotted. Peak concentrations are especially important for some drugs, such as the anti-infectives. For other drugs, such as anti-inflammatory medications, the total amount of drug absorbed is most important. The total amount of drug absorbed is determined by measuring the dotted area under the curve and applying mathematical formulae.

tines. Most drugs, however, exert their effects after absorption into the bloodstream and distribution to the target organ(s).

The standard way of measuring bioavailability is to analyze drug concentration in the blood over a specific time period and to plot it on a graph. The line obtained is called the "blood level curve" (Fig. 2-1). The time required to reach the peak serum concentration is important, since it is an indication of the time required for the drug to be absorbed after administraton by a certain route. The total amount of drug absorbed is the most important measurement; it can be determined mathematically, by measuring the total gray area under the curve (see Fig. 2-1).

DRUG BIOEQUIVALENCE

Bioequivalence is related to bioavailability. Bioequivalence studies are used to determine how different brands of the same generic drug compare clinically. The blood level curve is used. Each product is evaluated in terms of peak concentration, time required to reach the peak, and total amount absorbed. The existence of significant differences in any of these parameters is reason to judge the generic drugs of different companies not bioequivalent. For example, one product may not reach a desired peak concentration because of poor dissolution of its dosage form, thereby altering the drug's effectiveness.

FACTORS AFFECTING DRUG DISTRIBUTION
Concentration gradient

Were it not for the biological systems (for example, enzyme transport mechanisms) mentioned in Chapter 1, as well as in vivo solvents (such as plasma) and anatomical barriers such as the blood-brain barrier, drugs would rapidly distibute themselves uniformly throughout an animal's body. Initially, the highest concentration would be where the drug entered the body, and the drug would rapidly and passively diffuse from this entry depot into the rest of the system, in the same way that any solute mixes with a solvent. When solute movement is uninhibited in any system, biological or otherwise, nature will equalize the solute concentration throughout the system, by diffusion.

The rate of movement of drug molecules from one compartment to another (for example, bloodstream to target organ) is proportional to the difference between the drug concentrations in each compartment. This difference is referred to as the *concenration gradient*. *The greater the difference in concentration between two compartments, the greater the concentration gradient and the greater the propensity for the drug to move from the area of greatest concentration to the area of least concentration.* Movement of drug molecles in this direction has the tendency to equalize drug concentration throughout the system. Biological transport systems, solvents, and barriers moderate the concentration gradient effect, as will be discussed, so that different drug concentrations can persist for long periods of time in different biological compartments.

Plasma-binding ability

A major factor that moderates the concentration gradient principle is a drug's *plasma-binding ability*. Upon entering the bloodstream, drug molecules can be distributed in the aqueous or lipid phases of plasma. This distribution is not absolute; therefore some of the drug will be found in each phase, with a majority of the molecules being in one phase. The factor that determines where most of the drug will migrate is its lipid solubility.

After a drug has been absorbed into the bloodstream, its degree of lipid solubility is called its *protein-binding ability* or *plasma-binding ability* rather than its partition coefficient. A high plasma-binding ability indicates that a drug is very lipid soluble and will dissolve in the lipid portion of plasma. A low plasma-binding ability indicates that a drug is water soluble and will be transported in the aqueous plasma phase.

The amount of a drug dissolved in the lipid portion is called "bound drug" because it does not readily leave the lipid phase, despite its high concentration gradient as compared to extravascular tissue. Consequently it is not rapidly distributed over the body nor is it eliminated quickly by the kidneys. The clinical effect is that drugs with high plasma-binding ability remain in the body for long periods of time.

The amount of drug that dissolves in the aqueous portion of plasma is called "free drug" or "unbound drug" because it can readily leave the circulatory system, its rate of exit being largely controlled by the concentration gradient between bloodstream and extravascular areas. If the target organ is outside the circulatory system, then a low plasma-binding ability facilitates an effective drug concentration in the target tissue, providing it is not cerebral tissue.

Drug metabolism (detoxification) mechanisms

The extent of drug distribution is partly a function of how long a drug remains in the system. The liver is the primary organ associated with altering foreign substances, such as drugs, so that their removal is facilitated by the kidneys. Contemporary clinical terminology refers to foodstuff molecules as being "metabolized" by the liver, while drug molecules are "detoxified" by the liver. In fact, the same chemical reactions can occur whether a molecule is detoxified or metabolized. The term "detoxification" is left over from an obsolete theory that drug addicts suffer from an accumulation of toxins in the body.[3] As was mentioned in the first chapter, a drug that is administered orally must cross the gastrointestinal wall in order to reach the general circulation. However, before it reaches the general circulation, it must pass through the liver. Most drugs undergo metabolic transformation in the liver, although other tissues may also participate. It will be recalled that drugs with high partition coefficients (highly nonionized drugs) move easily across membranes. Consequently, they can diffuse readily from tubular urine, through the renal tubular cells, and back into the bloodstream, thereby avoiding elimination by the kidneys. Such drugs remain in the body for long periods of time. In addition, the kidneys are unable to excrete drugs with high partition coefficients, which further enhances their movement from tubule to systemic circulation.[4]

Drug-metabolizing mechanisms in the liver are mediated by enzymes located in the microsomal portion of the liver. *In nearly all cases these enzymes react with drug molecules to make them more water soluble (ionized), thereby enhancing their chances for elimination by the kidneys.*

A common measure of how long a drug remains active in vivo is "biological half-life" ($\tau\frac{1}{2}$), which is the time required to excrete half of an administered dose. Increasing the aqueous solubility of a drug decreases its lipid solubility, thereby inhibiting its passage across tubular membranes. This allows the kidneys to more efficiently excrete the drug and decreases the drug's biological half-life, which, in turn, affects distribution of the drug and dosage intervals.

The evolutionary explanation of the origin of drug-metabolizing enzymes is that they developed as adaptive mechanisms for life on land as opposed to life in the sea. Fish and other marine organisms generally lack some of the more sophisticated drug-metabolizing systems found in mammals. It has been postulated that as land life encountered more diverse foreign substances, hepatic enzymes and enzyme systems were developed to render these foreign agents less lipid soluble and therefore more easily excreted by the kidneys. Unlike mammals, fish have retained the ability to excrete lipid-soluble compounds into the water (across gill membranes).[4]

The amounts and types of microsomal metabolic enzymes differ between species; this fact accounts for the differing abilities of animals to metabolize foodstuffs and drugs. For example, cats lack glucuronide-forming enzymes and subsequently cannot efficiently biodegrade phenolic substances such as aspirin, many narcotics, and barbiturates. Accumulation of these compounds can cause toxicity, leading to the adverse clinical effects that have been observed[1,6]

Microsomal enzymes bring about many chemical reactions; however, there are four major types:

1. Oxidation, which causes a compound to lose hydrogen atoms
2. Reduction, which results in a compound gaining hydrogen atoms
3. Hydrolysis, or splitting of a molecule and addition of part of a water molecule to each of the split molecular potions
4. Conjugation, the most common reaction in which glucuronic acid is added to a molecule. Glucuronic acid is a highly water-soluble compound found in the liver. Microsomal enzymes attach glucuronic acid molecules to lipoidal substances, thereby increasing the lipid's ability to dissolve in water.

More than one of these reactions may be required to render a drug soluble enough for excretion. The efficiency with which hepatic enzymes bring about these and other chemical reactions determines the extent and duration of drug distribution throughout an animal's body. Drugs with high plasma-binding ability are protected from biodegradation by the liver and require many passes through the liver before their metabolic transformation to more water-soluble forms begins. Conversely, some mammals can remove up to 85% of an administered drug dose from the bloodstream after a single pass through the liver.[3] In some cases a drug is quickly eliminated by the kidneys; in other cases it is stored in the liver and then slowly released into the bloodstream. This storage capability illustrates another important function of the liver—its ability to initially store some foreign compounds (such as drugs) and foodstuffs (such as protein and carbohydrates) and then gradually release them back into the bloodstream. This results in more efficient utilization of food and protection of the animal from toxic substances. This storage function avoids "shocking" the system with large amounts of food or foreign matter, thereby allowing the body to gradually assimilate food and detoxify drugs.

Differences in liver function are responsible for the fact that metabolic capability varies according to age, state of health, and sex. Generally, young animals have little drug detoxification ability because they lack mature enzyme systems. Diseased livers, like advanced age, compromise hepatic detoxifiation mechanisms. The sex of an animal can be shown to influence drug detoxification rate; for example, female rats metabolize drugs slower than male rats.[1] Thus it is evident that an animal's general health, age, and sex should be considered when a dosage regimen is being formulated.

Constant exposure of the liver of a particular animal to certain molecules can make the liver more proficient in metabolizing those molecules and related molecules. This phenomenon, which is called *enzyme induction*, results in the animal having a higher concentration of the particular enzymes required to metabolize the molecules.

Fetal circulation

Studies of fetal drug levels during gestation are scanty; however, some information has been gained in regard to which drugs cross the placental membrane and enter fetal tissue. The data become more involved and less conclusive if one tries to correlate birth abnormalities (teratogenic effects) with the presence of drugs in fetal tissue. Until more conclusive data have been presented, it seems only reasonable that drug therapy in pregnant animals should be avoided whenever possible or at least kept to a minimum with respect to the number and types of drugs administered, their dosage amounts, and the duration of treatment.

Like other biological membranes, the placenta allows nonionized drug molecules to diffuse through it, thereby permitting movement of a drug from the maternal circulation to fetal tissue. *These nonionized drug molecules represent "free" drug (drug that is not bound to plasma); only these drug molecules cross the placenta into fetal tissue.* "Bound" drug remains in maternal plasma, and although it enters the fetal circulation, it does not leave the fetal vascular system.

The free drug concentration gradient between mother and fetus determines how much drug will be potentially available to enter fetal tissue. This gradient is rather small, because of the large difference between maternal mass and fetal mass. Equalization of the drug concentrations in the mother and the fetus therefore requires only a small amount of drug to enter the fetus. However, the movement of free, nonionized drug to the fetus is inhibited by the placenta, which decreases blood flow to the fetus as compared to other areas of the mother's body. Consequently the placenta decreases the amount of free drug available for possible fetal absorption.[4] Table 2-1 summarizes the ability of certain drugs to cross the placental membrane.

The presence of a fetus is not significant in terms of diluting a drug dose to the mother; however, it is of utmost concern in terms of the potential for teratogenic effects. The possibility of teratogenesis depends in part on maternal hepatic function. A healthy, mature liver detoxifies drugs more efficiently than a decompensated liver, thereby limiting both the concentration of a drug and the time the fetus may be exposed to the drug molecules.

TABLE 2-1

Some drugs that cross placental barriers

Chapter where discussed	Chemical or pharmacological classification	Drug name	Comments
Diuretics	Carbonic anhydrase inhibitors	Acetazolamide Dichlorphenamide Ethoxzolamide Methazolamide	Doses in excess of therapeutic amounts produced teratogenic effects in mice and rats
	Monosulfamyl type	Furosemide	Abortive and nonabortive deaths reported in mice, rats, and rabbits
Drugs affecting the central nervous system	Salicylate analgesics	Aspirin Sodium salicylate	No teratogenic or fetal deaths in normal dosage ranges
	Opiate analgestics Nonopiate analgesics Barbiturate anesthetics	Morphine Meperidine Thiamylal Thiopental	Major side effect is excessive CNS depression of the fetus
	Barbiturate hypnotics	Amobarbital Pentobarbital Phenobarbital Secobarbital	
	Phenothiazine-type tranquilizers	Acetylpromazine Chlorpromazine Perphenazine	All phenothiazine-type drugs cross placental barriers, teratogenic effects being reported in some cases
	Other tranquilizers	Chlordiazepoxide Diazepam	
	Anticonvulsants	Paramethadione	Inconclusive evidence as to whether it causes teratogenic effects

Continued.

TABLE 2-1—cont'd
Some drugs that cross placental barriers

Chapter where discussed	Chemical or pharmacological classification	Drug name	Comments
Anti-infective drugs and immunologicals	Cephalosporin-type antibiotics	Cephalothin Cephapirin Cephaloglycine Cephaloridine	Documented as crossing placental barriers in rabbits; all cephalosporin-type antibiotics should be considered capable of crossing placental barriers
	Aminoglycoside-type antibiotics	Gentamicin Tobramycin	All aminoglycoside-type antibiotics should be considered capable of crossing placental barriers
	Penicillin and semisynthetic penicillin-type antibiotics	Ampicillin Carbenicillin Cloxacillin Dicloxacillin Methicillin Penicillin G and VK	All penicillin-type antibiotics should be considered capable of crossing placental barriers
	Tetracycline-type antibiotics	Chlortetracycline Doxycyline Minocycline Oxtetracycline Tetracycline	All cross placental barriers and are deposited in fetal bone and teeth, causing discoloration of teeth
	Other antibiotics	Clindamycin	
	Sulfonamide-type anti-infectives	Salicylazosulfapyridine Sulfacetamide Sulfadiazine Sulfamethoxazole Sulfisoxazole	Most sulfonamides are capable of crossing placental barriers
	Piperazine-type anthelmintics	Piperazine salts	All phenothiazine-type drugs cross placental barriers, teratogenic effects being reported in some cases

Anti-inflammatory drugs	Glucocorticosteroids	Betamethasone Cortisone Dexamethasone Hydrocortisone Methylprednisolone Prednisone Prednisolone	Most serious potential side effect is secondary iatrogenic insufficiency (drug-induced adrenal atrophy)
	Nonsteroidal type	Ibuprofen Naproxen Oxyphenbutazone Phenylbutazone	Questionable whether all cross placental barriers, but they should not be given to pregnant animals since they can affect labor and parturition
	Phenothiazine-type antihistamines	Zomepirac Promethazine Trimeprazine	All phenothiazine-type drugs cross placental barriers; teratogenic effects have been reported in some cases
Cardiovascular drugs	Digitalis glycosides	Digitalis Digitoxin Digoxin	
	Cardiac depressants	Propranolol Quinidine	

Adipose tissue

Perhaps more than any other factor thus far considered, adipose tissue can have a dramatic effect on the distribution of certain drugs. The potential impact on drug distribution and blood concentration are proportional to the amount of fat tissue. The greater the amount of fatty tissue, the greater the potential effect on drug migration and consequently on blood concentrations.

Lipid-soluble, free drug molecules diffuse easily through capillaries and migrate to lipid tissue banks (such as the brain and adipose tissue). The molecules can remain stored in adipose tissue for relatively long periods of time. This storage, during which the drug molecules are dormant, occurs in adipose tissue because of its restricted blood supply as compared to cerebral tissue. The retention of drugs in cerebral tissue is transient because of the large volume of blood constantly supplying the brain. Conversely, since the blood supply to adipose tissue is minimal, shifts in its drug concentration do not occur rapidly in response to the concentration gradient existing between it and the bloodstream. Consequently, high concentrations of lipid-soluble, free drug molecules can be stored in adipose tissue; the more adipose tissue, the more storage sites for the drug. This nonproductive drug storage complicates dosage considerations, since a practitioner must compensate for it when determining a drug dosage schedule. If a drug does not penetrate fatty tissue, no dosage increase is needed.[1] Invariably, dosages of fat-penetrating drugs must be increased in proportion to the amount of adipose tissue. This increases the possibility that adverse side effects will occur once fat storage sites have become saturated with the drug. When these sites become saturated, the drug that had been stored begins to be reabsorbed into the bloodstream and new drug molecules cease to migrate into adipose tissue. The result is an increase in the blood level of the drug.[4] Unlike the situation with regard to other tissues, biodegradation of a drug does not occur to any significant degree while it is being retained in fatty tissue. Therefore, upon its reentry into the bloodstream the drug is still biologically active.

The fate of intravenous, ultra-short-acting, barbiturate anesthetics illustrates the hazard that exists when large amounts of drug migrate to and from adipose tissue. Shortly after injection the barbiturate moves from blood into fat, thus reducing both the blood and brain concentrations. (Central nervous system depression is caused by the presence of the drug in cerebral tissue; therefore as the drug's concentration diminishes, so does its ability to keep the animal sedated.) As more of the barbiturate is given to maintain the cerebral concentration, fatty tissue eventually becomes saturated and blood levels begin to rise, since no more drug can occupy adipose tissue receptor sites. As the drug is detoxified in the liver, more of the drug diffuses from adipose tissue to equalize the concentration gradient between adipose tissue and blood. If the amount of fatty tissue is great, the diffusion of the drug can be prolonged, thereby lengthening the recovery period from anesthesia.[6]

Blood-brain barrier

Certain anatomical barriers can influence drug distribution. Capillaries in the brain are much less permeable than capillaries elsewhere in the body. A layer of homogenous tissue, known as the blood-brain barrier, exists between cerebral capillary walls and cerebral tissue. The barrier's function is considered to be protective, since nutrients usually penentrate it with ease while foreign substances, such as drugs, are largely prevented from passing through it. The blood-brain barrier is composed of *glial* cells, which abut the basement membrane of the capillary endothelium. The glial sheath is dense (300 to 500 Å thick) and without visible pores. Drugs attempting to leave brain capillaries therefore have to pass through not only the capillary endothelium but also the glial sheath in order to reach cerebral interstitial fluid. Only the smallest ionized and nonionized, water-soluble drug molecules can pass through the glial sheath. Conversely, lipid-soluble molecules, regardless of size, pass easily and rapidly through this high-lipid-content barrier.[4]

Passage into cerebral tissue does not represent a usual route for most drugs. Therefore cerebral drug distribution is not a major consideration for many of the commonly used medications, unless the meninges of the brain become inflamed. Such inflammation dramatically increases capillary porosity and allows the passage of substances into the brain that normally would be excluded. In this situation the effects a drug may have on brain tissue must be carefully examined and weighed against the benefits of therapy. The same is true for drugs that are able to pass intact blood-brain barriers; these drugs generally are used to treat pathological conditions affecting the brain or spinal column.

Nutritional status

An animal's nutritional status has a major, but less than obvious, effect on drug distribution and consequently on the clinical efficacy of most drugs. If an animal's diet is quantitatively or qualitatively deficient, the animal's protein, carbohydrate, and fat stores will not reflect normal ratios with each other. This situation affects the relative amounts of drug that can be stored in each body compartment, which in turn affects the drug's blood concentration and the duration of effect. A deficient amount of proteinaceous tissue, including plasma, decreases the total amount of drug that can be bound to plasma. It has been theorized that drugs become bound to plasma by occupying drug receptor sites on plasma molecules. If an inadequate diet results in less plasma formation, then fewer sites will be available. As a result, the recommended dose of a drug may not only saturate all receptors, but leave more than the normal amount of free (unbound) drug in the bloodstream. In the case of sulfonamide (sulfa drug) administration, this situation can lead to precipitation of the unbound drug in renal tubules (a condition known as crystalluria), with resultant renal damage. This phenomenon will be reviewed in more detail in Chapter 5.

Excessive adipose tissue, formed as a result of an unbalanced diet, can serve as a reservoir for lipid-soluble drugs such as the barbiturates. Since these drugs are pooled in nontarget tissue, therapeutic blood levels may not be reached with normal doses; thus dosages must be increased. If fatty tissue sites become saturated as a result of higher doses, free (unbound) drug will immediately migrate from these stores into the bloodstream. As a result, toxic free-drug levels may be reached without warning.

Excessive hydration (edema) increases the amount of extravascular, nontarget fluid for drugs to be diluted in, thereby decreasing the chances that the required peak serum drug levels will be reached. In contrast, even marginal dehydration reduces the distributive area for a drug, which leads to higher-than-calculated blood or target-tissue drug concentrations once the drug becomes absorbed. This greatly increases the potential for side effects. Depending upon the cause of the dehydration, accompanying systemic alkalosis or acidosis may be present.

Shifts away from a physiologic pH range may also affect a drug's detoxification rate, which, in turn, will affect its duration of action and its distribution within the animal's body.

Summary

The rate of transfer of drug molecules from bloodstream to tissue depends on the concentration gradient of free (unbound) drug.[4] When a drug is first given, the blood concentration of free drug rises; the concentration then decreases as the drug moves to extravascular sites, whether they be target tissue or storage sites such as adipose tissue. Protein binding slows this migration of drug from the bloodstream and provides a depot of bound drug, which eventually dissociates from plasma proteins to replace free drug that has been lost through hepatic detoxification and excretion. Once tissue depots have been saturated with drug, the blood concentration increases. In an attempt to equalize the concentrations in blood and tissue sites as drug is lost from the bloodstream, drug also moves from tissue stores back to the bloodstream. Rarely will a drug remain in a dormant storage site for a significant time period. It is important to realize that *drug concentrations in all biological compartments are dynamic* and *transient and exist simultaneously*. Consequently a portion of an administered dose can be present in all biological compartments as well as in interstitial and extracellular fluid at the same time. Penetration of a drug can also occur in anatomical structures that are not discussed in detail in this book, such as bone and tooth tissue. It is fundamental to realize the potential distribution of a drug and the effect this distribution can have on animals, especially if they are immature. Only by appreciating the extent of a drug's distribution can a clinician determine if the drug is suitable for a particular animal and, if so, what the dose and administration interval should be.

ROUTES OF DRUG ELIMINATION

Drug molecules can be eliminated from the body either as metabolites or unchanged from their original chemical structures. In vivo enzymes and chemicals associated with food metabolism can react with most drug molecules to alter their original structure, the resulting forms being referred to as by-products or "metabolites" of the original drug. If a drug molecule is not chemically altered, it is eliminated as the same chemical it was given as; hence it is "unchanged." Depending upon how fast a drug is broken down, the total amount of drug given can be eliminated as (1) its metabolite(s), (2) unchanged, or (3) in both forms. Excretion by the kidney, biliary system, intestines, and lungs accounts for the majority of drug elimination. The kidney is the most important route. Small amounts of drug can also be found in secretions such as saliva, sweat, milk, and semen. Although the last two routes account for very little excretion, their importance with respect to reproduction and developing offspring should not be underestimated.[4]

Kidney excretion

Drugs or their metabolites, like other unneeded products of metabolism, are eliminated by two normal renal secretory mechanisms. Regardless of which mechanism is used, the kidney cannot remove lipoidal, nonionized drug molecules, since they will readily pass through renal tubular epithelium and be reabsorbed into the systemic circulation. Only free, ionized drug molecules (either anions or cations) in the aqueous portion of plasma are normally filtered and excreted by the kidneys.

Glomerular filtration

If the molecules of a drug are not too big, they can be filtered by the glomerulus, enter Bowman's capsule, and pass along the tubules. If the drug is in the nonionized form, it will be reabsorbed; ionized drug molecules are unable to diffuse back into the blood and will be excreted in the urine unless they are reabsorbed by an enzyme transport system.[4] Enzyme transport systems are responsible for reabsorption of ions, even when their concentration is higher in the interstitial fluid surrounding the tubules than in the tubules. In effect this reabsorption is reverse osmosis, since the normal flow of ions through a membrane is from areas of higher concentration (such as interstitial fluid) to areas of lower concentration (such as the tubular filtrate). If normal osmotic flow were allowed, reabsorption of needed ions would be inefficient, since as many would be eliminated as would be reabsorbed. Furthermore, the tubular anatomy does not allow passive diffusion of electrolytes from interstitial fluid to tubular fluid. Consequently the only movement of ions occurs against the concentration gradient, by means of energy-utilizing enzyme transport systems. Some nutrients reabsorbed by this system are glucose, amino acids, proteins, and most of the electrolytes, including sodium, magnesium, and calcium. Amino acids, glucose, and protein are almost always totally reabsorbed, while electrolyte reabsorption is variable, depending upon an animal's qualitative and quantitative needs. Electrolyte reabsorption is governed by hormones, most of which are secreted by the adrenal glands. The hormones selectively stimulate different enzyme transport systems to reabsorb electrolytes, thereby expending energy to carry them through tubular epithelium walls and return them to the bloodstream.[5]

Anions and cations are handled by different enzyme systems. As was discussed previously in this chapter, a common hepatic detoxification reaction is to conjugate glucuronic acid with drug molecules, thereby increasing their water solubility. One of the normal functions of the anion-secreting enzyme system is to eliminate these negatively charged glucuronide metabolites through the kidneys.

If drug anions and cations are compatible with the activated transport enzymes, they, like nutrient electrolytes, can be reabsorbed, consequently increasing their duration of activity. If the drug ions are not reabsorbed, they will be excreted in the urine.

Tubular secretion

In most warm-blooded and cold-blooded animals, hydrogen ions, a few electrolytes such as potassium, and some organic acids like penicillin and the cephalosporin drugs bypass the glomerular filtration route and are secreted directly from the bloodstream into the tubules via enzyme transport systems. These enzymes function like their counterparts just discussed, but in the reverse direction (they transport ions from blood to tubular fluid). In some fishes, tubular secretion is the only method for removal of waste products.[5]

The rate of drug elimination depends on renal efficiency. Obviously, if renal activity is decompensated as a result of disease or injury, filtration and excretion of drugs will be affected. What the exact effect will be depends on the nature of the pathological conditions. For example, if glomerular filtration is not affected but reabsorption mechanisms are, a drug could be secreted more quickly than anticipated, thereby reducing its duration of activity. If filtration is inhibited, a drug could maintain its blood level longer than anticipated, thereby prolonging its duration of action.

Concurrent administration of drugs must also be considered. If an animal is being given a diuretic drug, the effect of many other drugs could be less than anticipated, since the possibility for reabsorption is largely negated. The pharmacological activity of diuretics will be explained further in the next chapter.

Biliary excretion

Some drugs can be excreted by liver cells into bile and eventually pass into the intestines. If the properties of a drug (pH, partition coefficient, degree of nonionization) favor reabsorption from the intestines, a cycle (enterohepatic) can result in which the drug is continually reabsorbed from the intestines after biliary secretion until enough of the drug passes through the liver to render it sufficiently water soluble for urinary excretion.

Examples of such drugs include steroidal hormones which are partially excreted in bile but largely reabsorbed from the intestines. Digitoxin, a cardiac drug, and meralluride (Mercuhydrin), a diuretic, are two drugs that are excreted in the bile of rabbits, rats, and dogs. Antibiotics such as penicillin, streptomycin, and the tetracycline group are found in significant concentrations in the bile of most animals.[4]

Intestinal excretion

Aside from a few drugs secreted via bile into the intestines and then eliminated, most drugs eliminated by the intestines are not absorbed following oral administration. These drugs include those used for treatment of pathological conditions of the intestines. For example, drugs used to treat diarrhea, parasitic infections of the gut, and constipation are not usually intended for systematic distribution.

Minor routes

Although the amount of a drug eliminated by tissue not generally associated with excretory processes (salivary, perspiratory, mammary, and male genital glands) may be small in proportion to the amount eliminated by the kidney, this amount can increase noticeably when such glands are stimulated. Strenuous activity by an animal will increase the amount of drug lost in sweat. Excessive salivation will increase the amount of drug lost in saliva, although this route is not as significant or variable as perspiration.

Excretion of a drug in milk has resulted in side effects in offspring, since significant quantities of a drug can be eliminated by this route and nursing animals do not have highly developed detoxification or elimination mechanisms. Consequently, a drug can accumulate in a nursing animal. More often than not, this accumulation has had harmful results, such as bilirubin accumulation, which can lead to the death of the infant. However, proper and cautious administration of a drug to a nursing mother can be a physiologic, continuous way to provide drug therapy to the offspring, as is done in the oral inoculation of suckling piglets.[6]

Another consideration is the effect drug therapy may have on spermatoza formation. Admittedly, little is known about drug penetration into seminiferous tubules or the effect on the stored sperm. However, it seems likely that some of the anti-infective drugs that affect DNA structure and activity would also affect the genetic coding carried in the sperm. Because of the lack of definitive information, and the possibility of teratogenesis resulting from drug treatment of a sire, the administration of a highly potent anti-infective drug to a male prior to breeding does not seem indicated.

DETERMINATION OF DOSE AND FREQUENCY OF ADMINISTRATION

An understanding of the principles of drug distribution and elimination has a practical application when a drug's dosage schedule is determined. In the treatment of disease, the initial goal is to achieve an adequate response to a drug by ensuring that an adequate concentration of the drug reaches the target tissue(s). A proven method to determine whether enough drug is reaching the target tissue is to measure the blood concentration of the drug and relate it to biological responses that indicate whether the drug is effective.

This chapter has already outlined the general patterns of drug distribution and elimination and the factors that alter them. However, an understanding of the unique characteristics of each drug's distribution patterns allows a practitioner to prescribe

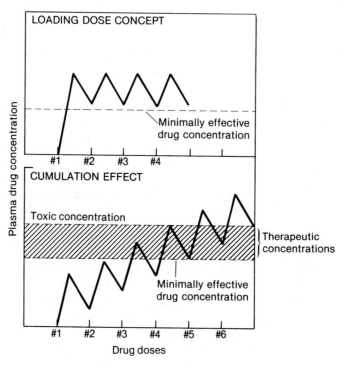

Fig. 2-2. Methods of dosing. *Top,* The loading dose concept is used almost exclusively in clinical practice. Once an effective blood level is established, periodic dosing with an amount smaller than the loading dose is enough to temporarily replace what is lost through elimination. Prolonged, high concentrations of drug in the blood are avoided, thereby reducing the potential for side effects. *Bottom,* the cumulative effect results from drug leaving tissue stores, not being adequately eliminated, and therefore accumulating in the blood. Consequently blood drug levels continue to rise with successive doses, possibly causing systemic toxicity. Cumulation can be an indication of poor renal function or too frequent doses.

a dosage schedule that will ensure an effective blood concentration. A satisfactory duration of drug action can sometimes be achieved through the use of such dosage forms as sustained-release medication or implants. However, the most common way to extend duration of action is to repeat doses at the proper intervals.

Drug clearance

Removal of a drug from the blood is called drug clearance. A drug does not have to be eliminated from an animal to be cleared. For example, diffusion of a drug into fatty tissue or into any extravascular area can be considered removal from the bloodstream. Obviously the distributive pattern of a drug, as well as how rapidly it is detoxified by the liver, has a dramatic effect on how quickly it is cleared from the blood. The more efficiently a drug is cleared, the shorter the interval between doses.

Knowing the distribution scheme of a drug can help a practitioner to determine not only the interval between doses but also the amount of the dose. One practice is to administer a high initial dose ("loading dose"), which theoretically saturates tissue receptors, and to follow it with doses that replace only the portion of the loading dose that is lost through binding (to plasma or tissue), metabolism, and excretion. This regimen, which is commonly used for anti-infective medication such as antibiotics and sulfonamides, is illustrated in Fig. 2-2, *top*. When clearance occurs as a result of storage of a drug in body tissues (including plasma) rather than elimination, then saturation of storage sites leads to a rapid increase in blood concentration. If degradation of the drug is slow, then elimination is retarded, which further contributes to prolonged, high blood drug levels. If subsequent doses are not decreased and/or the interval between doses is not increased a dose will not be eliminated before the next is administered. Consequently, drug concentration in the body will increase with each successive dose. This process, called "cumulation," is illustrated in Fig. 2-2, *bottom*. Cumulation can ensure high drug blood levels if critical situations warrant it. A significant hazard associated with this dosage regimen, however, is that drug concentrations are more likely to rise to toxic levels, unless adjustments are made, than is the case with standard dosing technique.[1]

Multiple drug therapy

In order to gain a greater clinical response than can be provided by one drug, two or more drugs can be given simultaneously. Administering two drugs may also reduce drug toxicity by avoiding high doses of a single drug. If the clinical effect is equal to the sum of each drug's individual effects, then "summation" has taken place. If the response is more than equal to the sum of each drug's individual effects, then "synergism" has occurred. Oftentimes synergism results from the liver not having adequate microsomal enzyme levels to detoxify both drugs within the time it takes to detoxify one of the drugs. Consequently neither drug is cleared as fast as when each is administered separately. Synergistic responses may offer the advantages of reducing the dose of each drug and/or increasing the time between doses, without sacrificing clinical response, and avoiding the possibility of drug-related toxicity. However, multiple drug therapy can also lead to a decreased drug response, because two or more drugs may be chemically incompatible, leading to destruction of one, both, or all of them. For example, mixing penicillin and aminophylline (a bronchodilating drug) in the same intravenous-administration bottle results in the destruction of the penicillin. Biological antagonism between drugs can also occur, in which case the pharmacological action of one drug interferes in vivo with the action of the other. Concurrent administratin of a bacteriocidal drug, such as penicillin, and a bacteriostatic drug, such as a sulfonamide, is not recommended, since the bacteriocidal drug is effective only during mitosis, which is inhibited by the bacteriostatic drug.

The use of a mixture of drugs for a single indication introduces variables—whether good or bad—into dosage considerations and the clinical response. Because of the advent of potent medications indicated for specific conditions, the prudent use of single medications for each indication oftentimes is preferable to the use of multiple drug, or "shot gun," therapy, the effects of which are frequently untraceable.

Therapeutic index

Wide margins of safety between effective and toxic doses are desirable for all drugs. While the outstanding toxic effect of CNS depressant drugs, namely respiratory depression, is clinically obvious, other drugs cause toxicities that are not so apparent. In order to ensure that a commercially available drug would not be dangerously toxic (especially in ways that are not apparent to the practitioner) when it is given in therapeutic doses, the concept of the *therapeutic index (TI)* was established.

The index is a numerical value that represents the relationship between the dose that is effective in 50% of animals tested (ED_{50}) and the dose that is lethal in 50% of animals tested (LD_{50}). The LD_{50} is obtained through laboratory testing in which a number of animals are given a drug in increasing amounts until the dose is lethal in 50% of the test animals. Because of biological variances among animals of the same species, some will exhibit toxic symptoms before others. As the dose increases, the animals that have toxic manifestations first will die first. Statistically, of the 50% remaining, only a few, if any, will not demonstrate at least one toxic symptom. In similar fashion the ED_{50} is determined when the desired end point is reached in 50% of test animals (for example, induction of sleep for CNS depressants, a significant drop in blood pressure for antihypertensive drugs, or eradication of pathogens for an antibacterial drug).

The therapeutic index is determined by means of the following equation:

$$TI = \frac{LD_{50}}{ED_{50}}$$

As the value of the TI increases, a wider margin of safety exists between the two doses. The greater the TI value, the safer the drug. For example, if drug A had an LD_{50} of 40 mg/kg and an ED_{50} of 4 mg/kg, its TI would be 10. If drug B (used for the same indication) had an LD_{50} of 16 mg/kg and an ED_{50} of 4 mg/kg, its TI would be 4. Thus it can be said that drug B is potentially 2½ times more toxic than drug A, or that drug A is 2½ times safer than drug B. All other variables not considered, if a company were considering marketing one of these two drugs, they obviously would choose drug A.

Generally, a minimum TI value of 4 is required by the Food and Drug Administration if a human prescription drug is to be made commercially available and not restricted to investigational use by designated clinicians. Many drugs having low TI values are used as anticancer agents (antineoplastics). Since these drugs are toxic to both cancer cells and normal cells, they traditionally have elicited serious hematological side effects, which are responsible for their low TI values.

Drug interactions

Knowledge about drug interactions is important in the determination of doses and administration intervals. Interactions are almost always a result of multiple drug therapy. The concept of drug interaction was first comprehensively discussed for practitioners during the Symposium on Clinical Effects of Interactions Between Drugs, presented in England by the Royal Society of Medicine, in April 1965. Since then the term "drug interaction" has appeared frequently in medical literature concerned with the side effects of multiple drug therapy.

"Drug interaction" can be defined as alteration of a drug's biological effect as a result of prior or concurrent administration of another drug(s) or substance(s).[6] The effect of an interaction can include anything from an absence of or a decrease in the expected clinical response to an exaggerated response. Although in practice the term has come to imply an unwanted effect, administration of more than one drug can be part of a planned drug therapy program designed to increase a drug's effect without increasing the drug's dosage to the point of risking toxic side effects. An example of a beneficial drug interaction is that produced by concurrent therapy with penicillin and probenecid, in which case the probenecid (used alone to treat gout and gouty arthritis) blocks tubular secretion of penicillin, thereby prolonging its blood level.

Interactions can occur as a result of chemical reactions between drugs or because of drug-induced alterations of biological systems. An example of a reaction between drugs is that which results from concurrent administration of a tetracycline-type antibiotic and a substance containing divalent (double-charged) ions. The chemical reaction forms a complex, composed of the tetracycline-type antibiotic and the ions, which markedly decreases antibiotic absorption. Divalent ions include calcium (Ca^{++}) and magnesium (Mg^{++}). Calcium can be found in dairy products such as milk and cheese, and magnesium compounds can be found in many antacids.

Drugs that alter the pH of various biological compartments, such as the gastrointestinal tract and the kidney, are responsible for chemical reactions that can influence the amount and rate of drug absorption and excretion. As was discussed in Chapter 1, pH changes in the gut affect the degree of drug nonionization and therefore the rate and degree of absorption. A drug that decreases urine pH will cause excessive excretion of basic drugs, since they will become more ionized (water soluble) and thus more readily excreted. As would be expected, drugs that increase urine pH promote the elimination of acidic substances, which become more ionized in higher pH ranges. It can generally be said that *acidic drugs promote the excretion of basic drugs, and vice versa.*

Another type of drug interaction results from differences in the relative lipid solubilities of different drugs and the effect of these differences on the drug-binding capacity of plasma. If drug A has a greater affinity for plasma than drug B, it can increase the concentration of free drug B by displacing drug B from plasma binding sites or inhibiting its uptake by plasma. Drug B thus is displaced when drug A is administered after it. Drug B is inhibited from binding to plasma by drug A when the two drugs are administered concurrently or when drug A is administered first. A clinically significant example of such a drug displacement type of interaction is the release of barbiturate molecules from receptor sites after their displacement by phenylbutazone molecules. Excessive concentrations of poorly water-soluble free drug resulting from plasma displacement can cause precipitation of the drug in kidney tubules as the fluid filtrate, but not the drug, is reabsorbed. Reabsorption of fluid makes less available to solubilize the drug, and when the drug's solubility constant is exceeded, precipitation results. Precipitation of sulfonamides in the kidneys, which can result when they are administered with the anticoagulant drug warfarin, is an example of such a displacement reaction. Sulfonamide precipitation in the kidneys, known as crystalluria, can cause proteinuria, hematuria, oliguria, and ultimately kidney failure, especially in carnivores.

The biological substances commonly involved in drug interactions are the liver microsomal enzymes responsible for drug detoxification. When the same enzymes are required to detoxify different drugs, they can initially be overwhelmed when a second drug is administered with the first. As a result, drug detoxification and excretion rates are temporarily decreased. Consequently the drugs maintain higher blood levels longer than anticipated. Clinically, it can be said that a drug interaction occurs that potentiates the activity of both drugs. In time, however, if concurrent therapy is continued, enzyme induction (see p. 28) usually occurs, resulting in decreasing detoxification time. If one drug is then discontinued, the elevated enzyme levels will detoxify the remaining drug more quickly than normal, resulting in lower than expected blood levels (because of enzyme induction), which can minimize therapeutic results.

Some drugs are believed to inhibit the action of secretory enzymes in the tubules, thereby prolonging blood levels of certain drugs. Probenecid (an enzyme inhibitor) acts in this manner to prolong penicillin blood levels. As indicated earlier in this discussion, food can be a factor in altering a drug's biological activity. Certain foods can react with drugs to decrease or delay their clinical effect. For example, concurrent ingestion of fatty foods and vitamin K, or other drugs having high partition coefficients, can result in delayed and decreased blood levels of this crucial vitamin, because its solubility in fat increases the time required for absorption and thus may prevent it from being entirely absorbed.

Specific drug interactions between commonly used drugs have been noted primarily as examples. The most practical approach to avoiding adverse drug reactions is to understand the general pharmacological and chemical characteristics of the drug groups discussed in this book. Memorization of individual interactions is both time consuming and temporary, but, more important, it does not provide one with the insight needed to evaluate the potential for interactions between any drugs and/or substances.

Be sure to review Appendix A, which provides an overview of interactions between intravenous medications.

• • •

This concludes the discussion of drug absorption, distribution, and elimination, which began with Chapter 1. Fig. 2-3 outlines the methods of administration and the possible routes a drug may travel, whether it is absorbed or not. As a review and study aid it would be beneficial to:

1. Consider all the principles discussed in the first two chapters that affect drug absorption and subsequent movement (kinetics) in animals
2. Decide the place(s) on the chart (Fig. 2-3) where these principles most appropriately apply
3. Determine the effects these principles have on the entire drug distribution pattern

For example, principles associated with the dissolution of oral dosage forms would most appropriately be listed between "Oral administration" and "Stomach," while the concentration gradient effect should be listed in all those areas of the chart where it affects drug kinetics.

The first two chapters have been intended to offer some fundamental insight into the complex in vitro and in vivo factors that govern drug kinetics and bioavailability. The intent of this brief exposure has been to give you an appreciation of

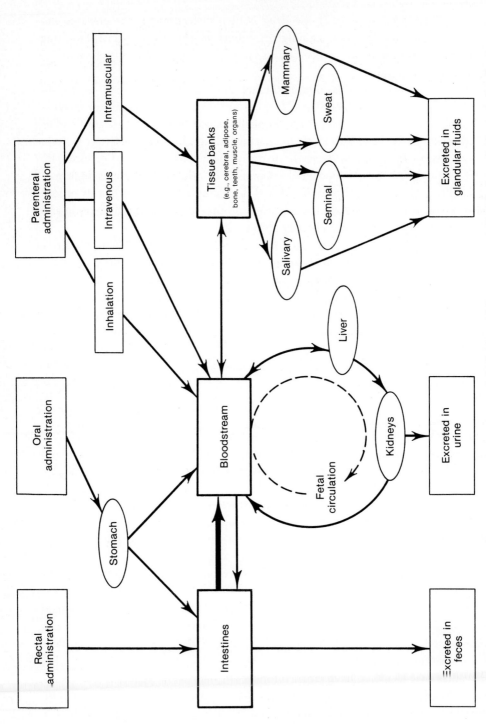

Fig. 2-3. Drug kinetics study outline—a schematic summary of the biological factors associated with drug absorption, distribution, and elimination, these three topics being collectively called "drug kinetics."

the factors that must be considered in developing a drug dosage form as well as dosage schedule. The remaining chapters of this book will primarily discuss the pharmacological activity of various drug classes, but it must be remembered that their biological impacts cannot be separated from the considerations thus far presented.

REFERENCES

1. Brander, G.C., and Pugh, D.M.: Veterinary applied pharmacology and therapeutics, ed. 2, London, 1971, Ballière Tindall.
2. Chodos, D.J., and DiSanto, A.R.: Basics of bioavailability and description of Upjohn single-dose study design, Kalamazoo, Mich., 1974, The Upjohn Co.
3. Dole, V.P.: Addictive behavior, Sci. Am. **243**(6):138, 1980.
4. Goldstein, A., Aronow, L., and Kalman, S.M.: Principles of drug action, New York, 1968, Harper & Row, Publishers, Inc.
5. Guyton A.C.: Functions of the human body, ed. 4, Philadelphia, 1974, W.B. Saunders Co.
6. Spinelli, J.S., and Enos, L.R.: Drugs in veterinary practice, St. Louis, 1978, The C.V. Mosby Co.

3

Diuretic drugs

PERFORMANCE OBJECTIVES

After completion of this chapter the student will:

- **Explain the mechanism of "obligatory water loss"**
- **List four factors that determine the relative potencies of diuretics that act by inhibiting tubular reabsorption of electrolytes**
- **Explain the difference between enzyme-inhibiting diuretics and osmotic diuretics**
- **List clinical situations that may be most suitable for each of the four major classes of diuretics**

Diuretic drugs

$\mathbf{D}$iuretics increase the volume of urine excreted by the kidneys. Urine excretion is directly proportional to the glomerular filtration and tubular secretion rates
(although the latter is not a significant factor) and inversely proportional to the
degree of tubular reabsorption. Therefore increasing the glomerular filtration rate
and/or decreasing the tubular reabsorption rate increases urine output. In practice,
increasing the glomerular filtration rate results in only a minor increase in urine output, since the animal still retains the ability to reabsorb electrolytes. Sodium and
chloride are the most abundant electrolytes, and consequently their location in the
body largely determines urine volume. When sodium and chloride concentrations
are highest in tissues outside the kidney, water diffuses from the tubular filtrate
into tissue as nature attempts to equalize the concentration of sodium on either
side of the tubular membrane. Water must migrate from the tubules, since in the
vast majority of animals tubular anatomy and physiology do not allow sodium to be
secreted from the bloodstream into the tubules. The higher the concentration gradient (the bigger the difference in electrolyte concentrations between filtrate and
tissue), the greater the movement of water from tubules and the smaller the amount
of urine excreted. A useful rule of thumb for determining routes of water migration
within a biological system is "Where sodium goes, water will follow." Fig. 3-1, *top*,

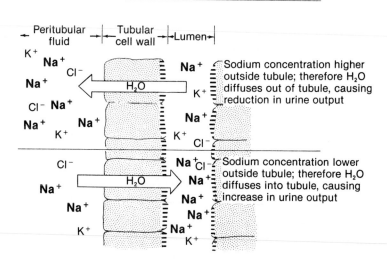

Fig. 3-1. Ionic concentration and osmotic flow. Passive water movement (osmosis) occurs as
a result of nature attempting to equalize different ionic concentrations on opposite sides of a
semipermeable membrane such as renal tubular cells. *Top*, Water migrates into peritubular
fluid to dilute its electrolyte concentration, which is composed mostly of sodium ions. *Bottom*, Osmotic flow occurs in the opposite direction when the electrolyte concentration is
higher in renal lumen fluid.

shows the dynamics of flow that are set up when sodium concentration is greatest outside the tubules; Fig. 3-1, *bottom*, illustrates the opposite condition. When tubular reabsorption is inhibited, electrolytes, especially sodium and chloride, are trapped in the tubular filtrate. As a result, larger quantities than usual of these ions remain in the tubules. Collectively they exert great osmotic pressure (concentration gradient effect), which opposes water reabsorption from the tubules. In addition, since these substances cannot leave the tubules, water is obliged to migrate, via osmosis, from other tissue into tubules in an attempt to dilute the filtrate so it can approximate body tissue concentrations. This osmotic flow of water into tubules is called "obligatory water loss"; it is responsible for lessening edematous conditions by increasing urine output. Diuretics that inhibit tubular reabsorption mechanisms are most commonly used clinically, since they are very effective and can be administered orally. The relative strengths of the drugs in this class of diuretic depend upon the following factors:

1. Number of enzyme reabsorption mechanisms that are inhibited.
2. Whether or not a drug also acts directly on tubular tissue to inhibit reabsorption (besides inhibiting enzymes).
3. The area of tubular inhibition. Reabsorption occurs all along the tubular surface, in proximal and distal tubules as well as the loop of Henle. Therefore the more area inhibited, the greater the diuretic effect.
4. The distribution and excretion properties of a diuretic.

The following discussion of drugs that act by inhibiting tubular reabsorption marks the first consideration of a drug category in this book. It should therefore be pointed out that chemical (including drug) nomenclature is based on structural similarities of compounds. Compounds sharing similar "core" structures are grouped together. Generally, drugs with similar chemical structures have similar pharmacological activity, potencies, and side effects. If one learns to connect nomenclature with drug categories and becomes familiar with the potencies that characterize the various categories, one will be able to predict an unfamiliar drug's biological effect.

TUBULAR REABSORPTION INHIBITORS
Carbonic anhydrase inhibitors

Carbonic anhydrase inhibitors (CAIs) are the least potent of the tubular inhibitors. They are rarely used as diuretics, since their administration causes little increase in urine output and chronic use oftentimes leads to metabolic acidosis. These drugs are indicated for the treatment of selected types of glaucoma (elevation of intraocular pressure), in which they reduce intraocular pressure without significant increases in diuresis. The mechanics of this pressure reduction in animals are not totally understood, but are currently presumed to be related to the inhibition of the enzyme carbonic anhdrase in the eye and a resultant reduction in the concentration of bicarbonate ions in the eye.[5]

Carbonic anhydrase is also present in tubular epithelium, where it is responsible for reabsorption of sodium as sodium bicarbonate. Carbonic anhydrase catalyzes the conversion of water and carbon dioxide (CO_2) in tubular filtrate to carbonic acid (H_2CO_3). Carbonic acid then immediately dissociates into bicarbonate ions (HCO_3^-) and hydrogen ions (H^+). The bicarbonate ions, having a negative charge, are attracted to free sodium ions present in the filtrate, to form the nonionized substance sodium bicarbonate ($NaHCO_3$). Since sodium bicarbonate is nonionized, it can be carried by transport enzymes through the tubular epithelium and into the bloodstream, thereby causing reabsorption of the sodium ion. This pathway is illustrated in Fig. 3-2. Since this mechanism is not a major pathway for sodium reabsorption, its inhibition does not significantly increase diuresis.

Carbonic anhydrase inhibitors are absorbed well from the gastrointestinal tract, with peak serum levels being reached in 1 to 3 hours. They are distributed throughout body tissue, concentrating in liver, muscle, eyes, central nervous system tissue, and especially the kidneys. Most drugs of this type can cross placental membranes,

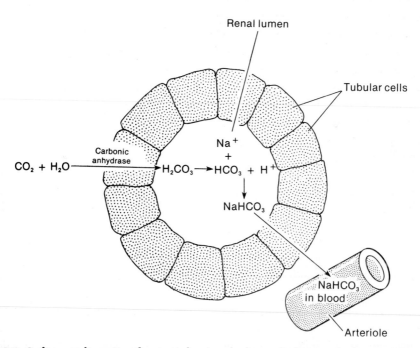

Fig. 3-2. Sodium reabsorption due to carbonic anhydrase. Carbonic anhydrase catalyzes the formation of carbonic acid, which in turn dissociates into hydrogen (H^+) and bicarbonate HCO_3^-) ions. Bicarbonate combines with sodium, forming sodium bicarbonate ($NaHCO_3$), which is reabsorbed. Interference with carbonic anhydrase results in copious diuresis of bicarbonate, sodium, potassium, and water.

and some have been recovered in the milk of lactating dogs. Teratogenic and embryocidal effects have been demonstrated in rats and mice that have received doses far above those used clinically.[1] Even though a cause-and-effect relationship has not been definitely established between clinical doses of these agents and developmental abnormalities, use of these drugs in pregnant or lactating animals should be discouraged if other agents can be substituted.

Diarrhea, malaise, and fatigue are the usual side effects that result from long-term CAI administration. Malaise and fatigue occur slowly and can go unnoticed unless one is familiar with how active an animal was prior to therapy. These side effects are associated with the development of systemic acidosis, which if not corrected will lead to further central nervous system complications, such as dizziness. Acidosis occurs because inhibition of carbonic anhydrase decreases the formation of bicarbonate, which is an in vivo alkalizing agent. Most side effects are dose related, and a reduction in dosage usually leads to a lessening of the side effects. The average dosage range for most small animals is 5 to 15 mg/kg once or twice daily.[7] However, since this group of diuretics as only marginal benefits at recommended doses, unless they are being used to treat glaucoma a reduction in dose can abolish any diuretic effect. The names of carbonic anhydrase inhibitors contain the ending "-amide" because they are derivatives of sulfon*amides*. The following are the commonly used CAIs; note the structural similarities between them.

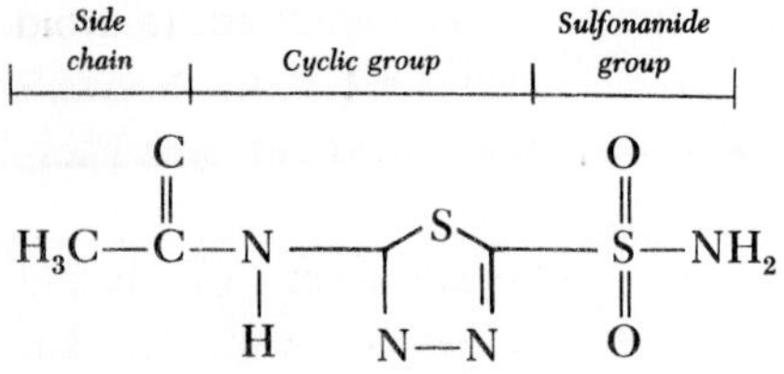

Acetazolamide

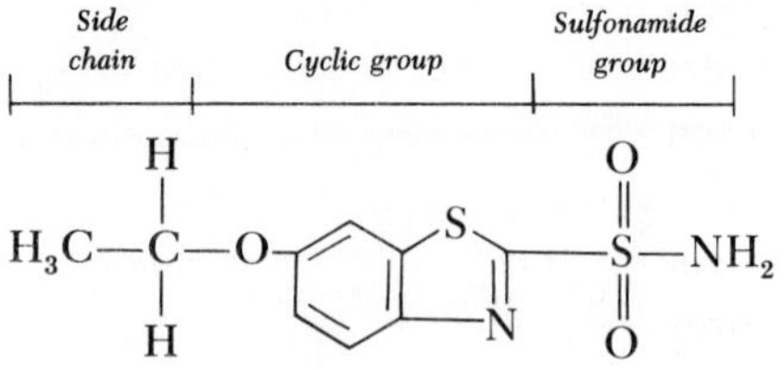

Ethoxzolamide

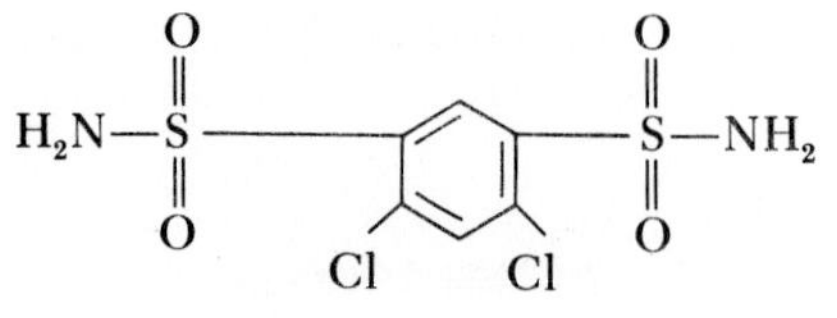

Dichlorphenamide

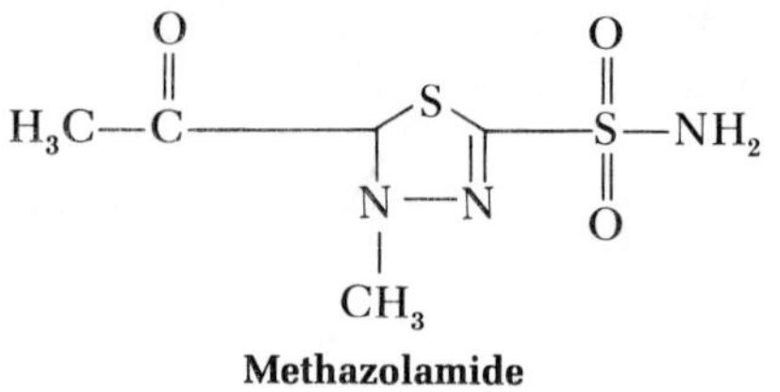

Methazolamide

The most important requirement for carbonic anhydrase inhibition by these drugs seems to be the presence of the sulfonamide group. If one or both of the sulfonamide hydrogen atoms are replaced, all carbonic anhydrase inhibiting action is lost. The presence of different cyclic groups and their side chains seems more for reduction of side effects than for increasing or decreasing potency.

Thiazides

Thiazide diuretics are used most commonly, since side effects are minimal and oral doses are highly effective. Like CAIs, most thiazides inhibit carbonic anhydrase, but they also act directly on the proximal tubules to depress sodium reabsorption.

Systemic acidosis, seen with use of the CAIs, is not as common with the thiazides, since depression of proximal function favors chloride excretion (as well as sodium excretion).[2,7] Loss of chloride, an in vivo acidifier, lessens the possibility of hyperchloremic acidosis.

Since both sodium and chloride are excreted, thiazides are more potent than the CAIs. Long-term thiazide use causes excessive potassium secretion (although less than sodium or chloride), which can lead to hypokalemia (deficient potassium) and resultant cardiac dysfunction. To prevent such electrolyte imbalance, foods or food supplements rich in potassium should be given concurrently with thiazide diuretics.

Thiazides are efficiently absorbed from the gastrointestinal tract after oral administration, with diuresis usually occurring within 1 hour and lasting from 12 to 24 hours, depending upon the excretion rate of the particular drug used. These drugs are distributed throughout extracellular fluid but do not concentrate in tissues or organs other than the kidneys.

If the edema is life-threatening a loading dose of double the normal dose can be given, but the dose should be reduced as soon as the animal has improved, to avoid excessive potassium loss. After the dose has been stabilized, some practitioners recommend occasionally skipping a dose to assure adequate potassium blood levels.[7]

Aside from the fact that side effects are minimal, another advantage of thiazide diuretics is that their effect is not diminished with prolonged use, a quality that precludes the need for dosage increases and thus reduces the potential severity of side effects such as potassium loss.

Hydrochlorothiazide can be considered the standard for thiazide drugs; its dosage range is as follows:

Parenteral	Small animals	12.5-25 mg IM
	Horse	50-150 mg IM or IV
	Cow	100-250 mg IM OR IV
Oral	Small animals	1.25-2.5 mg/kg
	Horse, cow	500 mg first dose; 250 mg daily thereafter[2]

Since hydrochlorothiazide is the standard for thiazide therapy, it can serve as a guide for determining doses of other drugs of this group. The relative potencies of other thiazides as compared to hydrochlorothiazide are as follows[2]:

Hydrochlorothiazide 1.0

Benzhydroflumethiazide	0.2	Methylcothiazide	0.08
Benzthiazide	2.0	Polythiazide	0.04
Chlorothiazide	10.0	Thiabutazide	0.75
Hydroflumethiazide	1.0	Trichlormethiazide	0.08

For example, 1 mg of hydrochlorothiazide has the clinical effect of 10 mg of chlorothiazide, while only 0.2 mg of benzhydroflumethiazide is equivalent to 1.0 mg of hydrochlorothiazide. Another way of interpreting these data is that it takes ten times more chlorothiazide than hydrochlorothiazide but only two tenths as much benzhydrofluomethiazide as hydrochlorothiazide to produce equivalent clinical results. Polythiazide is the most potent thiazide diuretic, since it requires only one twenty-fifth the dose of hydrochlorothiazide to effect the same clinical response.

The reason for benzhydroflumethiazide's high degree of potency is the presence of fluoride in its structure, as indicated by the syllable "flu" in its name. Fluoride-containing drugs are potent enzyme inhibitors, which accounts for the strong diuretic effect of this drug. In addition, most compounds containing fluoride are not easily detoxified by the liver's microsomal enzymes, since they too are inhibited by fluoride. This results in prolonged drug levels for most fluoride-containing drugs, including diuretics. Generally, fluoride-containing drugs within any class of drugs are the most potent agents.

As a group, thiazide diuretics have a low order of toxicity; daily oral doses of hydrochlorothiazide of up to 1000 mg/kg (400 times greater than the recommended dose) have been given to dogs for months without anatomical or physiological ill effects.[2]

Thiazide diuretics belong to a chemical group known as benzothiadiazides, and therefore all drugs in this category have the ending "-thiazide" in their names.

Furosemide

Although furosemide has structural similarities to both the thiazides and the carbonic anhydrase inhibitors, it is classified chemically as a monosulfamyl-type compound.[3] Like the carbonic anhydrase inhibitors, it is a sulfonamide derivative, as indicated by its "-mide" ending, but it does not inhibit carbonic anhydrase and therefore can be used in addition to the CAIs to increase urine output.

Inhibition of the tubular reabsorption mechanism by furosemide results in marked excretion of the following ions: sodium, chloride, potassium, hydrogen, calcium, magnesium, bicarbonate, ammonium, and possibly phosphate. Since all these ions are trapped in the tubules, the osmotic flow from tissue to tubule is pronounced, accounting for the effectiveness of this drug. Furosemide inhibits reabsorption of these electrolytes in the ascending portion of the loop of Henle as well as in the distal and proximal tubules. In addition to tubular reabsorption inibition activity, intravenous administration of furosemide initially causes a significant increase in renal blood flow, thereby increasing the glomerular filtration rate.[1] This effect may, in part, explain furosemide's rapid onset of activity. Because the drug is very potent, frequent blood electrolyte determinations are recommended, as well as periodic electrocardiograms to avoid hypokalemia-induced cardiac problems.[7] Side effects such as dehydration and sodium, hydrogen, potassium, and chloride depletion can occur rapidly.

Furosemide is absorbed well after oral administration, and even though 95% of the drug is bound to plasma protein its results are evident within 30 to 60 minutes and peak within the next 2 hours. The duration of activity is from 6 to 8 hours and can be expected to be longer if an animal has hepatic or renal dysfunction.[1]

As with all diuretics administered by an owner, rather than by veterinary personnel, doses should be given so that urination occurs at a convenient time for both the owner and the animal. Furosemide can be given to small animals (cats and dogs) at a rate of 1 to 2 mg/kg intravenously or 3 to 5 mg/kg orally, every 12 to 24 hours. Larger animals (horses and cows) may receive intravenous or intramuscular doses of 250 to 300 mg.[7]

Because of its rapid onset of action and the large increase in urine output, furosemide is usually reserved for alleviation of serious edematous conditions involving the heart and lungs. Once the threatening edema has been reduced, it may be preferable to start long-term treatment with thiazides, since side effects relating to electrolyte imbalances would not be as probable. If tolerance to the thiazides developed, however, most animals would still respond to furosemide therapy.

During reproductive studies in mice, rats, and rabbits, the administration of furosemide has been linked to unexplained abortions as well as to maternal and nonabortive fetal deaths.[1]

ORGANOMERCURIALS

Any mercury-containing compound, when absorbed, will cause diuresis during excretion through the kidney. This action is a result of the mercury separating from the organic portions of the compound and, like other heavy metals (such as iron and zinc), inhibiting specific enzyme systems that reabsorb sodium and chloride. Current mercurial diuretics are organic mercury-containing compounds; earlier, inorganic mercury drugs were found to be too toxic. The organic salts still produce mild kidney irritation in therapeutic doses and severe nephritis in higher doses. Mercurial diuretics are therefore reserved for emergency situations in which the animal has not responded to other diuretics. Since absorption after oral administration is erratic, mercurials are most often given by the parenteral route. Deep intramuscular injection is preferred, since injection of the drug close to the skin surface results in irritation and tissue sloughing because of liberated mercury. The intravenous route may also be used provided the adminstration rate is slow. Too rapid infusion results in cardiac damage.

The names of diuretics containing mercury usually begin with the "mer-" prefix, as in mercaptomerin, meralluride, and mercurophylline. The last two drugs contain mercury combined with the organic diuretic theophylline. The combination or concurrent administration of theophylline and mercury appears to reduce mercury toxicity and to increase the diuretic effect.[2]

ETHYL ALCOHOL (ETHANOL)

Administration of ethanol by the parenteral route causes a pronounced diuretic effect; ethanol acts as a general enzyme inhibitor, thereby preventing electrolyte reabsorption. Oral administration produces quick blood levels, since ethanol's high partition coefficient allows it to be absorbed directly from the stomach. Since oral administration to animals is not convenient because of ethanol's form and taste, veterinary use is usually limited to parenteral administration when other agents have proved unsuccessful. Ethanol is a central nervous system depressant, and therefore an animal's vital signs should be monitored during ethanol infusion and until the animal exhibits signs of increased activity.

SPIRONOLACTONE

Although spironolactone does not directly inhibit reabsorptive enzyme systems or act directly on tubular epithelium, it does inhibit reabsorption mechanisms in an indirect manner. The adrenocortical hormone aldosterone is responsible for activating enzyme systems in the distal tubules that reabsorb sodium, chloride, and consequently water. Potassium reabsorption is not affected. Spironlactone blocks receptor sites on these enzymes that are normally activated by aldosterone, so that aldosterone cannot activate them to perform their reabsorptive functions. Nonactive enzymes are called "proenzymes," so it may be said that spironolactone prevents the conversion of certain proenzymes to enzymes, the result being increased excretion of sodium, chloride, and water. In clinical cases of edema it is more expensive to use spironolactone instead of other diuretics—and less effective, since it is little more potent than carbonic anhydrase inhibitors. Thus spironolactone is usually reserved for special cases.

OSMOTIC DIURETICS

The diuretic effect of osmotic diuretics results from their physical property of being able to create large osmotic pressures, rather than from any chemical interaction with enzymes that are responsible for reabsorptive actions. Osmotic diuretics thus differ from the diuretics discussed thus far.[4] Osmotic diuretics are filtered by the glomerulus and largely retained in the tubules; thus their concentration in the tubules creates a large osmotic gradient between the filtrate and other body tissue. Since osmotic diuretics are poorly reabsorbed (if at all, as in the case of mannitol), they are administered by intravenous infusion and in high concentrations so that their concentration in the filtrate exceeds the kidney's capacity to reabsorb them.[6]

As a result, a major portion of these nonelectrolytes remains in the tubules, creating a large concentration gradient with respect to other tissue. The net effect is movement of cellular and interstitial fluid from tissues into tubules in an attempt to minimize the filtrate's concentration gradient, as illustrated in Fig. 3-3. These drugs elevate the osmotic pressure of the filtrate to such an extent that reabsorption of electrolytes such as sodium, potassium, and chloride is also inhibited.[1]

The effectiveness of osmotic diuretics is therefore due to the fact that they are not able to efficiently cross biological membranes and as a result stay in membrane-bordered compartments (such as the kidney), exerting a significant osmotic gradient effect. The osmotic effect causes water to flow out of other tissues and into the compartment.

Since osmotic diuretics do not cross membranes well, the only way to get high concentrations into the kidney is by intravenous infusion. When administered orally, some of these drugs remain largely in the gut because of their inability to penetrate intestinal walls effectively and gain access to the bloodstream; thus their effect is cancelled. As these hyperosmolar drugs circulate in the bloodstream prior

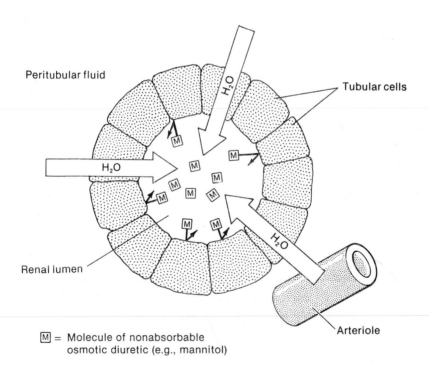

Peritubular fluid

Tubular cells

H_2O

H_2O

H_2O

Renal lumen

Arteriole

M = Molecule of nonabsorbable osmotic diuretic (e.g., mannitol)

Fig. 3-3. Diuretic effect of nonabsorbable molecules. High concentrations of nonabsorbable molecules in tubular fluid cause large amounts of water to move from peritubular areas and the bloodstream into the renal lumen. The resultant dilution of the nonabsorbable molecule concentration in the lumen leads to obligatory water loss.

to being filtered at the glomeruli, they cause similar osmotic fluid flow from other tissues. This phenomenon is the reason why osmotic diuretics are used to treat acute cases of elevated intraocular pressure resulting from glaucoma. The presence of hyperosmotic diuretics such as mannitol, urea, or glycerol in the serum increases the serum's osmotic pressure, which in turn causes fluid to flow from the vitreous portion of the eye. This reduces pressure and avoids irreversible damage to the optic nerve, which can result in blindness. Hyperosmotic agents are best used for acute glaucoma, since they are not as effective when used continually.[7]

Because of their administration route, quick onset of activity, and high degree of potency (which can lead to rapid electrolyte imbalances), osmotic diuretics are best administered by veterinary personnel and used only for emergency situations.

Mannitol

Since only a negligible amount of the mannitol that appears in glomerular filtrate is reabsorbed, it serves as an excellent agent to increase osmotic pressure in the tubules.

In mammals mannitol concentrates in the kidneys, as well as crossing the placenta, penetrating the eye, and probably appearing in the milk of nursing animals.[1]

Mannitol is available as a sterilized 25% parenteral solution; it should be warmed prior to use to ensure that any crystals of mannitol, which can form during storage, are dissolved.

Since so little mannitol is absorbed after oral administration, it is often used as a low-calorie sweetening agent in human foods.

Urea

Urea is a less desirable osmotic diuretic than mannitol, since it is generally less effective and more expensive. Like mannitol, urea causes water to be drawn from tissue masses—first into the blood and then from the blood into the renal tubules. Unlike mannitol, urea is a natural waste product and therefore is distributed in vivo more widely than mannitol. For this reason urea is not favored as a first-choice osmotic diuretic. In addition, high doses add to urea concentrations already in the bloodstream and may bring them to toxic levels. When administered orally, urea, unlike mannitol, is rapidly absorbed from the intestines and distributed in extracellular and intracellular fluids, including cerebrospinal fluid and blood.

Diuretic doses for smaller animals range from 0.5 g to 12 g; for larger animals, such as horses, doses range from 60 g to 250 g.[2]

Since solutions of urea are unstable, they are best stored under refrigeration (2° to 8° C). A kit containing a bottle of sterilized urea powder and a bottle of 10% invert sugar solution is available. This allows storage of the urea (in dry form) for at least 2 years. The solution is mixed with the urea when the drug is needed.

• • •

If diuretics are indicated for long-term therapy, such as in chronic congestive heart disease or chronic kidney dysfunction, it is helpful to maintain the animal on restricted-sodium or low-sodium diets. This can be done through the use of commercial food products that are designed to be low in sodium. These products usually contain moderate amounts of potassium, to avoid hypokalemia, as well as proper levels of other needed electrolytes, such as calcium and phosphates, to offset the amounts that are lost as a result of prolonged diuretic drug therapy.

REFERENCES

1. American Society of Hospital Pharmacists: Hospital formulary, vol. 2, 40:28, Washington, D.C., 1980, The Society.
2. Brander, G.C., and Pugh, D.M.: Veterinary applied pharmacology and therapeutics, ed. 2, London, 1971, Baillière Tindall.
3. DiPalma, J.R., and Rodman, M.J.: Basic readings in drug therapy, Oradell, N.J., 1972, Medical Economics Book Div., Inc.
4. Goldstein, A., Aronow, L., and Kalman, S.M.: Principles of drug action, New York, 1968, Harper & Row, Publishers, Inc.
5. Havener, W.H.: Ocular pharmacology, ed. 4, St. Louis, 1978, The C.V. Mosby Co.
6. Martin, E.W., and others, editors: Remington's pharmaceutical sciences, ed. 13, Easton, Pa., 1965, Mack Publishing Co.
7. Spinelli, J.S., and Enos, L.R.: Drugs in veterinary practice, St. Louis, 1978, The C.V. Mosby Co.

4

Drugs affecting the central nervous system

PERFORMANCE OBJECTIVES

After completion of this chapter the student will:

- Explain differences and interrelationships between the three sensory functions of the central nervous system

- List the events that occur in a neuron during polarization, depolarization, and repolarization

- List the biological sites of action for nonnarcotic and narcotic analgesics

- Name, in order of their appearance, the expected clinical symptoms manifested by animals that receive morphine in (1) recommended doses and (2) higher than recommended doses

- Describe the pharmacokinetics of ultra-short-acting barbiturates in terms of onset and duration of activity

- List two clinical differences between hypnotics and ultra-short-acting barbiturate anesthetics

- Calculate the therapeutic index, given the effective dose and the LD_{50} of a drug

- List two clinical differences between tranquilizing drugs and hypnotics

- Explain the etiology of convulsions and how anticonvulsant drugs alter it

Most drugs that alter central nervous system (CNS) activity depress such activity to one degree or another. Clinically these drugs are used for the following purposes:

1. To decrease pain without inducing sleep (nonnarcotic analgesics)
2. To decrease or totally block pain, with accompanying sleep (narcotic analgesics)
3. To cause localized loss of sensation, without sleep (local anesthetics)
4. To cause systemic loss of sensation, with accompanying sleep (general or systemic anesthetics)
5. To depress central nervous system activity to produce a state similar to sleep (hypnotics)
6. To alter behavioral patterns without inducing sleep (tranquilizers)
7. To correct abnormal brain activity (anticonvulsants)

All drugs discussed in this chapter have a common focal point of action—the central nervous system. However, not all of these drugs must cross the blood-brain barrier to exert their phramacological action (the local anesthetics, for example, need not do so). In order to understand and predict the clinical effects of CNS drugs, it would be helpful to briefly review the physiology of the CNS.

PHYSIOLOGY OF THE CENTRAL NERVOUS SYSTEM

The activity of the CNS can be conveniently divided into two major categories: sensory (reception) and motor (reaction). The sensory functions include receiving stimuli originating from inside or outside an animal's body, collecting them, and, finally, if they are complex enough, interpreting them. Once stimuli have been interpreted, motor neurons stimulate tissue masses to produce appropriate action.

The sensory functions of reception, collection, and interpretation are performed by neurons, which are the working units of both the sensory portion of the CNS and the motor portion. Receptor neurons are capable of converting energy, pressure, or chemical-related stimuli into electrical impulses, which ultimately can be collated and interpreted in higher sensory centers in the brain. *Preganglionic* receptor neurons convert in vivo or externally originated stimuli into electrical impulses. *Postganglionic* receptor neurons conduct electrical impulses. The strength of an impulse is proportional to the intensity of the stimulus (the more intense the stimulus, the stronger the electrical impulse).

A special type of receptor neuron is required for each of the three major types of stimuli. Energy stimuli (for example, heat and light) are received by *energy receptors*. Pressure (including sound waves) is received by *pressoreceptors* as varying amounts of force or percussion against body areas (such as the tympanic membrane in the case of sound waves). Physical properties (for example, wetness) and chemical properties (such as irritability) of substances are received by *chemoreceptors*. Receptor neurons are located throughout an animal's body but are concentrated on body surfaces such as the skin and hair follicles. Concentration of sensory neurons on the periphery is a result of evolutionary development, since more stimuli that are potentially harmful originate from the environment surrounding the body than from within the body. Receptors located on the skin and hair follicles are called *exteroceptors* (they include pressoreceptors, energy receptors, and chemoreceptors). *Proprioceptors* are located in tendons, muscles, joints and inner structures, while *visceral receptors* are located in the most internal areas of an animal, such as the stomach or the intestines. Thus sensory neurons can be classified according to the type of stimuli they receive as well as their location.

Chemoreceptors located in exteroceptive areas could be activated, for example, by chemicals released from damaged skin. Chemoreceptors in proprioreceptive areas could cause the perception of pain as a result of an accumulation of lactic acid in overexercised muscles. Chemoreceptors in visceral areas such as the stomach might elicit a nauseous feeling as a result of the presence of toxic substances or excessive amounts of hydrochloric acid.

Not all sensory receptors produce a conscious awareness of stimuli. In fact, a majority of responses to stimuli, such as increased heart rate during exercise, are subconscious motor reactions resulting from subconscious sensory interpretations. The farther up the brainstem impulses travel, the more complex they are and the closer to consciousness the motor reactions become. Complex stimuli elicit many types of sensations, which are called "modalities." The many modalities that can arise from simultaneous stimulation of energy receptors, pressoreceptors, and chemoreceptors (a situation that would result from the presence of a multifaceted stimulus) are loosely collected and crudely understood in the midbrain area. Full appreciation of the origin and intensity of a stimulus requires that the modalities it produces be passed on to the cerebral cortex, which is the true conscious area of the brain. The cortex, located in the upper portion of the brain, is the storehouse of information relating to past experiences.[6] It may be that reinforcement of these memories, as a result of the repetition of similar experiences, enables an animal to become more efficient in interpreting modalities. This would result in a quicker motor response each time a particular stimulus, or one similar to it, was received.

Since judgmental decisions made by animals are, in part, based on memory (acquired knowledge), it is not surprising that neurons associated with the measure of an animal's intelligence are found in the cerebral cortex. Unlike humans, who must accumulate most of their knowledge, lower animals are born with the type of inherited knowledge that enables them to stand, walk, and search for food. Generally, a major portion of the useful knowledge of many lower animals is inherited. The ability of a species to accumulate knowledge is proportional to its degree of cerebral development. Primates accumulate more knowledge than felines, and porpoises more than dogs.

Like stimuli, drugs that affect the activity level of the CNS exert their effect on its functioning unit, the neuron. The most common drug effect is an inhibitory action in the neuronal cycle, which is responsible for transmission of stimuli. Depression of neuronal activity, in turn, has a depressant effect on the entire CNS.

Discussion of the pharmacological activity of CNS drugs will be facilitated by the presentation of an overview of the neuronal activity associated with impulse conduction. Impulse conduction requires that (1) an electrical difference, called the *membrane potential,* exist between the inside and the outside of the neuronal membrane and (2) that the membrane be able to accommodate sudden shifts in electrolyte concentrations inside and outside the neuron. The membrane potential results from the concentration of positively charged ions being greater outside the neuron than inside (see Fig. 4-1). Although positively charged potassium ions are present inside the neuron, the amount of positively charged sodium ions outside is so great that the inside of the neuron becomes electronegative in comparison to the outside. It is this difference in electrical charges across the membrane that creates the electrical gradient (membrane potential) needed to facilitate impulse conduction along the axon when the neuron is stimulated.

When this condition of high sodium concentration outside the neuron exists, the neuron is said to be "polarized" or "resting." Stimulation of the neuron causes a change in the membrane permeability, which allows sodium ions to rapidly move inward. The rush of sodium ions into the neuron to offset the relatively negative

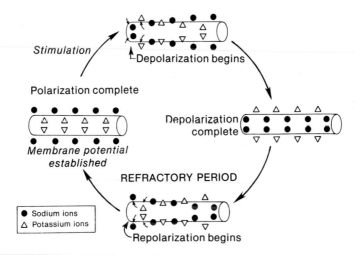

Fig. 4-1. Neuronal cycle of polarization, depolarization, and repolarization. A stimulus potent enough to depolarize a sensory neuron is conducted as an electrical current whose strength is proportional to that of the stimulus. Conduction along a neuron does not affect the entire neuron simultaneously but usually begins at one end and depolarizes the neuron as it travels its length. Depending upon conduction speed and neuron length, a neuron can be simultaneously undergoing depolarization at one end and repolarization at the other.

condition creates an electrical current, which is the impulse. As the area of permeability spreads along the axon, followed by the rush of sodium inward, the impulse is conducted and a reversal of the polarized condition occurs. Consequently this phase of neuronal function is called "depolarization." Immediately after the impulse passes, the inside of the neuron is positively charged because of the large number of sodium ions present (see Fig. 4-1). The membrane now becomes impermeable to continued sodium ion passage. Since potassium ions can freely diffuse across the membrane, they readily move to the outside of the neuron because of their high relative concentration inside. The loss of positively charged potassium ions completes the depolarization phase (see Fig. 4-1). The neuron now enters the refractory period, which can last from $\frac{1}{2500}$ to $\frac{1}{250}$ second.[6] During this period even a strong electrical impulse will not depolarize the neuron; hence the term "refractory period." As the refractory period continues, sodium ions that have entered the neuron during depolarization and potassium ions that have exited it must return to their original sites—a process known as "repolarization"—if the neuron is ever to become stimulated (depolarized) again. The reshifting of sodium ions is accomplished by the "sodium pump," which actively transports most sodium ions through the neuronal membrane and into interstitial fluid, thereby reestablishing the original resting membrane potential (see Fig. 4-1). The sodium pump is not necessary for membrane repolarization after the conduction of every impulse, since this is accomplished by the movement of potassium ions to the outside. The pump acts as a backup mechanism to potassium diffusion, to ensure that the process of reestablishing ionic concentrations is constantly occurring and to offset potential decreases in membrane potential that can be caused by a large number of impulses traveling along a neuron during a shorter period of time. The sodium pump operates only by expending cellular energy.

ANALGESICS

Analgesics (see Fig. 4-2) are not intended to be curative medication. Instead, they function to decrease the intensity of perceived pain by interfering with the functioning of sensory neurons.

Nonnarcotic analgesics

Nonnarcotic analgesics are used less frequently in animals than in humans. This may be due to the fact that unless an animal exhibits some sign of discomfort, the owner has no way of knowing that the animal is in pain. The most commonly used nonnarcotic analgesics are derivatives of salicylic acid, and therefore are called salicylates, or of aniline—for example, acetaminophen. A frequently used group consists of the pyrazolone derivatives, which have marked anti-inflammatory activity in addition to analgesic action. Other nonnarcotic analgesics are structually similar to morphine, while the remainder of such drugs represent a variety of chemical entities.

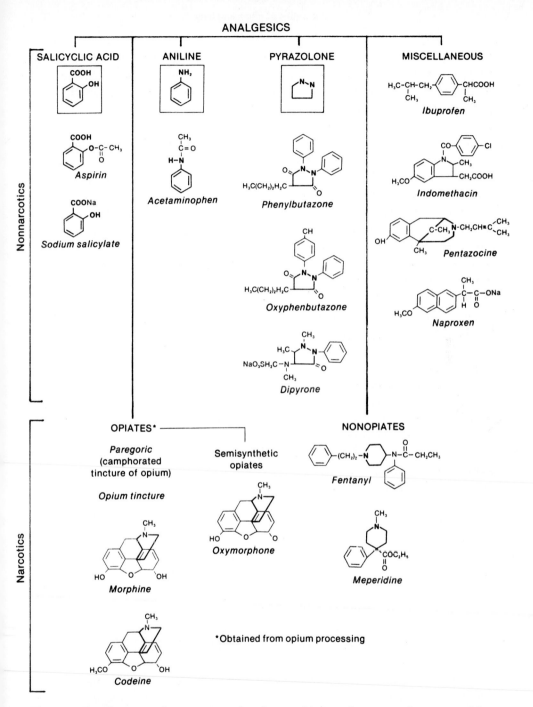

Fig. 4-2. Classification and comparison of analgesics. Most analgesics are derivatives of four core structures—salicylic acid, aniline, pyrazolone, and opium. It seems reasonable to suspect that the piperidine ring (outlined in darker print) present in pentazocine, fentanyl, and meperidine is at least partially responsible for their analgesic effect, as it is in the opiates and semisynthetic opiates. The newer analgesic, anti-inflammatory drugs, such as ibuprofen, indomethacin, and naproxen, appear to be structurally unrelated to each other.

Salicylates

The ability of salicylates to alleviate certain types of pain is related to their depressant action on the CNS. Experiments in animals suggest that collection and crude interpretation of pain impulses occur in the thalamus, which is located in the lower brain to midbrain region in most animals. Because salicylates do not cause mental disturbances, sleep, or changes in modalities of sensation other than pain, it is believed that they do not act in the higher, cortical regions of the brain. The exact mechanism by which salicylates block pain is unclear; however, it seems probable that they combine with neuronal membrane tissue to make it less permeable to the entrance and/or exit of sodium ions. Inhibiting the entrance of sodium would inhibit the speed and intensity of impulse conduction; inhibiting the exit of sodium would extend repolarization time, thereby reducing the number of impulses carried by a neuron per unit of time. There is also evidence that a portion of the pain relief offered by salicylates is due to a peripheral effect that may occur at receptor neurons.[5]

Salicylates also exert an anti-inflammatory effect; their ability to relieve pain by acting outside the brain could be related to this anti-inflammatory ability. During inflammation, in vivo chemicals such as histamine are released. Chemoreceptors—exteroceptive, proprioceptive, or visceral, depending on the location of the inflammation—can be depolarized by chemicals such as histamine and transmit pain impulses. Salicylates depress the inflammatory process by inhibiting the production of histamine, prostaglandins, and other endogenous chemicals. This inhibition reduces painful neuronal stimulation and prevents further tissue damage as a result of direct contact with histamine. (See Chapter 6 for a detailed review of the inflammatory process.)

Salicylates also exhibit antipyretic activity (fever reduction), which is attributed to their acting centrally in lower brain areas, especially the hypothalamus. The hypothalamus regulates body temperature by controlling heat production and heat loss. Rather than decreasing heat production, salicylates apparently act on the hypothalamus to stimulate mechanisms for heat loss. Loss of heat is thus facilitated by increased peripheral blood flow and sweating, both functions being mediated by salicylate-induced hypothalamus activity. Salicylates, like other antipyretics, therefore reduce fever by acting mainly on the CNS and not peripherally on blood vessels or sweat glands. The antipyretic activity is rapid and effective only when an animal's temperature is elevated and is rarely demonstratable when the temperature is within normal ranges.[5]

Because of their pH (4 to 5), salicylates are significantly ionized in the stomach; thus some absorption occurs there. Most absorption, however, takes place in the small intestine. Salicylates are rapidly distributed to all tissues, including lungs, heart, brain, and skeletal muscle (concentrations are small in the last two). Traces are found in bile, sweat, and feces. Salicylates cross placental barriers into fetal tissues. In situations in which salicylates need to be excreted quickly (such as salicylate intoxication), administration of systemic alkalizing agents such as sodium bicarbonate or sodium acetate hastens their excretion.

Acetylsalicyclic acid (aspirin). Use of aspirin is limited in veterinary medicine. Aside from problems of gastric irritation, some animals, especially members of the cat family, are overly susceptible to aspirin toxicity. Aspirin toxicity is manifested by loss of appetite, vomiting, and loss of balance; if allowed to continue, it causes anemia, bone marrow depression, severe ulceration of mucous membranes (especially in the upper gastrointestinal tract), shock, and finally hemorrhagic death. Aspirin's exaggerated toxicity in cats results from the inability of cats to detoxify an equivalent human dose efficiently. Unless the dosage is correct, high serum concentrations are prolonged, causing the adverse side effects. The following comparison of dosage levels illustrates the inefficiency with which cats detoxify aspirin:

> Bovine: 100 mg/kg every 12 hours
> Dog: 25 to 35 mg/kg every 8 hours
> Cat: 10 mg/kg every 52 hours, up to 25 mg/kg every 24 hours[10]

Sodium salicylate. Sodium salicylate is rarely used in veterinary or human practice; it exhibits the same adverse effects as aspirin, but they are often more pronounced. In addition, its analgesic and antipyretic actions are equal to or less than those of aspirin.

Sodium salicylate is usually reserved for use in larger animals, such as horses and pigs. To reduce gastric irritation, it is recommended that this drug be administered as an enteric-coated tablet or with food.

Acetaminophen (*N*-acetyl-*p*-aminophenol, APAP)

Acetaminophen is a derivative of *p*-aminophenol, which, in turn, is a derivative of aniline, as indicated in Fig. 4-2. Although other analgesics, such as phenacetin and acetanilid, are also derivatives of *p*-aminophenol, their use has been largely discontinued because of liver and kidney toxicity. In addition, their detoxification yields a metabolite, phenylhydroxylamine, which is responsible for methemoglobin production.[8] Unlike phenacetin and acetanilid, acetaminophen does not form phenylhydroxylamine. Like salicylates, acetaminophen is not used extensivly in veterinary practice, since it is effective only in treatment of mild to moderate, nonvisceral pain, which oftentimes is not evident to an animal's owner.

Frequently, drug metabolites have greater biologic activity than the "drug" itself. As a result the clinical actions of some drugs are due to their metabolites, the drugs themselves being largely innocuous. Acetaminophen is a classic example of this situation, since it is a metabolite of phenacetin and is largely responsible for the analgesic and antipyretic activity previously attributed to phenacetin. Detoxification of acetaminophen by hepatic microsomal enzymes forms a glucuronide conjugate, which is very water soluble and thus is eliminated rapidly by the kidneys. It should also be noted that toxic side effects of a drug can be due, in part or in toto, to drug metabolites rather than the administered drug.[4]

Acetaminophen produces analgesia and antipyresis through mechanisms similar to those of the salicylates. Unlike the salicylates, acetaminophen does not exhibit anti-inflammatory activity. Like the salicylates, acetaminophen is rapidly and almost completely absorbed from the gastrointestinal tract and quickly distributed to most body tissues.[4]

The major advantage of acetaminophen over the salicylates is that it does not irritate gastric mucosa and thus can be administered in high doses for extended periods of time. Prolonged use of excessive doses, however, can cause hepatic toxicity.

Acetaminophen is used as an analgesic and antipyretic in smaller animals; it is tolerated better than aspirin by cats. Maximum daily amounts are 900 mg for dogs and 300 mg for cats.[3]

Pyrazolone derivatives

Pyrazolone derivatives exhibit mild to moderate analgesia as well as significant anti-inflammatory effects in tissue outside the CNS, the precise mechanism probably being similar to that of salicylates. Pyrazolone drugs, like the salicylates, cross the blood-brain barrier to produce analgesia by inhibiting impulse transmission in midbrain to lower brain sites. Like salicylates, these drugs cause antipyresis by acting on the hypothalamus, with heat dissipation being increased as a result of vasodilation and increased peripheral blood flow.

The most common use for pyrazolone-type drugs is to provide symptomatic relief of pain, and the inflammation that oftentimes accompanies it, associated with musculoskeletal disorders such as capsulitis, bursitis, arthritis, an uncomplicated lameness.[2,10] These drugs are not curative medications; irreversible damage can result if an animal exercises too strenuously before the disorder is corrected.

These drugs are readily and completely absorbed from the gastrointestinal tract, with noticeable clinical effects occurring within 45 minutes in single-stomached animals. In smaller animals peak plasma levels are reached in 2 hours and the duration of activity can be up to 5 days (except in dogs, in which it is considerably shorter). This prolonged activity is a result of high plasma-binding ability. As a result, increasing the dose does not result in a proportional increase in the amount of free drug or in the clinical effect. Only when plasma sites are saturated will the free drug concentration increase upon subsequent doses. In such a situation, unless dosage is regulated the sudden increase in the amount of free drug can have adverse hematological effects.

Pyrazolone derivatives are notorious for interacting with many other commonly prescribed drugs. One common case for these interactions is the pyrazolone drugs' high plasma-binding ability. These drugs displace previously or concurrently administered drugs (such as anticoagulants and sulfonamides) bound to plasma, causing excessive free drug blood levels. Displacement of anticoagulants and sulfonamides can cause hemorrhaging and crystalluria, respectively. Other frequently used drugs, including selected barbituates, antihistamines, tranquilizers, and steroids, are reported to diminish the effect of pyrazolone-type drugs during concurrent therapy. Presumably this is due to elevated amounts of the particular microsomal enzyme(s) required to detoxify all these drugs. Since they all utilize the same enzyme system(s), concomitant administration of at least any two will stimulate excessive production of the enzyme(s), resulting in quicker detoxification.[2]

Like the salicylates, pyrazolone derivatives are significantly irritating to the gastrointestinal tract and therefore should not be given with salicylates. (Be sure to review Appendix A for drug interactions involving these agents.) Since pyrazolone drugs can cause serious adverse effects in addition to those associated with drug interactions, they should not be the first drugs of choice and should be used only for conditions that are unresponsive to an adequate trial with salicylates.

Phenylbutazone. Phenylbutazone is the most widely used drug of the pyrazolone group. It produces an anti-inflammatory response while simultaneously depressing CNS activity associated with pain impulse transmission. It is slowly metabolized in cats, and dosage schedules that are not adjusted for this fact can lead to fatalities resulting from drug accumulation. Even in dogs, which can rapidly metabolize the drug, cases of anemia (presumably due to drug accumulation) have been reported. In most animals toxic symptoms include loss of appetite, resultant weight reduction, dehydration, and severe depression. Suggested doses for cats range from 6 to 12 mg/kg daily; in dogs the suggested dose is 10 to 15 mg/kg three times a day, with a maximum dose of 800 mg daily. Recommended oral doses for larger animals such as horses range from 2 to 4 gm/450 kg one to three times a day; the intravenous dose is 1 to 2 gm/450 kg.[10]

Oxyphenbutazone. Oxyphenbutazone is the most recent addition to the pyrazolone series. Although this drug has approximately the same effectiveness in terms of analgesic and anti-inflammatory action as phenylbutazone, it is claimed to be less irritating to mucosal tissue.

Dipyrone (Methampyrone). Like other drugs in the pyrazolone series, dipyrone also has the "-one" ending. It is reported to have an analgesic effect equivalent to that of phenylbutazone and oxyphenbutazone, but it is most prudently used for its antipyretic and anti–equine colic activity. Dipyrone should be used for its antipyretic effect only after adequate results with salicylates and/or acetaminophen have not been achieved. The drug can be used for dogs and cats as well as horses and cattle, but because of its great potential for side effects its use should be discontinued within a few days if desired results are not obtained.[5,10]

Pentazocine (Talwin)

Pentazocine has structural similarities to morphine. As a result it is a strong analgesic, without anti-inflammatory activity, and it is effective in musculoskeletal as well as visceral pain.[10]

Since pentazocine causes dizziness and occasional mental confusion in humans and temporary uncoordination in animals, it probably inhibits impulse transmission in cortical as well as lower brain areas. Like morphine, it exhibits depressant activity on motor impulse transmission and therefore is helpful in the treatment of muscular spasms such as those resulting from equine colic.[10] Pentazocine was originally designed to be dose equivalent to morphine but without the marked CNS depression that accompanies the use of morphine. However, there seems to be a maximum analgesic effect with pentazocine, so that increasing its dose does not produce an analgesic effect greater than that obtained with approximately 10 mg of morphine.[5] The drug can be administered orally or by intramuscular injection, but never intravenous injection. In dogs, intramuscular doses range from 0.5 to 1 mg/kg. Pentazocine is not recommended for use in cats.[5]

Despite initial claims by the manufacturer that the drug cannot be abused, significant amounts are used illicitly and practitioners are apprehensive about stocking it, especially in view of its questionable advantage over morphine or other narcotic analgesics.

Ibuprofen, indomethacin, meclofenamic acid, naproxen

These are all relatively new drugs producing analgesic and anti-inflammatory activity. Even though they are chemically dissimilar to each other, they all exhibit gastrointestinal irritation upon oral dosing and, like salicylates and the pyrazolone derivatives, should not be given in the presence of gastrointestinal disturbances or on an empty stomach.

Salicylates—most notably, aspirin—remain the standard for analgesic and anti-inflammatory activity, and therefore the literature for newer drugs claiming to have these pharmacological actions compares their relative potencies to the potency of aspirin. Only further clinical experience with these newer drugs will indicate whether their degree of pharmacological activity (both beneficial and adverse) in comparison to aspirin justifies their added expense.

Narcotic analgesics

Unlike nonnarcotic analgesics, narcotic analgesics induce sleep as well as abolish the types of pain generally seen in clinical situations. Narcotics can be classified by their origin. The opiate narcotic analgesics are either extracted from naturally occurring opium or derived in part from opium, with the remainder of the molecule being synthetically manufactured. Nonopiate narcotic analgesics are manufactured synthetically; usually only those portions of the opiate molecules that are believed to possess analgesic activity are duplicated. Morphine remains the most commonly used narcotic analgesic. Use of synthetic narcotics, such as meperidine, is increasing dramatically because of their decreased number and intensity of side effects as compared to morphine.

Opiate analgesics

The opium group of narcotic drugs contains among the most powerful and clinically useful drugs for the production of sensory and motor CNS depression. These drugs are used as analgesics and sedatives, because of their sensory depression activity, and as antispasmodics, to relieve a variety of spastic gastrointestinal tract conditions. Unfortunately, the CNS depression induced is not limited to the correction of pathological conditions but can progress to inhibit life-sustaining functions such as respiration. Prolonged administration of opiates leads to tolerance, possibly because of enzyme induction, so that the dose must be increased periodically. This is not usually experienced in veterinary practice, however, since morphine is most commonly used only as a preanesthetic medication.

As can be seen in Fig. 4-2, opiates share a mutual central structure known as the phenanthrene portion (three fused phenyl rings), and therefore they are sometimes referred to as phenanthrene narcotics. Interestingly enough, work with nonopiate analgesics has indicated that the phenanthrene moiety is not necessary for analgesia but that the piperidine portion, which contains the nitrogen atom, is required.[4]

Basic substances, such as opiates, found in plants are called alkaloids. Opium is the crude extract obtained from the plant *Papaver somniferum*, which contains the opiate (or phenanthrene) alkaloids. On the average, opium contains 11.6% morphine and 2.2% codeine, along with other opiate alkaloids of lesser medicinal significance. Although the largest producers of opium are Turkey, Yugoslavia, Iran, and India, only opium from the first two countries is used for medicinal preparations, because of its higher yield of morphine.[9]

Because of their potent CNS depressant effect, opiates inhibit all aspects of sensory and motor impulse conduction. They seem to interfere with sodium and/or potassium movement across neuronal membranes throughout the CNS (including higher cortical areas) and at neuromuscular junctions. This latter site of action could account for the marked antispasmodic (depressant) activity opiates exert on gastrointestinal musculature. It is also believed that opiates have a direct depressant effect on the sodium pump. Depression of the sodium pump, along with inhibition of ionic movement across neuronal membranes, would significantly increase the refractory period, thereby abolishing the conduction of pain impulses.

The activity of the opiates at motor and sensory ganglionic synapses is associated with their inhibition of acetylcholinesterase. This enzyme is responsible for destroying acetylcholine, which is released at synapses to carry an impulse from presynaptic to postsynaptic neurons. If acetylcholine is not destroyed after performing this function, its presence keeps the postsynaptic neuron in the refractory state. By inhibiting acetylcholinesterase, opiates prolong the contact of acetylcholine with postganglionic neurons, thus increasing the refractory period. An analogous situation occurs at selected neuromuscular junctions where acetylcholine is released. At these junctions, the muscle tissue remains refractory to further stimulation and muscular quiescence results.

In addition to the depressant effect on sensory and motor function, it also appears that the opiate alkaloids have a direct inhibiting action on intestinal smooth muscle.[7]

Tincture of opium. Tincture of opium consists of air-dried, naturally occurring opium exudate mixed with water and alcohol. As was mentioned earlier, crude opium contains all the opiate alkaloids, and presumably it is this mixture of alkaloids that allows opium tincture to be used not only as a good analgesic but an especially effective gastrointestinal antispasmodic. Tincture of opium contains 1% morphine, which is primarily responsible for its analgesic effect; however, its main use is for intestinal relaxation. It acts centrally as well as having a direct depressant effect on intestinal tissue; both actions cause closure of sphincters and decreased peristalsis and produce more prolonged constipating effects than morphine.

Tincture of opium is not recommended for use in cats, because of prolonged stimulatory effects, and it is generally not as reliable in large animals as it is in dogs. An additional drawback to its use in larger animals is that high volumes are required (for example, up to 120 ml in cows); such volumes increase the chance of excessive CNS depression. Depending upon the size of the animal and the condition being treated, doses in dogs usually range from 0.3 to 2 ml.[3]

Although not as potent as narcotics, nonnarcotics such as diphenoxylate should be used to decrease gastrointestinal motility in cases of diarrhea or gastric enteritis, when narcotics may not be indicated. Narcotics should be used for intestinal spasms only after nonnarcotics have proved unsatisfactory.

Paregoric (camphorated tincture of opium). Like tincture of opium, paregoric owes its antispasmotic and analgesic activity to a mixture of opium alkaloids; it is used for less severe conditions than tincture of opium. It is vital to remember that *paregoric contains only one-fortieth as much morphine as opium tincture; care must be taken not to confuse the two products.* In dogs the usual dose of paregoric is 2-6 ml. If opium tincture were mistakenly used in place of paregoric, the animal could receive a toxic amount of opiate alkaloids.

• • •

Use of both tincture of opium and paregoric may diminish drastically if newer, nonnarcotic analgesics and antispasmodics, which offer more predictable behavior in terms of both pharmacological response and animal acceptance, prove equally effective. Since these newer agents, such as nalbuphine hydrochloride, are nonnarcotics, a practitioner is not required to maintain purchase and utilization records or to provide a locked storage area, as must be done with narcotics.

Morphine. Morphine has remained the analgesic agent to which all others are compared. It has excellent analgesic and antispasmodic properties, although its use is primarily indicated for pain rather than hypermotility of the intestine. Morphine functions as the classical opiate analgesic; it exhibits central depressant activity, possibly by inhibiting the movement of sodium and potassium ions across neuronal membranes as well as inhibiting acetylcholinesterase and the sodium pump. Studies in dogs indicate that morphine freely penetrates the blood-brain barrier and that it is distributed to all regions of the brain and cerebrospinal fluid.[4] In addition to its central activity, morphine seems to exert a depressant effect directly on intestinal tissue.

In most cases, an animal receiving morphine will experience an initial, transient excitatory episode, resulting in involuntary salivation, urination, defecation, vomiting, and panting, accompanied by peripheral vasoconstriction. This paradoxical stimulatory phase is believed to be due to CNS receptor sites first becoming stimulated when they are exposed to morphine and then becoming depressed as the concentration reaches therapeutic levels. This supports the theory that opiates, if not all narcotic analgesics, cause CNS depression by accumulating on receptor sites, thereby blocking impulse transmission along neurons. The excitatory phase can be dangerous if an animal has food in its stomach, since it can aspirate the vomitus, causing life-threatening pneumonia. Defecation and urination are obviously problems, especially when morphine is used as preoperative medication. The most effective way to circumvent them is by following routine fasting procedures for animals that are scheduled for surgery. In cases of unanticipated surgery, preoperative administration of morphine can be used to quickly evacuate the entire gastrointestinal tract. CNS depression in dogs and other animals in which morphine is predictably effective follows directly after the stimulatory phase and is characterized by peripheral vasodilation, sedation, and shallow breathing.

The excitatory phase is exaggerated and prolonged in some animals, such as goats, horses, mules, and sheep, and therefore the use of morphine in these animals is not recommended; if it is used, it should be given with extreme caution. Traditionally morphine has also not been recommended for cats, because the extended hyperactivity it produces. This excitation seems to be primarily due to cats' inability to detoxify morphine as efficiently as certain other species can. As a result, the drug accumulates, leading to adverse clinical effects. It has been reported that since the effects are dose related, reducing the dose to 0.1 mg/kg giving it by intramuscular or intravenous injection result in analgesia without excitation. This is one-tenth the intravenous or intramuscular dose required for dogs.

Excitatory behavior in other animals may not be dose related but instead may result from a genetically determined peculiarity *(idiosyncrasy)* that causes it to react abnormally to the drug.[4] Most idiosyncratic responses result in adverse clinical manifesations, as is the case with morphine. However, the term is also used to include a marked reduction in biological response to a drug—or absence of a response—that is not due to enzyme induction or any other readily apparent reason. Administration of morphine, or any drug, in an animal that exhibits a true idiosyncratic response is *contraindicated* (not justified).

Morphine is not predictably absorbed after oral administration; when given by this route, it causes nausea and oftentimes vomiting. Thus intramuscular or subcutaneous administration is recommended. Morphine should never be administered by the intravenous route, since this causes exaggeration of the excitatory stage, which can lead to convulsions and death. In addition, the onset and intensity of the depressant phase are unpredictable when morphine is administered intravenously.

Upon reaching the bloodstream, morphine, like most narcotic analgesics, rapidly leaves and is distributed, in decreasing order of concentration, in skeletal muscle, kidneys, liver, intestinal tract, lungs, and brain. It is primarily detoxified in the liver, by conjugation, to form its diglucuronide salt; in the liver morphine also undergoes hydrolytic and oxidative degradation reactions. As is true of other drugs that are detoxified in the liver, blood levels of morphine will be prolonged in the presence of hepatic dysfunction. Morphine is also detoxified in CNS tissue, the kidneys, and the lungs. It is excreted mostly in the urine, with a small amount being excreted in the feces. Small amounts probably enter the milk of nursing animals. No developmental abnormalities have been reported as a result of animals that have been weaned on milk containing morphine.

Fatalities associated with morphine overdosage are due to respiratory depression leading to respiratory arrest. It seems probable that impulses from vascular chemoreceptors, which normally inform the respiratory center in the brain of the carbon dioxide level in blood, are inhibited or abolished. Since motor responses are proportional to sensory input, any signal reaching the depressed respiratory center could, at best, evoke only a minimal stimulation of intercostal muscles. Since morphine is distributed to skeletal muscle, it can be expected that the intercostal muscles will also be directly depressed by the drug. The resultant effect is decreasing respiration in the face of increasing carbon dioxide blood levels. Ultimately respiration ceases because of lack of central stimulation and possibly because of direct inhibition of the intercostal muscles.

Drugs that act to displace morphine from tissue receptor sites can be used as antidotes (antagonists) in cases of morphine toxicity. Two such drugs are nalorphine and naloxone. If such a drug is administered in time, it promptly reverses all the narcotic effects and causes marked stimulation of respiration.[4] When morphine is used preoperatively, it is usually given with atropine, a drug used to decrease salivation and prevent bradycardia (excessive cardiac depression).

Since morphine, like all narcotic analgesics, has such a profound impact on CNS activity, concurrent use of other depressant drugs usually increases its depressant activity. Refer to Appendix A for a listing of drugs that interact with morphine and the other narcotic analgesics.

Codeine. This opium alkaloid is approximately one-sixth as potent as morphine. Unlike morphine, codeine fails to produce proportionately greater narcotic effects as the dose is increased. Consequently, if recommended doses do not relieve pain, larger doses are unlikely to do so. Like morphine, codeine produces cortical and respiratory depression, but serious degrees of either are rare. In cases of acute codeine intoxication, nalorphine is the specific antidote. As would be expected, codeine is less likely to cause nausea, vomiting, or constipation than morphine. Similarly, the initial stimulatory effects of codeine in dogs are minimal, if clinically demonstrable at all. Codeine is effective when given orally; it should be administered with food or milk to lessen gastric mucosal irritation.

Codeine is commonly used as a cough suppressant, since it seems to suppress the cough reflex center in the brain. Its use should be limited to dogs. For pain 2 mg/kg should be given every 6 hours by subcutaneous injection; for cough 5 mg (per dose) should be given every 6 hours by mouth.[7]

Semisynthetic opiate analgesics

In an effort to obtain analgesics that possess the advantages of morphine but not its disadvantages, chemists have modified the structure of the natural opium alkaloids. Interestingly, it was this type of molecular manipulation that produced not only more potent analgesics than morphine but also the morphine antagonist nalorphine.

Oxymorphone. As indicated in Fig. 4-2, oxymorphone is a semisynthetic opiate analgesic that retains the phenanthrene moiety. Oxymorphine is approximately 8 to 10 times stronger in intensity of analgesia than morphine. It is somewhat less constipating and usually does not cause vomiting or defecation. The overall incidence and severity of side effects, including respiratory depression, are considered to be somewhat less than for morphine. Oxymorphone is used as a preoperative and analgesic medication for cats and dogs; the dose for both species is 0.1 to 0.2 mg/kg, given subcutaneously, intramuscularly, or intravenously.[7,9]

Nonopiate analgesics

The many undesirable side effects of natural and semisynthetic opiates, as well as the dependence on Mediterranean and Near Eastern countries for opium supplies, has stimulated the search for synthetic drugs having the analgesic abilities of morphine but fewer side effects and less addiction potential.

It is generally agreed that an ideal analgesic should (1) not cause the development of tolerance, (2) not be habituating or addicting, (3) have a large difference between its analgesic dose and its toxic dose, (4) be effective against all types of pain, (5) exhibit quick onset and long duration of activity, (6) not affect sensory modalities, (7) not depress respiratory, cardiac, or gastrointestinal activity, (8) be quickly reversible in its action, upon administration of a proper antidote, (9) be effective by all routes of administration, and (10) be relatively inexpensive.[9] The synthetic narcotic analgesics (nonopiates) represent an attempt to meet some of these criteria.

Meperidine hydrochloride. At first glance the structure of meperidine (see Fig. 4-2) seems to have little in common with that of morphine. However, both contain the piperidine group (in darker print in Fig. 4-2), which is essential for analgesic activity. Generally, meperid ι.e is indicated for all the uses of morphine, except as an antispasmodic agent. In dogs it causes less analgesia, respiratory depression, and sedation than morphine. Likewise, vomiting and defecation are not expected when meperidine is administered to dogs.

In cats the use of meperidine is not predictable because they rapidly detoxify it, even at doses bordering on toxic amounts. As a result the normal dose for a cat is 3 mg/kg; the dose should not exceed 11 mg/kg, since toxic excitatory symptoms can be precipitated. Administration to cats is limited to intramuscular injection, since the contact of meperidine with oral mucosa may trigger reflex salivation and intravenous administration can cause toxic reactions.

Doses for dogs approximate the maximum for cats—10 mg/kg, by subcutaneous or intramuscular injection.[7,10]

Fentanyl citrate, fentanyl citrate with droperidol. Fentanyl is reported to be over 100 times more potent on a weight basis than morphine and to be equivalent to morphine in its respiratory depressant activity. It does not produce vomiting in dogs when it is given in recommended doses (0.02 to 0.04 mg/kg) as a preanesthetic medication. The use of fentanyl is not recommended in cats because of its hyperstimulatory effects; however, these side effects can be reduced through concurrent administration of the proper tranquilizing medication.[7,10]

A product containing fentanyl citrate and droperidol (Innovar-Vet) is used to produce a smoother state of analgesia and sedation, since droperidol, a tranquilizer, potentiates the action of the narcotic analgesic. Excitatory actions such as defecation and transient diarrhea still occur when the combination product is used, as they do with fentanyl alone. Even though the tranquilizer droperidol is present, Innovar-Vet is still contraindicated for use in cats, because of excessive stimulation.

Unlike the situation in regard to fentanyl, the depressant effects of the combination product are not totally reversible by administration of nalorphine hydrochloride or naloxone. These narcotic antagonists can reverse the respiratory depression caused by Innovar-Vet, but the tranquilizing symptoms can be eliminated only through detoxification and excretion of droperidol. Innovar-Vet can be administered intramuscularly in doses of 0.1 to 0.14 ml/kg; unlike morphine, it can also be given by the intravenous route—up to 0.09 ml/kg in dogs.[7]

• • •

The narcotic analgesics can be used as preoperative medications; they calm an animal, significantly reduce the amount of anesthetic drug required, and promote a smoother induction period. In addition to relieving severe pain, they are helpful for animal management in certain diagnostic or painful therapeutic procedures, such as bone resetting.

Endogenously secreted analgesics

Recent investigational work indicates that all vertebrates, regardless of their degree of evolutionary development, have receptors specific to opiate or opiate-like molecules located in the limbic portion of their brains. The limbic area consists of evolutionarily primitive regions in the core of the brain that are primarily involved with smelling in lower animals and emotions in humans. The fact that the receptors in the limbic area did not develop in response to opiate drugs suggests that they are normally concerned with receiving some molecule(s) that has remained unchanged throughout evolution.

Two investigators (Hughes and Kosterlitz) have isolated a morphine-like chemical from pig brains; they named the chemical "enkephalin," from the Greek "in the head."[11] Subsequently many variations of enkephalin have been isolated, all having potencies equivalent to that of morphine. Enkephalins appear to be produced at nerve endings of brain cells; like opiate drugs, they inhibit the rate of neuronal depolarization by making postganglionic fibers more resistant to sodium ion influx and potassium ion efflux.

Other investigators, at the University of California, have isolated a chemical from pituitary glands of camels that also exhibits a high degree of analgesic activity; it is 3 to 48 times more potent than morphine, depending upon the route of administration. They named this chemical alpha-endorphin (for endogenous morphine). Two other, chemically similar endorphins, beta-endorphin and gamma-endorphin, were subsequently isolated from the hypothalamus and pituitary glands of pigs at the Salk Institute. Interestingly, beta-endorphin has analgesic and tranquilizing effects in animals, while gamma-endorphin has been found to induce violent behavior in rats.

Further research in the area of enkephalins and endorphins holds the possibility that their in vivo production could be enhanced so that animals and humans could synthesize larger amounts than usual in response to pain stimuli. The advantage of in vivo production is that such agents are nonallergenic and, it is hoped, nonaddicting. It may also be possible to commercially manufacture these chemicals—or similar chemicals that, when injected, would mimic the in vivo response without necessarily causing a dependence upon the drug once it was no longer needed to manage pain.[11]

Comparison of analgesic potencies

The relative potencies of analgesics—both narcotics and nonnarcotics—are tested by a simple method known as the "tail flick" response. Constant heat is applied to a rat's tail so that in approximately 10 seconds the tail is flicked away from the heating coil. After injection of an analgesic into the rat, the flick is delayed or sometimes even abolished. Since the extent of delay is both drug and dose related, the potencies of different analgesics can be compared; the longer the delay, the more potent the drug.[5]

• • •

Since opiates and other narcotic analgesic drugs can create a nonmedical dependence, their use and distribution are closely governed by federal regulations enforced by the Drug Enforcement Agency (DEA). Refer to Appendix B for a summary of the regulations affecting the use of narcotic drugs.

ANESTHETICS

Two classes of anesthetics are discussed in this book: (1) local anesthetics, which abolish sensory perception only from that part of the body to which they are administered and do not produce clinical systemic CNS depression, and (2) general anesthetics, which abolish sensory perception and motor activity throughout the entire body. The general anesthetics are classified according to route of administration—either inhalation or intravenous injection.[9] Fig. 4-3 summarizes the categories of anesthetic agents discussed in this chapter, listing the individual drugs in each group and their routes of administration.

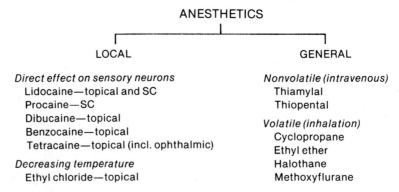

Fig. 4-3. Categories of anesthetics and usual routes of administration. Local anesthetics affect only the immediate area of their application. If a surgical procedure is to be done, restraint of the animal is required. General anesthetics result in total immobilization of the animal and require monitoring of vital signs.

Local anesthetics

Local anesthetics diminish or abolish pain perception from localized, peripheral areas by one of two related methods: rapidly lowering body temperature in the area of application or decreasing nerve transmission from the area. Most commonly used local anesthetics are applied as topical solutions, creams, ointments, or ophthalmic solutions. Parenteral solutions intended for subcutaneous injection can also be used. It is important to remove hair and organic debris from the area of application so that the topical anesthetic has direct contact with the peripheral tissue.

Ethyl chloride

The only clinically used drug that functions by lowering tissue temperature is ethyl chloride. When sprayed on skin, it evaporates rapidly (because of its extremely low boiling point and the temperature of the skin), drawing heat from the tissue and causing it to become insensible to stimuli. The actual reason why insensibility develops may be the inability of enzymes involved in shifting electrolytes across the neuronal membrane to function in the low-temperature environment. If the anesthesia produced is viewed as the result of a dysfunction in enzymatic activity that prevents depolarizing of nerve membrane, then the pharmacological effect of ethyl chloride can be considered very similar to that of other local anesthetics, the only difference being the way it is achieved. Ethyl chloride inhibits enzyme-mediated depolarization by a decrease in temperature, while other local anesthetics chemically react with neuronal enzymes to inhibit depolarization.

Ethyl aminobenzoate (Benzocaine), dibucaine, lidocaine, procaine

It has been theorized that these local anesthetics (which are listed in Fig. 4-3) prevent depolarization of nerve membrane, an event that is necessary for transmission of an impulse. As in the case of ethyl chloride, this can be the result of interference with the enzymatic activity associated with the exchange of sodium and potassium ions across cell membranes. As a result, the membrane potential needed prior to impulse transmission does not develop and the neuron cannot enter the depolarized (conductive) stage. Most local anesthetics do not cause vasoconstriction at the site of application or injection. As a result some practitioners may also apply or inject a vasoconstrictor such as epinephrine in a strength of 1 part epinephrine to 200,000 parts diluent. Some commercial anesthetic products contain a vasoconstrictor, usually epinephrine 1:200,000 or 1:100,000, along with the anesthetic. Vasoconstrictors increase the duration of anesthesia by impeding absorption of the anesthetic through inhibition of blood flow to the area of injection or application. Any potential toxicity (especially to the heart) that an anesthetic agent may have is also reduced by the vasoconstricting activity, since it slows down entry of the drug into the cardiovascular system. Use of any local anesthetic injection containing epinephrine is not recommended for extremities (that is, paws), since the circulation can be excessively reduced causing gangrene-like, irreversible tissue destruction. The opposite effect—that is, increasing the area of local anesthesia without multiple injections—can be produced by using hyaluronidase in conjunction with the local anesthetic. Hyaluronidase is an enzyme that, by modifying the permeability of connective tissue, allows an injected anesthetic to markedly spread out from the area of its injection, thereby increasing its sphere of activity. As would be expected, the use of hyaluronidase greatly diminishes the duration of anesthesia. This can be obviated, however, by the addition of epinephrine, without affecting the spreading action.

$\bullet$ $\bullet$ $\bullet$

A requirement for any local anesthetic is that it should not cause tissue damage in the wake of its activity, especially when applied to the eye.[8] Preparations such as clove oil and eugenol have long been used as local anesthetics, especially in dentistry. However, in view of their potential for mucous membrane irritation and their questionable clinical results, their use is not recommended.

General anesthetics

A major difference between narcotic analgesics and general anesthetics is the degree of CNS depression induced by therapeutic doses. Narcotics, in addition to abolishing painful stimuli, induce a degree of CNS depression that is similar to sleep; general anesthetics induce a state of greater CNS depression, termed "unconsciousness." The stupor produced by narcotics can be interrupted by sufficient stimulation, while the unconscious state cannot. Another distinction between narcotic analgesics and general anesthetics is that when sleep terminates after a narcotic analgesic has been administered, the sensation of pain is missing, while termination of the unconscious and sleep stages induced by a general anesthetics is accompanied by pain perception. Methoxyflurane is an exception to this generalization.

Intravenous anesthetics

All injectable anesthetics are derivatives of barbituric acid, which, strangely enough, is not a CNS depressant (see Fig. 4-4). Substitution of different organic groups on carbon 5 either increases or decreases the partition coefficient of the drug molecule as well as giving it hypnotic activity. To a point, as the number of carbon atoms attached to carbon 5 increases, so does the molecule's lipid solubility. The partition coefficient can also be markedly increased by replacing the oxygen on carbon 2 with a sulfur atom. As was discussed in Chapter 2, increasing the partition coefficient of free drug molecules facilitates their movement across any membrane, including the blood brain-barrier. The more lipid soluble a barbiturate is, the easier

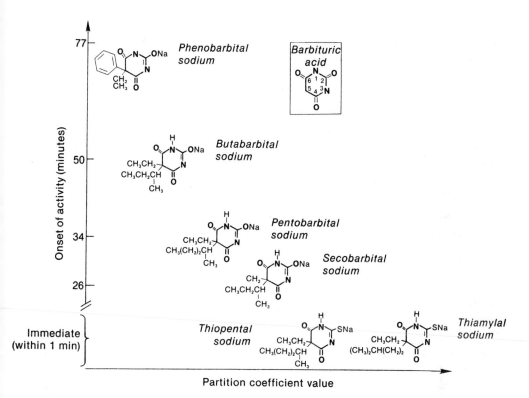

Fig. 4-4. Structure-activity relationships between barbituric acid derivatives. The addition of organic groups to carbon 5 of barbituric acid (insert) imparts CNS depressant activity to the molecule. When these groups are straight-chained and/or branched aliphatics rather than cyclic molecules (such as the phenyl ring of phenobarbital), the partition coefficient is high. As the total number of aliphatic carbon atoms on carbon 5 increases, the time required for onset of activity decreases. In addition, if sulfur replaces oxygen on carbon 2, anesthetic activity is immediate, because of the dramatic increase in partition coefficient and the resultant ease with which these molecules pass the blood-brain barrier.

(and quicker) it can cross the blood-brain barrier, the quicker its onset of activity, and the shorter its duration of action. Barbiturates are classified according to duration of activity: long-acting, medium-acting, short-acting, or ultra-short-acting. As would be expected, the ultra-short-acting barbiturates have the largest number of carbon atoms attached to carbon 5 and a sulfur atom on carbon 2, while the long-acting barbiturates have the smallest number of carbon atoms attached to carbon 5 and an oxygen atom on carbon 2. Barbiturates that have a sulfur atom on carbon 5 are referred to as "thiobarbiturates" ("thio" means sulfur), while the other barbiturates, all of which contain oxygen on carbon 5, are called "oxybarbiturates."

Pharmacological activity and distribution. The ultra-short-acting barbiturates are used for induction of general anesthesia. Upon intravenous administration their extremely high partition coefficient allows immediate penetration across the blood-brain barrier and into brain tissue. They appear to act, in part, at the level of the thalamus to inhibit conduction of impulses to cortical areas. As a result these areas receive minimal input from stimuli, activity drops to a baseline, unconsciousness follows. The rapid onset of activity is due to the route of administration as well as the partition coefficient value. However, the brevity of their apparent duration is related to the redistribution of these drugs, by the bloodstream, from cortical areas into noncerebral areas, which is facilitated by their high partition coefficient rather than detoxification by the liver.[1] Awakening therefore does not mean that all effects of the anesthetic have worn off; animals, particularly if they are obese, oftentimes remain drowsy or asleep for extended periods of time, especially if multiple doses of an ultra-short-acting barbiturate were used to maintain anesthesia.

In order to understand the effect adipose tissue has on anesthetic action, it would be helpful to trace the fate of an ultra-short-acting barbiturate once a single dose is injected. Because of its high lipid solubility, a large amount of the drug becomes temporarily inactivated by being bound to plasma protein. This forms one depot from which the anesthetic will later be released to replace free drug removed from the bloodstream by distribution into extravascular tissue. Since brain tissue is lipoidal and highly vascularized, there is no delay in the onset of anesthetic action; effective doses usually induce sleep in the time required for blood to travel from the injection site to the brain. As free drug continues to be carried by the bloodstream, it is deposited in areas of the body in proportion to blood supply (the larger the blood supply, the more drug deposited). Consequently, cerebral uptake occurs first, followed by increasing visceral concentrations, and finally uptake by lean body tissue (muscle) occurs. Assuming the animal is not obese, adipose tissue concentrations of anesthetic increase gradually (since blood supply to adipose tissue is minimal) until the drug begins to diffuse from muscle tissue. At this time, drug concentration in fat increases more rapidly. Fig. 4-5 provides a chronological summary of the distribution of the anesthetic thiopental into different body tissues. As a result of extravascular distribution, anesthetic tissue concentration quickly equilibrates with

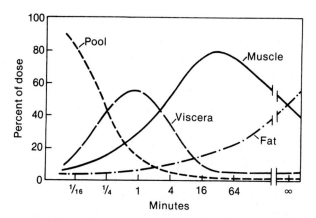

Fig. 4-5. Distribution of thiopental after injection. The time required to reach peak concentrations in each tissue area depends on the rate of blood flow to it. The "pool" refers to the amount of drug in cortical areas. Once anesthetic starts leaving cortical areas, peak concentrations are first reached in the viscera, where blood flow is abundant, then in muscle, and finally in fatty tissue, where blood perfusion is lowest. (Modified from Abbott Laboratories: A professional guide to the use of Pentothal, publication no. 97-0919/R2-35, April 1975.)

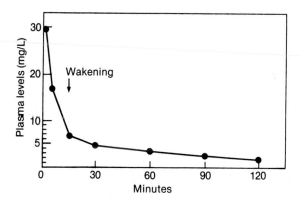

Fig. 4-6. Thiopental plasma levels following administration. This graph illustrates the decline in plasma concentration of the ultra-short-acting barbiturate thiopental (Pentothal) that occurs after administration of a 400 mg dose. Initially plasma levels of the drug decrease to replace free drug in the aqueous blood phase. Once whole blood concentrations of the drug fall below tissue levels, the drug rapidly leaves tissue sites, such as the brain, and migrates to the blood. Unless more drug is given, plasma and free drug levels continue to drop until enough drug leaves the brain so that the animal can be awakened. Awakening in this case occurs approximately 15 minutes after administration of the thiopental. (Modified from Abbott Laboratories: A professional guide to the use of Pentothal, publication no. 97-0919/R2-35, April 1975.)

the free drug concentration in blood. As free drug in the aqueous portion of the blood diminishes, plasma-bound drug diffuses out in an attempt to equalize the concentration between the two blood phases. When the total blood concentration falls below the concentration in the tissue, the direction of anesthetic distribution reverses in an attempt to reach equilibrium between tissue and bloodstream. At this point the cerebral anesthetic concentration decreases to less than that required to maintain anesthesia; unless more anesthetic is administered, the animal will begin to regain consciousness. Fig. 4-6 illustrates graphically the typical rapid decline in blood levels of an intravenous ultra-short-acting barbiturate after a single injection.

It is important to be aware that in nonobese animals in which an intravenous anesthetic is predictably effective, maximum cerebral tissue concentrations of drug are reached within 1 minute of a single injection. Because the vascularization of the muscles is less than that of the brain, anesthetic distributed to them requires longer to diffuse out. Therefore anesthetic will continue diffusing out and equilibrating with the blood concentration even after the animal first awakens. This is why, as was previously mentioned, the duration of anesthetic effect is more a function of drug redistribution (from brain to bloodstream) than liver detoxification and kidney excretion.[1]

The amount and distribution of adipose tissue dramatically affects anesthetic induction and especially recovery from anesthesia. If fatty tissue is excessive, more of the anesthetic will migrate into it, thereby prematurely reducing free drug blood levels. This results in the anesthetic diffusing out of cerebral tissue quicker than normal, which in turn decreases the period of anesthesia. In order to sustain anesthesia, more of the drug must then be administered, ultimately resulting in higher drug concentrations in adipose tissue. It should be remembered that the low vascularity of adipose tissue will cause gradual diffusion of drug out of fatty tissue in order to equalize blood–adipose tissue concentrations. The more adipose tissue, the more drug that can be stored in it and consequently the longer elevated blood levels of the drug will persist. The clinical result is a prolonged recovery period from the effects of the anesthetic drugs, especially if multiple doses were necessary.

If enough anesthetic is administered to saturate adipose tissue storage sites, free drug will most probably enter cerebral tissue at an accelerated rate, thereby causing rapid and excessive CNS depression. Furthermore, drug will continue to diffuse from the saturated adipose tissue sites to other tissue. This causes even more anesthetic to enter cerebral tissue. In practice this rapid, dynamic redistribution of drug in obese animals makes it difficult to maintain a steady state of anesthesia. Since more drug always has to be administered to compensate for that transiently lost in fatty tissue, the potential for dangerous degrees of CNS depression resulting from redistribution of drug is greater than it is in lean animals. In addition, a significant, but unknown, amount of drug will be gradually released from adipose stores, causing extension of the recovery period.

The administration of barbiturates must be monitored extremely closely when they are used in thin, muscular breeds (such as greyhounds) or in emaciated animals. Since less than the "normal" amount of noncerebral tissue is available for drug distribution in these animals, it can be expected that much smaller doses will be required to maintain anesthesia. Once cerebral uptake occurs, the barbiturate begins to equilibrate with other body tissue by migrating from the brain. Since the amounts of adipose and muscle tissue are low, less drug is required to leave cerebral areas before equilibration with other tissue is achieved. Consequently, anesthetic dosages of thiobarbiturates as well as oxybarbiturates should be drastically reduced from normal ranges for these animals, since it can be expected that cerebral barbiturate concentrations will endure for longer than normal periods of time.

Besides distribution to muscle and fatty tissue, ultra-short-acting anesthetics enter all body tissues; they readily cross the placental barrier, and have been found in milk, although no abnormal developmental patterns in offspring have been attributed to their presence.[2]

Detoxification. Although detoxification does not play a major role in the duration of anesthetic effect, it cannot be overlooked entirely. For many years it was believed the detoxification rate of the ultra-short-acting barbiturates was very slow. It is now generally recognized that detoxification occurs more rapidly than was formerly realized and that it may, in part, be responsible for early reduction in free blood drug levels and early awakening, along with the redistribution phenomenon.[1]

Barbiturates are detoxified mainly in the liver and primarily by oxidation of the carbon 5 side chains. The larger the chains the quicker the oxidative detoxification (which accounts in part for the extremely short duration of effect of ultra-short-acting anesthetics). Another detoxification process, which renders a drug molecule less fat soluble and more prone to excretion, is the removal of the sulfur atom (desulfuration).[2]

Thiopental sodium and thiamylal sodium. Chemically these ultra-short-acting barbiturates differ only in one of the carbon groups attached to carbon 5, with thiopental having an ethyl group (CH_3CH_2—) and thiamylal having an allyl chain (CH_2=$CHCH_2$—) as shown in Fig. 4-4. Clinically the two drugs can be considered equivalent in onset of activity, distribution, length of action, and rate of elimination.

Since these drugs are supplied as sterilized powders, only sterile water for injection (USP) (never bacteriostatic water for injection) should be added, aseptically, to reconstitute the powder and make solutions of varying strengths. Customarily a 2% solution is administered to both dogs and cats. Higher concentrations increase the risk of perivascular irritation and skin sloughing. Diluents containing bacteriostatic agents such as methylparaben, propylparaben, benzyl alcohol, and metacresol jeopardize solubilizing the drugs, with the possibility that a precipitate could be formed. In addition, they represent potential allergens, which could elicit dramatic anaphylactic reactions when administred directly into the bloodstream.

Unless these thiobarbiturates are administered with a muscle relaxant, tranquilizer, or other suitable preanesthetic sedative, they should not be administered to horses. Use of the anesthetic alone in horses induces anesthesia, but heavy falls may occur. In addition, Cheyne-Stokes breathing (characterized by a cyclic pattern of gradually increasing respiratory depth, and sometimes rate, followed by periods of apnea, with each cycle lasting approximately 30 seconds) is common when the anesthetic is used alone, and violent recovery periods are frequent. Because the rate of injection is directly proportional to the onset of anesthesia and inversely proportional to the duration of anesthesia, rapid injection of the calculated dose in horses premedicated with a CNS depressant will cause anesthesia in 20 to 30 seconds, with the effect lasting 3 to 4 minutes. If anesthesia is to last longer, it is customary to maintain it with volatile anesthetics.[3]

As was mentioned earlier, both thiopental and thiamylal are supplied as sterilized powders to which only sterile water for injection (USP) is added to make a solution of the desired concentration. Since these solutions are strongly alkaline (pH 10.5), they have been considered to have an innate bacteriocidal effect. However, bacterial challenge testing indicates they are not bacteriocidal against all microorganisms; therefore aseptic technique should be used during their preparation. When sterile water for injection is used as the diluent and the solution is stored in closed glass bottles or capped glass syringes, it will remain physically stable for a few days at room temperature, and longer if refrigerated. Nevertheless, it is recommended that solutions be used promptly after reconstitution and that unused portions be discarded after 24 hours to guard against microbial contamination.[1]

Volatile anesthetics

Volatile liquids and gases are commonly used to induce anesthesia; the amount of anesthetic in the inspired air is progressively increased, ultimately increasing the concentrations in blood and brain. Like administration of nonvolatile, intravenous anesthetics, the use of volatile anesthetics results in progressive depression of the CNS, which can be preceded by varying degrees of excitation, depending upon the animal. These drugs initially depress the cerebral cortex and then the basal ganglia and cerebellum. This is followed first by sensory and then motor paralysis of spinal cord functions, starting from below and moving up the cord.[9] The clinical manifestations of these biochemical responses are classified as "stages of anesthesia."

Pharmacology, distribution, and excretion. Volatile anesthetics lack obvious common molecular features, yet all produce very similar effects on cerebral tissue. Like the ultra-short-acting barbiturates, they all have high partition coefficients, and it is postulated that they may dissolve in the lipoprotein portion of neuronal membranes and somehow inhibit their electrical impulse–conducting abilities. Volatile anesthetics may also alter the structure of enzymes involved in membrane permeability to sodium and potassium in a way that negates or largely inhibits their activity.[4,5]

Volatile anesthetics produce their effect regardless of how they are administered, as long as they reach the CNS. The standard method of administration is inhalation. Because they have high partition coefficient values, their distribution from the lungs and into tissues follows the same principles of distribution as the injectable anesthetics. Consequently volatile anesthetics distribute themselves out of the blood according to lipid solubility characteristics and the relative blood supplies to different tissue masses. The higher the concentration of drug (expressed as "volume per cent" or "partial pressure") in the inhaled mixture, the quicker the onset of anesthesia. As long as arterial blood contains a concentration of drug that is higher than the concentration in the tissue, the anesthetic continues to pass from blood to tissue faster than it passes from tissue to venous blood. Ultimately, an equilibrium is established when the anesthetic leaves and enters the tissue at the same rate. This condition is referred to as "anesthetic equilibrium," and, as is true with the use of the injectable anesthetics, it is seldom experienced in practice.

When the mask is removed, and drug administration thus discontinued, the following events occur in rapid succession:

1. The partial pressure (concentration) of the drug in the inhaled air is reduced to zero.
2. Arterial blood ceases to carry any anesthetic drug.
3. Tissue concentrations of anesthetic drug become higher than blood concentrations, so the drug moves from tissue to venous blood, thus reducing the cerebral drug concentration below the level needed to continue anesthesia.
4. Drug continues to diffuse out of muscle and fat stores in proportion to their relative supplies of blood.

Volatile anesthetics are excreted, largely unchanged (not detoxified), in the exhaled air, although small amounts may also be excreted in urine. The rate of exhaled excretion is different for each drug; it depends on many variables, such as concentration in blood, partition coefficient, respiration rate, and lung capacity. The general pattern of excretion, however, is about the same for most agents given to nonobese animals: approximately half of the drug is excreted in the first 30 to 60 minutes after cessation of anesthesia. The remainder is excreted more slowly as it diffuses from poorly vasacularized areas.[8]

HYPNOTICS

The term "hypnotic" refers to the production of sleep. Hypnotic drugs are used to induce sleep when sleeplessness is not the result of a definite stimulus, such as pain. When pain is present, hypnotics in therapeutic doses do not usually cause sleep. If sleep is desired in such conditions, then other CNS depressants, such as narcotic analgesics, can be used, or the doses of hypnotics can be increased. Conversely, a low dose of hypnotic drugs can be used to achieve a "sedative" state. Sedation refers to the production of a calm condition, characterized by rest and relaxation but not necessarily sleep.

Hypnotics may be divided into two classes: barbiturates and nonbarbiturates. The former group consists of long-acting, medium-acting (or intermediate), and short-acting drugs. Clinically, barbiturate hypnotics differ from ultra-short-acting barbiturate anesthetics in that the former (1) require a longer time before their activity is apparent, (2) do not depress CNS activity to as great a degree, and (3) have a longer duration of action.

Barbiturates

Like the ultra-short-acting barbiturates, the long-acting, medium-acting, and short-acting barbiturates are derivatives of barbituric acid. Their classification by duration is rather arbitrary; comparisons of clinical data relating to duration of activity show considerable variation among different investigators, even when the same animal model is used.

Identifying the animal(s) used for such studies is of utmost importance, since considerable differencs in duration of sleep can be noted between species. For example, when the barbiturate hexobarbital is adminisered to various animals on an equal milligram-per-kilogram basis, laboratory mice sleep for an average of 90 minutes, rabbits for about 49 minutes, and dogs for approximately 315 minutes.

Responses to the barbiturates, as well as to any drug, by different species or breeds of animals are determined by the interplay between many factors. Rate and characteristics of absorption, rate and degree of detoxification, and excetion rate, all discussed in Chapters 1 and 2, affect the response of a particular species or breed to a particular drug. In addition, the type and amount of body tissue characteristic of each species and breed govern how animals respond to a drug. Differing responses among species are largely the result of differing absorption, detoxificaton, and excretion mechanisms (for example, the relative inability of cats to respond favorably to barbiturates). The fact that reactions to a drug vary among breeds is mainly the result of differences in tissue type and dispersement (for example, larger doses, on a milligram-per-kilogram basis, of a barbiturate are needed for a husky than for a greyhound).

It is also important to use the same route of administration when the actions of barbiturates are being compared. The onset time of a long-acting barbiturate such as phenobarbital can be somewhat decreased when the drug is given by intravenous injection rather than the oral route.

Any classification of barbiturates according to onset and duration of activity must therefore specify the animal model and the route of administration and be based on equivalent milligram-per-kilogram doses. Only when these factors are taken into account can any meaningful distinctions be made about onset or duration of pharmacological effect. An example of such a comparison appears in Fig. 4-7, which compares six barbiturates in terms of duration of effect and time required for the disappearance of all drug-related symptoms. The test animals were dogs, and all doses were administered orally and in equivalent amounts. Duration of activity can be determined by measuring the horizontal distance on the dotted line between the curves of each drug line. Time required for disappearance of symptoms can be obtained directly fom the "hours" axis. It is generally agreed that for many animals secobarbital *(line A)*, pentobarbital *(line B)*, amobarbital *(line D)*, and its sodium analogue *(line C)* are considered short-acting barbiturates while barbital *(line E)* and phenobarbital *(line F)* are long-acting drugs

The drug partition coefficient is a major factor in determining the onset and duration of action. The higher the partition coefficient, the quicker the onset and the shorter the duration. As would be expected (see Fig. 4-4), the ultra-short-acting barbiturates have the highest partition coefficient, with this value decreasing as the onset time increases. As a result, the long-acting barbiturates have the lowest partition coefficients of the four groups.

Like the ultra-short-acting barbiturate anesthetics, the barbiturate hypnotics are derived from barbituric acid. Unlike the ultra-short-acting anesthetics, however, all other barbiturates contain the suffix "-barbital" in their names.

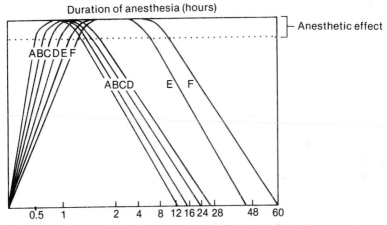

Fig. 4-7. Duration of activity for certain barbiturates administered to dogs. Secobarbital (line *A*), a short-acting barbiturate, requires approximately 30 minutes (0.5 hours) to induce anesthesia, which lasts 45 minutes. In comparison, the long-acting barbiturate, phenobarbital (line *F*) requires approximately 70 minutes to induce an anesthetic state, which lasts for about 96 minutes. The time required for disappearance of symptoms is proportional to both rapidity of onset and duration of effect; the longer the onset time, the longer the duration of activity and the longer the time required for complete disappearance of all barbiturate symptoms. For example, short-acting secobarbital requires 12 hours for disappearance of drug symptoms, while longer-acting phenobarbital requires 60 hours. Line *B*, Pentobarbital. Line *C*, Amobarbital sodium. Line *D*, Amobarbital. Line *E*, Barbital. (Adapted from Krantz, J.C., and Carr, C.J.: Pharmacological principles of medical practice, ed. 6, Baltimore, 1965. The Williams & Wilkins Co.)

Pharmacology, distribution, and excretion

The principal response evoked by a hypnotic barbiturate is depression of the CNS to a degree that causes sleep. Generally, most barbiturates are absorbed well from the gastrointestinal tract, but their absorption route and maximum attainable blood levels are affected by the presence of food. As is true of most drugs, the quickest action can be obtained if they are given on an empty stomach. The hypnotic barbiturates act upon the cerebral cortex, most probably in the thalamus, to interfere with the conduction of sensory impulses to the cortex. When these agents are given orally in therapeutic doses, their effect on respiration is slight. This is probably due to the wide distribution these drugs have throughout an animal's tissues. Being less fat soluble than the thiobarbiturates, they can equilibrate themselves into relatively more muscle mass. A dose thus is more uniformly distributed throughout the biological system rather than immediately being concentrated in cerebral lipids. Like the ultra-short-acting agents, hypnotic barbiturates rapidly cross placental tissue after administration and may appear in milk. Generally, the hypnotic drugs follow the same distributive pathways as the injectable thiobarbiturates, with the relative amounts of drug that dissolve in cerebral tissue and nonlipid tissue being functions of the drugs' partition coefficients.

If large enough doses of a hypnotic are administered, the respiratory function will become paralyzed as a result of central depression. The dose of hypnotic barbiturates that would be required to produce respiratory arrest is much greater than would be needed with the ultra-short-acting barbiturates.[8]

The long-acting barbiturates (such as phenobarbital) are absorbed and excreted slowly in urine. In some animals up to 85% is eliminated unchanged, indicating that the organic groups attached to carbon 5 are resistant to oxidative detoxification by the liver. This also accounts for their prolonged duration of activity.[3]

Medium-acting (intermediate) barbiturates (such as butabarbital) are seldom used clinically, since a genuine need for them instead of the longer-acting drugs rarely exists.

Secobarbital and pentobarbital are short-acting barbiturates that upon intravenous injection can be used as surgical anesthetics, their onset being quicker and their duration being longer than those of the ultra-short-acting barbiturates. If sedation or hypnosis (rather than anesthesia) is desired, secobarbital and pentobarbital are routinely given orally. They are also used as preoperative medications to reduce the amount of anesthesia needed and to lessen an animal's anxiety. These drugs are detoxified more rapidly than the longer-acting drugs (but slower than the ultra-short-acting barbiturates), with detoxification occurring primarily in the liver. Unlike the situation in regard to the ultra-short-acting barbiturates, whose duration of effect is determined largely by drug redistribution, the hepatic detoxification rate is the primary factor governing the duration of action for short-acting barbiturates. Consequently, if hepatic and/or renal disease is present, it can be expected that the duration of their activity will be increased. In such a situation the dose should be appropriately reduced if administration is intended to continue for long periods.[3,8] When secobarbital and pentobarbital are used as injectable preanesthetic medications, there is a tendency to mix other drugs, such as the phenothiazine-type tranquilizers, with them in the same syringe. This is not advisable, since the injectable short-acting barbiturates have a pH of approximately 10. If the pH is lowered by addition of acidic drugs, precipitation of the barbiturate will result.

Generally, barbiturates can be administered to dogs and cats as well as to larger animals. The possibility of producing excessive excitaton is greater in cats than in dogs, and intravenous injection for sedative purposes in horses results in prolonged, significant CNS depression.

Nonbarbiturates

The use of older, nonbarbiturate drugs to induce sleep is rapidly on the wane. These drugs often took the form of "cocktails" composed of numerous CNS depressant drugs, such as paraldehyde, chlorobutanol, and chloral hydrate. Although these mixtures were effective, concern about their potential for cardiac, liver, and kidney toxicity resulted in their being replaced by newer, single-entity drugs, the effects of which can be measured more definitively.

Chloral hydrate

Chloral hydrate still is of value as a hypnotic (when administered by the oral route) or as an anesthetic (when given intravenously). Sleep results from depression of higher cortical areas, with the lower cerebral areas (which are responsible for vital functions such as respiration) not being affected unless doses are very high.

Since the hepatic detoxification of chloral hydrate requires conjugation with glucuronic acid, it is not recommended as a first-choice drug for use in the cat family. As was discussed in Chapter 2, cats do not have hepatic conjugation abilities for glucurnoic acid.

Concurrent administration of chloral hydrate and any drug containing a significant amount of ethyl alcohol is not advisable, since their mutual CNS depressant actions can produce unconsciousness rapidly. Mixtures of chloral hydrate and alcohol were originally called "Mickey Finns" or "knockout drops."

Sedative doses administered orally range from 0.3 to 1 gm for dogs, from 0.12 to 0.6 gm for cats, and from 15 to 45 gm for horses.[3]

Ethinamate, ethchlorvynol

These drugs, which are not related to each other structually, induce sleep for most animals within 20 to 30 minutes, the duration of action being about 4 hours. Both drugs have demonstrated a low order of toxicity in various laboratory animals. Organs such as the brain, bone marrow, and kidney showed no clinical toxicity after prolonged ingestion of either drug. It appears that the liver is not involved with the detoxification of either drug, and thus the effect of either is not potentiated or prolonged when administered to animals having impaired liver function. Unlike the situation with regard to the barbiturates, animals do not seem to develop a tolerance to these drugs, and therefore increasing the dose after long-term therapy is not usually required.[8]

Flurazepam

Structurally flurazepam belongs to a group of chemicals known as the "benzodiazepines," which are widely used as animal and human tranquilizers. The two most publicized drug in this group are chlordiazepoxide (Librium) and diazepam (Valium).

Flurazepam's exact mechanism and site of action are not known, but the drug appears to inhibit impulse conduction at subcortical levels of the CNS to produce not only sleep but also skeletal muscle relaxation.[2] This indicates that flurazepam may affect motor as well as sensory portions of the CNS. Flurazepam also exhibits anticonvulsant effects in many animal species.[2]

After oral administration the drug is rapidly absorbed from the gastrointestinal tract, with a sleep-like state occurring in most animals within 30 minutes. Animal studies indicate that flurazepam and its metabolites are distributed throughout all tissue. No data are presently available relating to flurazepam's penetration of placental tissue or whether it appears in milk. The drug is rapidly detoxified (probably in the liver, by conjugation), with its glucuronide metabolites being excreted in the urine. As is true of phenacetin, the metabolites of diazepam are pharmacologically active and probably contribute somewhat to its hypnotic effect.[2] Because, like chloral hydrate, flurazepam probably requires hepatic conjugation for at least one detoxification method, its use in cats should be monitored closely.

•   •   •

Nonbarbiturates are rapidly replacing the barbiturates as hypnotic drugs. All the nonbarbiturates that have been mentioned here require much higher relative doses than the barbiturates before respiration is significantly depressed; therefore, a wide margin of safety exists between the effective and toxic doses of nonbarbiturate hypnotics.

TRANQUILIZERS (ATARACTICS)

Before the advent of tranquilizers, animals were usually "sedated" by altering the dose of an intermediate or long-acting barbiturate. If sedation was intended for short periods, this was, and still is, an acceptable use for the barbiturates. If sedation was needed for extended periods to manage a behavioral problem, the barbiturates were, and are, less than satisfactory. Long-term barbiturate therapy for management of behavioral problems requires, when possible, constant modifications in dosage amounts and intervals. Excessively high blood levels of barbiturate(s) cause an animal to become lethargic, dizzy, and confused, while subtherapeutic levels do not manage the symptoms and may cause paradoxical excitation.

Like barbiturates, tranquilizers are CNS depressants. They differ from the intermediate-acting barbiturates, long-acting barbiturates, and nonbarbiturate hypnotics in that they do not produce sleep or excessive inhibition of voluntary movement, nor do they depress respiratory or cardiac function when they are given in therapeutic doses.[10]

Tranquilizers are derived from a wide variety of chemical compounds, which generally produce marginal CNS depression, thereby making an animal less responsive to external stimulation.[3] Clinically, a calming effect is manifested in the animal's behavior, accompanied, in most instances, by a loss of conditioned reflexes.

Pharmacology

It has been theorized that most tranquilizers act by at least one of the following, related mechanisms.

Alteration of concentrations of CNS neurotransmitters

A number of chemicals found in the brain have been identified as being necessary for transmission of nerve impulses throughout the CNS, the most prominent being dopamine, epinephrine, and norepinephrine. These are called catecholamines. Catecholamines are believed to facilitate, and probably potentiate, nerve impulse transmission. If neuronal impulses entering the brain are potentiated by excessive concentrations of catecholamines, and as a result normal impulse inhibitory mechanisms are overpowered, the brain becomes hyperstimulated, leading to fearful or aggressive behavior. It is believed that some tranquilizers, such as the members of the phenothiazine group, may act in the brain stem area to decrease the concentration of catecholamines, possibly by inhibiting enzymes responsible for their production or interfering with dopamine receptor sites. As a result, impulse transmission into cortical areas is depressed.[8,10]

Alteration of biochemical activity

Like any living tissue, the CNS, especially the brain, requires oxygen and glucose (an energy source) to power biochemical reactions. CNS depressant drugs can reduce the availability of oxygen and glucose to nervous tissue by a number of mechanisms, which are still not fully understood. Diminished oxygen and glucose supplies to cerebral tissue inhibit oxidative metabolic processes that are necessary for such reactions as the synthesis of catecholamines.[8] Since catecholamines facilitate impulse conduction, a reduction in their concentration should retard impulse transmission. It can likewise be expected that decreased catecholamine levels would reduce impulse intensity, thereby making an impulse's interpretation by an animal less traumatic.

Investigations in this area that have involved the administration of insulin (which reduces blood glucose levels) has demonstrated significant reductions in cerebral activity in hyperactive animals. As a result the animals become more manageable and even-tempered during a variety of stressful situations.

Alteration of CNS electrical functions

Preceding sections of this chapter have indicated that electrical activity within the CNS can be altered by certain drugs. These alterations are measured by implanting electrodes in the brain of restrained, conscious animals. In these experiments special attention has been given to measuring electrical activity in the "ascending reticular formation" of the lower brain, which is responsible for receiving impulses from all stimuli, both within and outside an animal's body. The recticular formation sorts and relays these input sensory impulses to appropriate higher cortical areas. It as been proposed that the impulses passed on from the reticular formation are essential to keep the cerebral cortex in a "waking state." As the number of impulses decreases, the cortex becomes less awake. It follows that the progressive depression of recticular activity will result in progressive CNS depression, the clinical effects being tranquilization, hypnosis, anesthesia, and death, in that order. Some tranquilizers are able to inhibit the activity of certain portions of the reticular formation, resulting in selective portions of the cerebral cortex not becoming affected while others show varying degrees of general depression.[8]

Inhibition of only those impulses originating from stimuli outside an animal's body is the most desirable tranquilizing effect, since internal stimuli, such as those involving respiration and cardiac function, would not be affected. No tranquilizing drug yet exists that depresses impulses from only environmental stimuli. It is the aim of drug manufacturers, however, to create a drug that primarily depresses impulses from stimuli originating from outside an animal rather than from within. Such a drug would moderate an animal's reaction to its surroundings without affecting vital internal sensory and motor activities.

• • •

The three mechanisms just discussed cannot be considered to operate independently of each other. For example, alteration of biochemical activity affects the concentration of neuronal transmitters as well as the degree of reticular activity. These mechanisms have been discussed individually here only for the sake of clarity and academic classification. All functions of the CNS, like the effects of the drugs that alter its activity, must be considered closely interrelated.

Phenothiazines

Phenothiazine-derived drugs cause a number of pharmacological responses other than tranquilization, such as moderate antihypertension, mild antihistaminic activity, and anthelmintic action. The phenothiazine molecule is a relatively unusual entity in medicine, being a triple-ring structure that incorporates a nitrogen atom and a sulfur atom, with various organic groups being attached to the nitrogen:

(tranquilizer, antihistamine, anthelmintic, or antihypertensive)

The composition of the organic group attached to the nitrogen atom largely determines the pharmacological effect of the entire molecule. If three aliphatic carbon atoms attached to another nitrogen atom (—C—C—C—N—) are bonded to the core nitrogen, the molecule will exhibit tranquilizing activity. If one of the carbons is removed, the effect of the molecule will be predominately antihistaminic. Other organic groups attached to the nitrogen will cause the molecule to have primarily anthelmentic or antihypertensive activity. Drugs derived from the phenothiazine molecule all contain the ending "-azine" as an indication of their origin.

Originally the phenothiazines were used as anthelmintics, but the CNS depressant side effects associated with their administration caused investigators to explore their use as tranquilizers. The phenothiazines are first-generation tranquilizers; they have represented a breakthrough over the use of barbiturates for animal and human management.

One interesting pharmacological effect most phenothiazines exhibit is the ability to reverse the biochemical effect of epinephrine. Normally epinephrine, like other catecholamines, acts to raise blood pressure. In the presence of phenothiazines, however, epinephrine causes a reduction in blood pressure.[10] Therefore epinephrine should not be administered to combat allergic reactions to a phenothiazine-type drug, since excessive hypotension (and possibly shock) can occur.

As was mentioned previously, phenothiazines appear to function in the brain stem area by reducing catecholamine levels. Whether this is accomplished by direct inhibition of enzymes responsible for catecholamine production and/or by depression of glucose and oxygen remains unclear.

Phenothiazine tranquilizers are also helpful in preventing nausea caused by motion (as in traveling) and agitated behavior resulting from minor stimuli such as itching. This is because these drugs depress not only stimuli from the environment surrounding an animal but also stimuli originating from within the animal, such as visceral regions.

Acetylpromazine, chlorpromazine, perphenazine, promazine, and trimeprazine

Acetylpromazine is useful in tranquilizing large and small animals and probably enjoys more use than the other phenothiazines as a preanesthetic medication. Although chlorpromazine and perphenazine are compatible in small animals, the results obtained are not as consistent as with acetylpromazine. Acetylpromazine should be used judiciously in male horses, because of the potential for irreversible paralysis of the retractor penis muscle. Neither chlorpromazine nor perphenazine is recommended for use in horses, since severe reactions such as excessive CNS excitation (especially with perphenazine) can occur. Perphenazine is especially potent in producing tranquilization in cattle.

Promazine has for many years been used for cats and dogs as well as for horses and cattle. Since promazine is excreted slowly, it accumulates in tissue. If an animal is used for human consumption, it is necessary to discontinue use of the drug within the prescribed period prior to slaughter. This avoids human uptake of the drug. Because promazine is excreted partially in milk, it cannot be administered to lactating animals.[10] The recommended behavior-modifying doses for the phenothiazines just mentioned are summarized in Table 4-1. (Preanesthetic phenothiazine doses are listed in *Small Animal Anesthesia,* the first volume of this series.)

TABLE 4-1
Recommended doses for commonly used phenothiazine-type tranquilizers

Drug name	Animal	Route of administration	Dose
Acetylpromazine	Cat	Oral, IM, IV, SC	1.1-2.2 mg/kg
	Dog	Oral	0.5-2.2 mg/kg
		IM, IV, SC	0.5-1.1 mg/kg
	Horse	IM, IV	2-4 mg/45 kg
Chlorpromazine	Cat, dog	Oral	3.3 mg/kg
	Cat	IM	1 mg/kg
	Dog	IM	1.1-6.6 mg/kg
		IV	0.5-4.4 mg/kg
Perphenazine	Cat	Oral	2 mg/kg
		IM, IV	1 mg/kg
	Cattle		
	Under 360 kg	IM, IV	10 mg/45 kg
	360-700 kg	IM	100-150 mg
		IV	75-125 mg
	Dog	Oral	1 mg/kg
		IM, IV	0.5 mg/kg
Promazine	Cat, dog	Oral, IM, IV	2.5-6.5 mg/kg
	Cattle, horses	Oral	1-2.5 mg/kg
	Cattle, horses, sheep, swine	IM, IV	0.4-1 mg/kg

The phenothiazine derivative trimeprazine is approximately 30% weaker than chlorpromazine and has a shorter duration of activity (approximately 1 hour after intravenous injection). Unlike chlorpromazine and the other phenothiazines, trimeprazine does not exhibit anti-epinephrine activity and has strong antihistaminic effects. Consequently its main use is in controlling agitated reactions to pruritis. Its mode of action in this condition is presumed to be generally like that of the other phenothiazines, with trimeprazine possibly being more specific for stimuli received by exteroceptors. Trimeprazine is recommended for use in all species of domesticated animals but is particularily indicated for horses and cattle, in both of which chlorpromazine and perphenazine are not usually the first drugs of choice. As is true of all the phenothiazines, concurrent use with barbiturates potentiates the CNS depressant activity of both drug groups. If members of the two groups are given concurrently, it is suggested that the barbiturate dose be reduced by 30%.[3] (Review Appendix A for the effects of concurrent administration of CNS drugs and other commonly used medications.)

Butyrophenones

This group of tranquilizers includes the drugs droperidol, dehydrobenzperidol, and azaperone. These drugs are considered potent tranquilizing medications, and they have proved very effective in pigs which are notoriously difficult animals to handle. They also are of benefit in animals that are not responsive to phenothiazines.

For most species of animals butyrophenones can also be administered intramuscularly as preanesthetic drugs.[3]

Benzodiazepines

The benzodiazepines are used extensively in both human and veterinary medicine. The most notable drugs in this group are diazepam (Valium) and chlordiazepoxide (Librium). Both chlordiazepoxide and diazepam exhibit tranquilizing and skeletal-muscle relaxant properties in animals, with diazepam being approximately five times more potent in most species. Both drugs have been used to tame wild animals that have been removed from their natural settings. In addition, both medications, especially diazepam, exhibit anticonvulsant activity. Diazepam has also been of limited value in the treatment of muscle spasms, although no evidence to date suggests it has selective depressant activity on the motor portion of the CNS. It has also been reported that chlordiazepoxide exhibits anti-inflammatory activity in some species; however, verification is thus far lacking.[8]

Doses of diazepam for dogs range from 2.5 to 20 mg, whether administered orally or by intravenous injection, and from 2.5 to 5 mg in cats, in which the drug is given by the same routes. Diazepam is most readily detoxified by glucuronide conjugation in the liver. Members of the cat family cannot detoxify it by this route, which accounts for the drug's lower recommended dose in cats.

Recently a new member of the benzodiazepine group, Lorazepam (Ativan), has been introduced; this drug is presently available for oral or intravenous administration.

"-diols"

Although at first glance meprobamate and phenaglycodal seem structurally unrelated, both contain two carbon atoms with oxygen atoms attached to them:

$$H_2N-\overset{\overset{\textstyle O}{\|}}{C}-O-CH_2-\overset{\overset{\textstyle CH_3}{|}}{\underset{\underset{\textstyle (CH_2)_2CH_3}{|}}{C}}-CH_2-O-\overset{\overset{\textstyle O}{\|}}{C}-NH_2 \qquad CH_3-\overset{\overset{\textstyle OH}{|}}{C}-\overset{\overset{\textstyle OH}{|}}{\underset{\underset{\textstyle Cl}{\bigcirc}}{C}}-CH_3$$

Meprobamate **Phenaglycodol**

Biotransformation of the molecules into similar metabolites produces a clinically similar CNS tranquilizing effect. In phenaglycodal the oxygen is part of a hydroxyl group (-OH), and therefore the molecule is a double alcohol. In meprobamate the two oxygen atoms are bonded to carbon atoms, and thus the molecule is considered a ketone. In vivo, ketones are potentially capable of converting to hydroxyl groups (alcohols).

Although uniformly distributed in the brains of animals, meprobamate and phenaglycodal seem to exhibit selective neuronal blocking, primarily in the thalamus area. The measurable effect is a reduction in the magnitude of strong sensory impulses entering the thalamus. These exaggerated impulses are reduced to "normal" magnitude once they pass through the thalamus (presumably by the action of the drugs) and continue to higher cortical areas. The clinical effect is that the animal becomes less aggressive and less fearful.

Meprobamate also has a marked skeletal-muscle relaxant ability. Whether this action is centrally mediated or a result of direct muscle blockade at neuromuscular junctions remains to be determined.

In contrast to the butyrophenones, the "-diols" are minor tranquilizers, exhibiting only a mild degree of CNS depression in therapeutic doses.

Both meprobamate and phenaglycodol are limited to oral administration. Phenaglycodal has a more rapid onset of activity. The long period (approximately 1 hour in many animals) before clinical effects are apparent with meprobamate is probably due to the time required to form pharmacologically active metabolites, which, as in the case of phenacetin, are probably responsible for the tranquilizing effect.[8] This theory is supported by the fact that only about 10% of the drug is excreted unchanged.

• • •

Much investigation is currently being devoted to developing or discovering chemical entities that alter selective CNS functions without causing excessive depression. The groups that have been discussed consist of established drugs derived from traditional chemicals that have predictable tranquilizing effects in most animals. Newer chemicals await clinical testing to determine whether they offer significant benefits over these time-tested drugs.

ANTICONVULSANTS
Etiology of convulsions

Although the clinical manifestations of convulsions can vary from loss of consciousness to uncontrollable skeletal muscle contractions, the causes of these seizures or "fits," regardless of their severity, are related to abnormal, isolated brain activity. For unexplained reasons localized areas (foci), consisting of a single cell or groups of cells, in the cerebral cortex emit intermittent, rapid bursts of high-frequency electrical impulses (up to 800 per second). These renegade impulses have no predetermined neuronal pathway to follow, and so they spread randomly over cerebral tissue. Their spread is followed by depolarization of cerebral cells, which in turn stimulate motor neurons originating in the involved area(s). Stimulation of motor neurons by impulses of such high magnitude results in the powerful, uncoordinated, smooth and/or skeletal muscle contractions typical of an epileptic episode.

The occurrence of a seizure, however, is not always marked by such dramatic movements. If the innate inhibitory mechanisms in the brain that are responsible for the suppression of "wandering" impulses are not overwhelmed by the abnormal impulse, the seizure can take the form of unconsciousness or of an isolated muscle mass contraction, such as that of the urinary bladder to cause urination or of the gastrointestinal tract to cause involuntary defecation. The ultimate manifestation of the seizure or convulsion therefore seems to be related to the magnitude of the renegade impulse and the path it follows through the cerebral cortex. If the impulse cannot be contained at its origin, dramatic clinical results such as those seen in status epilepticus result. If the impulse does not significantly stimulate surrounding cerebral tissue, symptoms ranging from abnormal behavior (dizziness, stupification, sudden excretory functions, and salivation) to loss of consciousness can occur.

No definitive explanation of the cause of these high-frequency firings in seizure foci cells exists. It appears that certain biochemical changes such as localized cerebral ischemia may predispose brain tissue to electrical hyperactivity while at the same time lowering the "threshold" for the spreading of electrical discharges.

The term "threshold" refers to the innate inhibitory effect that cells have for suppressing their reactions to electrical impulses. It serves as a protective mechanism not only for CNS tissue but probably for all other body tissue. If neuronal cells were depolarized by every electrical impulse (regardless of strength), cerebral circuits would be overloaded and thus not able to carry all the vital impulses. In addition, the brain could not cope with the vast number of impulses reaching it. By allowing only impulses of a certain strength to stimulate nervous tissue, the threshold mechanism ensures that many of minor (background) impulses are never realized and thus enables nervous tissue to concentrate on the more important stimuli. "Raising the threshold" means increasing cellular resistence to electrical impulses and thus necessitating that an impulse increase in magnitude before it can depolarize a cell. Conversely, "lowering the threshold" results in an increased cellular propensity for stimulation. Exactly how the threshold mechanism works remains a mystery; however, it seems reasonable to assume that cellular electrolyte concentrations are involved.

Some of the pathological conditions that appear to promote formation of seizure foci are cerebral infection, especially by neurotropic viruses; congenital defects; head injuries (for example, concussion or skull fracture); hypoxia, especially at birth; and inflammatory vascular changes related to some infectious diseases. In addition, it seems probable that some physiological changes that in themselves cannot cause seizures may aggravate existing seizure foci, causing them to "fire." Among such changes are blood glucose fluctuations, fatigue, change in the pH of plasma, endocrine changes, nutritional deficiencies, and emotional stress (for example, fear). Use of some drugs in animals with a history of seizures can precipitate convulsions. For example, administration of phenothiazines to seizure-predisposed animals makes them much more susceptible to epileptic-type seizures, although the mechanism for this is not known.[10] Concurrent use of some medications can potentiate or diminish the pharmacological effect of anticonvulsants, in the latter case enhancing the chance for seizures. (Review Appendix A in regard to anticonvulsant drugs.)

Since many factors contribute to brain-induced seizures, it can be expected that, species differentiation aside, not all animals will respond to the same medication in similar fashion. It becomes especially important to obtain detailed histories in these cases so that clues as to the reason for the convulsions may be used to decide on the medication(s) needed.

Pharmacology of anticonvulsant drugs

Prior to the late 1930s, treatment of epileptic seizures in humans and animals was confined mainly to the use of two drug types: barbiturates and bromides. The use of bromides was discontinued because of the multiple organ toxicities of these drugs. Research therefore centered around derivatives of barbituric acid. Many years before 1938, Arthur Dox, of Parke, Davis & Co., synthesized a derivative of barbituric acid that was named diphenylhydantoin (now called phenytoin). Unfortunately, he was interested in creating a more efficient and less toxic hypnotic barbiturate, so his evaluation of this drug did not indicate its ability to inhibit isolated cerebral stimuli. Since phenytoin had hypnotic effects only in extremely high doses, it was not viewed as a drug of any clinical value.

In 1938 two investigators (Merritt and Putnam) were evaluating anticonvulsant drugs by measuring their capacity to increase the threshold of the motor cortex of cats to electrical stimulation. They found that phenytoin offered excellent protection against electrically induced seizures in cats. In addition, they found that the drug did not cause hypnosis as did therapeutic doses of some barbiturates and bromides. The advantage of a nonhypnotic drug to treat epilepsy was apparent to them, and as a result phenytoin has been used for more than 40 years in the successful management of epilepsy.[8]

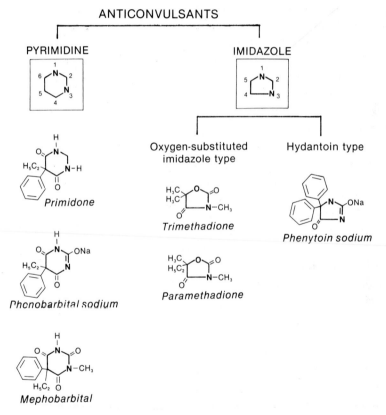

Fig. 4-8. Chemical classification of anticonvulsants. Pyrimidine-type anticonvulsants are made by adding molecules or atoms to the core pyrimidine structure. In contrast, some imidazole anticonvulsants substitute an oxygen atom for one of the core nitrogen atoms, thereby forming an oxazolidine ring. Generally, hydantoins are useful for managing major psychomotor seizures. Oxazolidines are beneficial for treatment of lesser seizures and are of no value for major episodes; in fact, they have been used to experimentally induce major convulsant episodes in animals.

The use of phenytoin in veterinary practice, however, has been limited, owing largely to the way it is detoxified by dogs and cats. Phenytoin has, however, served a purpose for veterinary medicine, since it demonstrated to researchers that the barbiturate molecule could be manipulated to produce anticonvulsant effects without hypnotic side effects. As a result primidone, which enjoys widespread veterinary use, was eventually discovered.

Anticonvulsant drugs do not cure epilepsy or conditions that cause seizures, but by depressing CNS activity, and sometimes specifically the seizure foci, these drugs can maintain conditions that are unfavorable to the initiation and/or spread of a high-intensity impulse.

Anticonvulsant drugs, which are all somewhat structurally similar, are either imidazole derivatives, such as phenytoin, or pyrimidine derivatives, such as primidone (see Fig. 4-8).

Imidazole-derived anticonvulsants

Also known as hydantoin drugs, imidazole-derived anticonvulsants do not markedly increase the seizure threshold of foci cells, but rather inhibit the degree of discharge spreading. Suppression of spreading seems related to these drugs' ability to deplete sodium from brain tissue.[8] Depletion of sodium can inhibit impulse conduction, since the strength and speed of an impulse depends on the magnitude of the sodium concentration gradient that exists prior to depolarization. By reducing the sodium concentration gradient (by reducing the sodium content) the hydantoin drugs thus decrease the electrical potential. It will be recalled from the initial discussion of impulse conduction that an electrical potential must exist before a neuronal cell can be stimulated, the magnitude of the cell's response to the stimulus being proportional to the magnitude of the gradient. Thus the lower the electrical gradient, the less, if any, the reaction of the neuron.

Phenytoin, paramethadione, and trimethadione are all derivatives of imidazole. In some of these drugs an oxygen atom has been substituted for one of the nitrogen atoms normally in the imidazole ring (see Fig. 4-8).

The use of phenytoin in dogs and cats is limited; dogs tend to have low plasma levels even when very large doses are given, while small doses in cats produce high plasma levels, leading to toxicity. Toxicity in cats is probably related to their relative inability to detoxify the drug, which results in its accumulation in the blood. Since constant adjusting of the dose is not practical for most situations, it is suggested that the hydantoin anticonvulsants be used in dogs and cats only when other drugs have been unsuccessful.

Trimethadione can be considered to be related to phenytoin, since both originate from the imidazole molecule; in trimethadione an oxygen atom is substituted for one of the nitrogen atoms. Like phenytoin, trimethadione has not had much use in dogs, although it has been effective in antagonizing chemically induced seizures in cats, guinea pigs, rabbits, and mice.[8]

Parmethadione is trimethadione in which one of the methyl ($—CH_3$) groups on carbon 5 has been changed to an ethyl group ($—CH_2CH_3$), as shown in Fig. 4-8. Parmethadione can be used in cases in which trimethadione has not proved satisfactory, and vice versa. Generally, paramethadione has proved successful in 65% of the cases that do not respond to other therapy. Vomiting, especially at the onset of therapy, is not uncommon with either drug and can usually be lessened or avoided if the drugs are given with food.[8, 10]

Pyrimidine-derived anticonvulsants

It is evident from Fig. 4-8 that mephobarbital, phenobarbital, and primidone, all of which are derivaties of pyrimidine, share the barbiturate core structure, with their differences being primidone's lack of an oxygen atom on carbon 2 and different groups on carbon 5 for each drug. These drugs seem to act directly on the CNS to elevate the seizure threshold.[10] For example, after an animal has received adequate primidone therapy, microelectrodes implanted in seizure foci of the brain must emit more voltage to cause "firing" of the foci than was required before therapy was initiated.

Barbiturates, especially the longer-acting ones such as phenobarbital and mephobarbital, still remain valuable medications for the treatment of seizures. Depending upon the intensity of the renegade discharge, the barbiturates can be used alone or as ancillary medications with either pyrimidine-type or imidazole-type anticonvulsants. Administration of mephobarbital to dogs is costly and unnecessary, since it is demethylated in the liver to form phenobarbital, which is the active metabolite. If phenobarbital, which is generally less expensive, is given initially, a detoxification step is avoided. In addition, better blood levels are obtained, since phenobarbital is absorbed more uniformly than mephobarbital from the gastrointestinal tract.[8] The pharmacological effect of phenobarbital on neuronal transmission was explained earlier in this chapter, and it is assumed that mephobarbital functions in an identical manner.

Primidone, another of the pyrimidine (barbiturate)-type anticonvulsants, differs from phenobarbital only in the loss of an oxygen atom from carbon 2. Primidone is widely used in dogs, where it is believed to act by increasing the seizure threshold.

Side effects of primidone include drowsiness and loss of balance, which is to be expected from a CNS depressant drug. Normally the oral dose of 55 mg/kg can be given once daily unless convulsions cannot be adequately controlled, in which case it should be administered every 6 to 12 hours. Since primidone is basically a barbiturate, its use is not recommended in cats because of their relative inability to detoxify the drug efficiently.[10]

In animals in which primidone is predictably effective, it has a high therapeutic index. For example, in laboratory rats its acute toxicity dose is 1.5 to 2 gm while the protective dose against electrically induced seizures is 0.005 gm. An index based on these figures is 300 to 400 (1.5/.005 to 2/.005). This is indicative of an even larger therapeutic index value, since the TI is a comparison of the effective dose and the LD_{50}, which is higher than the acute toxicity dose.

No single anticonvulsant drug is equally effective for all types of seizures in all species. Hence, anticonvulsant therapy should be individualized, with the drug therapy being selected according to seizure type and animal variety. Once the drug or drugs have been selected for an animal, administration should be started at a mimimum dose, which should be gradually increased until seizures are controlled or toxicity develops. If toxicity occurs without seizure control, the dose of the drug should be reduced to nontoxic levels and a second anticonvulsant drug administered concurrently, with the same procedure of increasing doses being followed. This practice allows for a body reservoir of two different anticonvulsant drugs, the combined action of which may be more effective and less toxic than a single drug given in an inordinately high dose. Whenever a new drug is added, previous medication should not be discontinued until an effective, nontoxic dose has been determined for the new anticonvulsant drug.[9]

CENTRAL NERVOUS SYSTEM STIMULANTS

Thus far we have considered CNS depressants, which have recognized indications for clinical use. Drugs such as dextroamphetamine (Dexedrine) sulfate, which evoke the opposite response, namely CNS stimulation, were once widely used—or, more accurately, misused. Although intended to suppress appetite, they were primarily used for their psychically uplifting side effects. Claims initially made as to their ability to increase mental awareness have been more than offset by later findings, which prove that general mental ability is impaired.

CNS stimulants, other than those used to combat CNS depressant drug effects, are interesting today only from an academic point of view. They apparently act to lower threshold values required for stimulation of neurons. While analgesics, anesthetics, hypnotics, tranquilizers, and anticonvulsants interrupt or inhibit impulse conduction, CNS stimulants facilitate biochemical reactions associated with impulse transmission. This can be done by decreasing the refractory period, thereby allowing conduction of more impulses per unit of time, and/or by acting on the neuronal membrane in such a manner that depolarization requires a lower threshold voltage. The "increased mental awareness" is due to the greater number of low-intensity impulses entering the brain. Since the brain becomes preoccupied with a multitude of these subliminal impulses (which it normally may never be aware of), the efficiency of higher cortical functions becomes compromised because of the extra work load. In humans this results in decreased deductive abilities, as well as impairment of long-term memory; in animals it causes exaggeration of fearful or excited behavior.

REFERENCES

1. Abbott Laboratories: A professional guide to the use of Pentothal, publication no. 97-0919/R2-35, April 1975.
2. American Society of Hospital Pharmacists: Hospital formulary, vol. 1, 28, Washington, D.C., 1980, The Society.
3. Brander, G.C., and Pugh, D.M.: Veterinary applied pharmacology and therapeutics, Oradell, N.J., 1972, Medical Economics Book Division, Inc.
4. Goldstein, A., Aronow, L., and Kalman, S.M.: Principles of drug action: the basis of pharmacology, ed. 2, New York, 1974, John Wiley & Sons, Inc.
5. Goodman, L.S., and Gilman, A.: The pharmacological basis of therapeutics, ed. 4, 1970, New York, Macmillan, Inc.
6. Guyton, A.C.: Physiology of the human body, ed. 5, Philadelphia, 1979, W.B. Saunders Co.
7. Kirk, R.W.: Current veterinary therapy, Philadelphia, 1980, W. B. Saunders Co., vol. 8, Small animal practice.
8. Krantz, J.C., and Carr, J.C. Pharmacologic principles of medical practice, ed. 6, Baltimore, 1965, The Williams & Wilkins Co.
9. Martin, E.W., and others, editors: Remington's pharmaceutical sciences, ed. 13, New York, 1965, Mack Publishing Co.
10. Spinelli, J.S., and Enos, L.R.: Drugs in veterinary practice, St. Louis, 1978, The C.V. Mosby Co.
11. Snyder, S.H.: Opiate receptors and internal opiates, Sci. Am., May 1980.

5

Anti-infective drugs and immunologicals

PERFORMANCE OBJECTIVES

After completion of this chapter the student will:

- State two differences between antibiotics and antibodies
- List three mechanisms by which microbes become resistant to some anti-infective drugs
- Differentiate between bacteriocidal and bacteriostatic drug activity
- Describe and classify (as bacteriocidal or bacteriostatic) the antibacterial action of the following:
  1. Penicillin and its semisynthetic derivatives
  2. Cephalosporins
  3. Macrolides
  4. Aminoglycosides
  5. Polypeptides
  6. Sulfonamides
- Name three common adverse side effects that could occur as a result of excessive antibiotic therapy
- List three principles relating to dosage determination and duration of therapy that should be followed when anti-infective drugs are used
- Explain the "competitive inhibition process," and name one group of anti-infective drugs that functions by it
- Name two specific groups of antibiotics and one unique potential adverse side effect of each
- State two differences between "active immunity" and "passive immunity," and name a class of immunologicals that confers each type

The number and variety of medications and chemicals that exhibit clinical anti-infective activity are staggering. It is the prerogative of each author writing on this subject, therefore, to decide how general, how detailed or how extensive his or her considerations will be. Consistent with the introductory nature of this book, this chapter will present basic information on selected anti-infectives that are suitable for administration to animals. Consequently it will be concerned with antibiotics, sulfonamides, anthelmintics, and immunologicals.

The information currently available on any of these subjects could fill volumes. The approach of this chapter will be to present basic pharmacological mechanisms of anti-infectives, the rationale for their classification, and therapeutic indications.

ANTIBIOTICS

The name "antibiotic" clearly defines the role of these drugs. It is derived from the Greek *"anti-,"* meaning "against," and *"biosis,"* meaning "life." In essence, antibiotics are designed and used to destroy simple forms of life (that is, microorganisms). Antibiotics are overwhelmingly effective against most bacteria, some fungi, and a few viruses. Usually antibiotics are obtained from microorganisms—most notably bacteria, actinomycetes, yeasts, and molds. Although some antibiotics have been isolated from tissues of higher plants and animals, the term generally has come to refer to life-inhibiting substances obtained from microbes. Another hallmark of antibiotics is that their inhibitory activity is demonstrable in very low concentrations. If these observations are combined, we can currently define antibiotics as substances that are produced by or derived from living bacteria and that in low concentrations have lethal or inhibitory action on microorganisms.

The antagonistic effect of one microorganism upon another has probably existed since creation. It seems reasonable to assume that the early environment of our developing planet favored excessive proliferation of microorganisms and that their abundant distribution eventually led to competition for food. Survival therefore depended on the ability of some microbes to kill or inhibit the growth of others. Apparently the survivors developed the ability to produce potent, toxic substances (endotoxins), which they secreted into their immediate surroundings. Adjacent microbes that were unable to survive in the presence of an endotoxin died, thereby facilitating the survival of the remaining microorganisms. The same phenomenon can be demonstrated today if a culture medium in a Petri dish is overrun by various microbes. For example, if certain strains of staphylococci exist with *Pencillium* mold, chances are the staphylococci will be killed by the endotoxin secreted by the *Penicillium* mold. Medicine has adopted this evolutionary phenomenon of killing microbes by exposing them to endotoxins obtained from other microbes. The endotoxins have been renamed "antibiotics," and the environment in which they are placed to exhibit their antimicrobial action has come to be called the pathogen's "host," be it animal, fish, fowl, or plant. Likewise, the designation "pathogen" is a man-made classification, since nature does not consider microbes good or bad.

Discovery, detection, and isolation of antibiotic-producing organisms

Since most antibiotics are obtained at least in part from secretions of naturally occurring microbes, the search for newer microbes capable of producing more potent antibiotics is constant. Since there is no formula for where such microbes can be found, drug companies are literally searching the world for strains of microbes that will produce clinically useful antibiotics. Searchers have collected samples of soil from the Amazon River banks to lawns in Orlando, Florida. They have scraped bacterial colonies from tree bark in the Philippines and from the insides of sewage drain pipes in Venice, the latter location resulting in the discovery of an extremely useful group of antibiotics known as the cephalosporins. The only rule generally followed is to look in areas where microbes must compete with each other to survive.

The detection of organisms that secrete antibiotics is based on their ability to inhibit test bacteria in vitro. The spectrum of antimicrobial activity for an antibiotic can be determined by using different test organisms. For example, the use of *Staphylococcus aureus* will make possible the detection of all antibiotics that inhibit that bacterium. Even though cross-sensitivity exists among microbes, it is necessary to test each organism with an antibiotic to determine absolutely whether it is sensitive to the antibiotic.

The screening method involves plating out thousands of serial dilutions from aqueous samples of soil or other natural collections of samples, using agar medium previously seeded with the test microbe(s). In a collection sample that contains multiple organisms, those secreting antibiotics are distinguished by a clear zone or "halo" around the colony. This clear zone indicates inhibition of the test organism's growth, which is normally demonstrated by marked cloudiness (turbidity) in the medium. The relative potencies of antibiotics and/or amounts produced can be compared by the width of the clear zone; the wider the halo, the more antibiotic produced and/or possibly the more potent the antibiotic.

Once an organism producing an antibiotic has been isolated, it is identified and conditions favoring its optimal growth, such as pH, temperature, culture composition, and age, are determined. Next the antibacterial spectrum is obtained. The term "spectrum" refers to the range of organisms, especially those considered pathogenic, against which an antibiotic may prove useful—for example, gram-positive bacteria, gram-negative bacteria, rickettsiae, viruses, and fungi. Antibiotics, like any antibacterial drug, are not effective against all microorganisms. Some antibiotics have a "narrow spectrum," being effective against relatively few bacteria, most of which are either gram-positive or gram-negative. "Wide-spectrum" antibiotics are effective against many bacteria, usually both gram positive ones and gram-negative ones.

If antibacterial data are promising, the therapeutic index of the antibiotic is determined. As was discussed in Chapter 2, the higher the TI value, the safer the drug. Consequently only low-toxicity antibiotics, especially those in which toxicity is inversely proportional to antimicrobial potency (toxicity decreases as potency increases), are of clinical interest. If clinical trials indicate that an antibiotic is safe and effective, attention then centers on large-scale manufacturing techniques.

Resistance (insensitivity)

The increased use of antibiotics for treatment and prophylaxis of disease, especially within the last few years, has created unanticipated problems in both human and veterinary medicine; these problems continue to increase, in both number and severity. An increasing number of organisms have developed that are resistant to traditional antibiotics. This is especially true of penicillin-type antibiotics, which are probably the most widely used, accounting for approximately 20%-25% of all antibiotics administered annually. One study indicates that in "closed populations" such as hospitals, 85% of staphylococci strains that were originally sensitive to penicillin mutated to form less sensitive or totally resistant strains. The term "drug resistance" refers to the inability of a drug to act as anticipated. This does not necessarily mean that the microbe has become resistant to the drug; the phenomenon can be due to accelerated drug detoxification and excretion by the animal, too low a dose, or any of the other reasons mentioned in Chapter 2. One reason, however, for drug resistance can be "acquired resistance," which results when microbes that were initially sensitive to a drug undergo a change, causing them to be less sensitive or absolutely resistant to the actions of that drug. Today this type of resistance plays the most clinically significant role in drug resistance problems.[5] The pharmacological action (bacteriocidal or bacteriostatic) by which an antibiotic exerts its effect may also be responsible for the development, if any, of microbial resistance to a drug.

The development of drug resistance is not universal. Not all microbes develop the ability to become insensitive to a particular antibiotic, regardless of how long they have been exposed to it. For example, even after more than 30 years, no clinical resistance to penicillin G has developed in *Streptococcus pneumoniae*. Conversely, use of the same antibiotic against a different organism, or against a strain of the same organism, can cause the immediate emergence of resistance.

Development of resistance by a microbe involves a *stable,* genetic change, a mutation, which is heritable to succeeding generations.[6] For many years it was believed that the presence of the drug triggered the mutation process. It is now evident that *acquired resistance to a particular antibiotic is not due to exposure of the microorganism to the drug*. Instead, a new strain, which differs genetically from the original microbial population, is *created, spontaneously, with resistance to the drug* (and usually to similar drugs), without having been exposed to it. Continued use of the drug eliminates the original microbial population (since it is still sensitive to it), thus favoring the establishment of the new, mutant strain.

The resistance in a mutation can result from one or more of the following mechanisms:

1. *The ability of the new strain to produce an enzyme that rapidly degrades the drug.* This process is most common in microbes that develop resistance to penicillin G or to antibiotics that are chemically or structurally similar to it. The enzyme produced is penicillinase, and it also makes the mutant strain resistant to ampicillin, amoxicillin, carbenicillin, hetacillin, and phenethicillin V, all of which are semisynthetic derivatives of penicillin G.[6,9]

2. *Alteration in the mutant's cell wall that decreases its permeability to the antibiotic (or other antimicrobial drug).* Certain minimal concentrations of the antimicrobial are needed to adversely affect the activity of the microorganism. If such concentrations are not attained (because insufficient amounts of drug gain access to the protoplasm of the organism), the microbe will be resistant to the action of the drug.

3. *Reduction in the number of drug receptor sites on the cell wall, or a change in their configuration.* In accordance with the "lock and key" theory of drug activity mentioned in Chapter 1, the antibiotic must first be able to conform to specific areas on the surface of the organism if it is to exert an effect. These areas are called "drug receptor sites," and their existence is theorized to explain the activity not only of anti-infective drugs and agents, but of all drugs that are capable of interacting with tissue. If receptor sites are reduced in number and/or changed in configuration, antibiotic molecules will not attach to them, or not attach as well, and therefore their pharmacological activity will be lost or lessened.[6]

4. *Decreased ability of the drug to convert to a more active form.* As will be discussed later in this chapter, many antibiotics adversely affect the deoxyribonucleic acid (DNA) or messenger ribonucleic acid (mRNA) of the microbe. In order to do so, they are oftentimes required to change from their administered molecular form. This change can be inhibited or prevented if the protoplasm of the microbe is altered. Sometimes a mutation involves the production of large-chain protein molecules that interact with the antibiotic to render it less effective. Or the creation of simpler substances, such as carbohydrates, can sometimes be enough to interrupt drug conversion. Whatever substance is produced in association with a mutation, a mutant cell can use this mechanism to inhibit conversion of some drugs to their more active forms.

Generally, microorganisms that are insensitive to a particular drug tend to be resistant to chemically or structurally related drugs of another chemical class. For example, staphylococci that are resistant to penicillin and semisynthetic penicillins

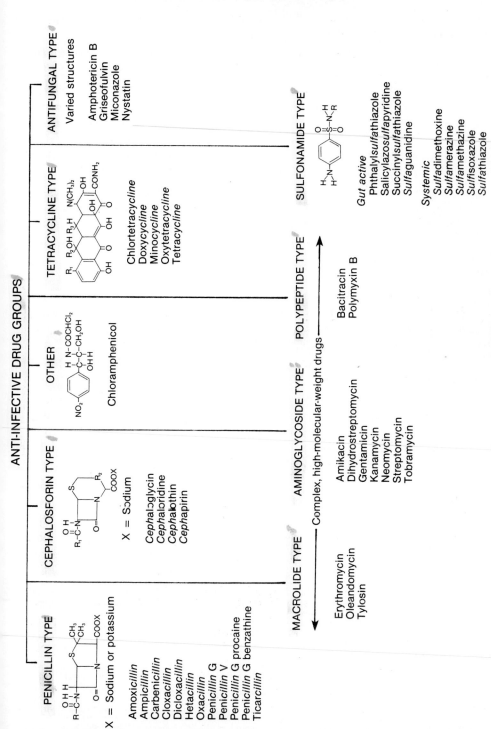

Fig. 5-1. Classification of clinically significant anti-infectives. Individual drugs listed under the respective structural formulas differ only in their R groups. For example, amoxicillin and ampicillin share the same core penicillin structure (beta lactam and thiazolidine rings) but differ in the composition of their R portions.

ANTI-INFECTIVE DRUG GROUPS

PENICILLIN TYPE

X = Sodium or potassium

Amoxicillin
Ampicillin
Carbenicillin
Cloxacillin
Dicloxacillin
Hetacillin
Oxacillin
Penicillin G
Penicillin V
Penicillin G procaine
Penicillin G benzathine
Ticarcillin

CEPHALOSFORIN TYPE

X = Sodium

Cephaloglycin
Cephaloridine
Cephalothin
Cephapirin

OTHER

Chloramphenicol

TETRACYCLINE TYPE

Chlortetracycline
Doxycycline
Minocycline
Oxytetracycline
Tetracycline

ANTIFUNGAL TYPE

Varied structures

Amphotericin B
Griseofulvin
Miconazole
Nystatin

MACROLIDE TYPE

Erythromycin
Oleandomycin
Tylosin

AMINOGLYCOSIDE TYPE

Amikacin
Dihydrostreptomycin
Gentamicin
Kanamycin
Neomycin
Streptomycin
Tobramycin

Complex, high-molecular-weight drugs

POLYPEPTIDE TYPE

Bacitracin
Polymyxin B

SULFONAMIDE TYPE

Gut active

Phthalylsulfathiazole
Salicylazosulfapyridine
Succinylsulfathiazole
Sulfaguanidine

Systemic

Sulfadimethoxine
Sulfamerazine
Sulfamethazine
Sulfisoxazole
Sulfathiazole

TABLE 5-1
Chemical and biological comparisons
of some commonly used semisynthetic penicillins

Substituted portion	Name	Acid stable*	Penicillinase resistant
General formula for penicillins $X=$ sodium or potassium			
	Ampicillin	Yes	No
	Carbenicillin	No	No
	Dicloxacillin	Yes	Yes
	Oxacillin	Yes	Yes
	Penicillin G	No (yes for dogs)	No
	Penicillin V	Yes	No

*Acid stability and penicillinase resistance are functions of the R group attached to the penicillin nucleus. With few exceptions, namely dicloxacillin and oxacillin, the organic group in the R position rarely confers both acid stability and penicillinase resistance. Oftentimes the conferring of penicillinase resistance results in a decrease in a drug's antimicrobial spectrum, and vice versa.

are also resistant to most cephalosporins (a group of antibiotics similar in structure to penicillins and semisynthetic penicillins). Occasionally, however, "cross-resistance" can occur—a microorganism becomes resistant to two or more unrelated anti-infective drugs. Prudent, simultaneous use of two antimicrobial drugs can greatly reduce the speed with which resistance develops, since microbes that are resistant to one of the drugs may still be killed by the other.[6]

Fig. 5-1 shows the anti-infective drug groups discussed in this chapter and, when possible, the structural similaries between these groups.

Penicillin and semisynthetic derivatives

This group of anti-infectives enjoys the largest use of any of the antibiotics. Penicillin G (benzylpenicillin) was the first penicillin to be used clinically.[9] Since its first use, over 40 years ago, more than 34 biosynthetic penicillin "salts" have been manufactured. Table 5-1 lists only some of the currently used semisynthetic forms. The term "salt" is used, since the nucleus of the penicillin structure (6-aminopenicillanic acid, also referred to as 6-APA) is an organic acid. When additions are made to an acid, the resultant molecule is called a "salt." 6-APA is composed of a thiazolidine ring fused to a beta lactam ring, as shown in Fig. 5-2. Like barbituric acid, which serves as the nucleus for the barbiturate depressants, 6-APA does not exhibit any anti-infective activity until organic molecules are attached to the "6-amino" position, indicated by "R" in Fig. 5-2.[1] Addition of various organic molecules to the 6-amino position has yielded semisynthetic penicillins that differ in the following ways:

1. Bacterial spectrum
2. Degree of resistance to degradation by gastric acid
3. Rate of absorption
4. Degree of resistance to pencillinase
5. Plasma-binding ability

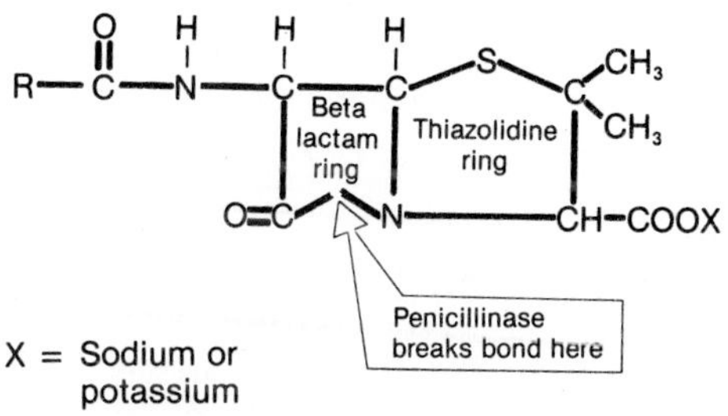

Fig. 5-2. Destruction of penicillinase-sensitive penicillins. Breaking the carbon-nitrogen bond destroys antibacterial activity of the molecule. It is theorized that the organic molecule on the R position of penicillinase-resistant penicillins is spacially arranged so that it "covers" the carbon-nitrogen bonding area, thereby preventing its contact with and destruction by penicillinase.

Originally the antibacterial activity of the penicillins was expressed in "units." However, the same weight of each penicillin was equal to a different number of units when compared to a standard. This led to confusion and errors when dosages were prescribed. Good medical practice currently dictates that dosages be expressed only in milligrams or grams of a particular penicillin salt.

In addition to the fact that some penicillin salts can undergo in vivo inactivation by penicillinase, penicillins also can be readily degraded in vitro by higher-than-normal room temperatures (in excess of 25° C) and by alkaline solutions. These conditions can be avoided by storing reconstituted solutions of penicillin salts in a refrigerator and by making sure that no medication having a pH higher than 4 is mixed with a solution containing a penicillin or one of its semisynthetic derivatives. (Review Appendix A to determine which drugs are incompatible with the penicillins as well as with other antibiotics mentioned in this chapter.)

Pharmacological activity

The penicillins may be either bacteriocidal or bacteriostatic, depending on their concentration at the infection site and the susceptibility of the pathogen. Penicillins act to inhibit biochemical functions needed for the synthesis and maintainance of the bacterial cell wall. Since penicillins suppress reactions associated with forming the cell wall, they are most effective in younger, maturing microorganisms, in which these drugs act in a bacteriocidal fashion to destroy the developing organism. Destruction is caused by the hypertonic protoplasm of the microorganism exerting an osmotic pressure against the disrupted cell wall and eventually causing it to lyse. Penicillins are most effective when cells are undergoing mitosis, since their developing cell walls are then most permeable to these agents. It is also during this phase that inhibition of wall formation is most disastrous to the developing microbe. Mature microbes are neither lysed nor killed by penicillins. Since their walls are established, the penicillins do not cause immediate destruction but rather act in a gradual (bacteriostatic) manner to retard further multiplication.[6,8]

If a penicillin is to be administered with another anti-infective drug, it is necessary to be sure the other drug is also bacteriocidal. Simultaneous use of a bacteriostatic drug with a penicillin will prevent microbes from undergoing mitosis and thus prevent the penicillin from exerting its optimal bacteriocidal effect.

Antibacterial spectrum and resistance

It should be remembered that in vitro sensitivity of an organism to a particular antibiotic may not occur in vivo. Physiological barriers created by the pathogens may exclude therapeutic concentrations of the antibiotic from reaching the microorganisms. For example, in staphylococcal and *Corynebacterium pyogenes*–induced mastitis large amounts of pus, edema, or fibrous tissue are produced, within which the pathogens multiply. Consequently systemic and even localized injections of antibiotics may not be effective against the organisms, since they cannot penetrate the organic debris surrounding the microbes.[2]

Generally, penicillins are active, in vitro, against gram-positive bacilli and against a very limited number of gram-negative cocci. Penicillin-sensitive, gram-positive bacteria that commonly infect domestic animals include *Bacillus anthracis, Actinomyces bovis,* and many strains of *Clostridium, Corynebacterium,* and *Leptospira.* In addition, some of the newer semisynthetic penicillins are effective against staphylococcus and streptococcus strains that produce penicillinase, although penicillin G is more active than the newer penicillins against *Erysipelothrix rhusiopathiae,* another common gram-positive organism that is pathogenic in domestic animals.[1,9]

The ability of some organisms, especially strains of the *Bacillus subtilismesentericus* group, to produce the enzyme penicillinase provides them with resistance to penicillin and to some of the newer semisynthetic penicillins. Penicillinase breaks the bond between the nitrogen of the thiazolidine ring and a carbon of the beta lactam portion, as indicated in Fig. 5-2. Once the 6-APA structure is broken, all antibacterial activity is lost.[8] Some of the newer penicillins are resistant to penicillinase, possibly because the organic molecules substituted on the 6-amino portion do not allow the enzyme to come into proper alignment with the molecule, so its active center cannot interact with the critical nitrogen and carbon atoms on the thiazolidine and beta lactam portions, respectively.

Generally, it appears that the addition of the side chain, in order to confer penicillinase resistance, decreases the potency of penicillins. Up to 50 times more of a penicillinase-resistant penicillin can be required in order to produce the same effect on a non-penicillinase-producing organism that penicillin G has.

The spectrums of activity of the newest semisynthetic penicillins differ dramatically from those of the older penicillins. Substitutions for the 6-amino portion increase the activity of these drugs against selective gram-negative bacilli. Unfortunately, these substitutions do not confer concurrent penicillinase resistance to the antibiotics; therefore what is gained in gram-negative killing potential is lost in ability to kill penicillinase-producing bacteria. Generally, the altered-spectrum penicillins (ampicillin, amoxicillin, hetacillin, carbenicillin, and ticarcillin) have gram-positive spectrums of action that are similar to the spectrum of penicillin but are also active against many gram-negative organisms.

Acid resistance

As has been mentioned, additions to the 6-APA molecule can increase the spectrum of activity or make a penicillin more acid resistant. Although penicillin G is considered acid stable, oral administration results in erratic blood levels for most animals except dogs. The acid-resistant penicillins (see Table 5-1), such as methicillin, nafcillin, oxacillin, cloxacillin, dicloxacillin, and penicillin VK, are more resistant to gastric acid because of the organic side chain on the 6-amino position. As a result, they are more completely absorbed and predictable blood levels are usually attained. Unfortunately the side chains do not significantly increase these drugs' spectrum of activity above that of penicillin G, and in the case of penicillin VK, the spectrum is narrower against some bacterial strains than is the spectrum of penicillin G.

Penicillin G

Since penicillin G is the most commonly used penicillin in veterinary practice, it is not surprising that it is available in many dosage forms. Oral tablets are generally suitable for dogs, but only on an empty stomach (when the acid content is low). Because of the high doses required, oral tablets are not practical for use in cattle, horses, or other large animals.[9] Injectable forms of penicillin G potassium as well as the sodium salt are available for parenteral use. Intramuscular injections are used if absorption is to be slower, and the dosage interval is increased. Intravenous administration results in such rapid excretion that unless the animal is hospitalized, it becomes impractical to maintain adequate blood levels. Suspensions of penicillin G salts, some combined with procaine, are available. When given by intramuscular injection, they produce prolonged blood levels. The two most common penicillin suspensions are procaine penicillin G and benzathine penicillin G. The use of procaine for extending the time between doses was discussed in Chapter 1. Benzathine pencillin G, like procaine penicillin G, is a suspension of penicillin particles, which are slowly absorbed into the bloodstream after injection. For certain indications, use of either penicillin preparation can be limited to a single injection every 24 hours. Larger doses are required for large animals such as horses. Regardless of the particular parenteral penicillin G used, it is not uncommon to have volumes of 70 ml injected into large animals. For comfort, multiple injections of up to 10 ml each should be made until the calculated volume is administered.

Normally, penicillin G does not pass healthy, noninflamed blood-brain barrier tissue. Likewise, unless massive intravenous doses are given, it is not usually found in milk. The highest in vivo concentrations are found in liver, bile, intestines, and skin. Because of their slower, more irregular absorption from the intestines, oral doses must often be from three to ten times larger than parenteral doses.

Absorption of orally administered penicillin G in dogs occurs primarily in the duodenum, with smaller amounts being absorbed in the stomach and trace amounts in the large intestine. In most animals, unabsorbed penicillin G is for the most part inactivated by colonic bacteria.

The limited in vivo distribution of penicillin G, as well as its low plasma-binding ability, comes as no surprise, since its partition coefficient is low. Thus it exists largely in ionized form in the bloodstream and as such does not pass membranous barriers (such as the blood-brain barrier)

Penicillin G is a narrow-spectrum antibiotic; it is primarily indicated for gram-positive bacilli and cocci, some rickettsiae, and a few viruses.

It is fundamental to realize that penicillin G, like all other antibiotics, cannot neutralize bacterial toxins. Like antibiotics themselves, bacterial toxins are endotoxins, produced within the microorganisms. Unlike antibiotics, they are oftentimes responsible for the clinical symptoms of a disease (for example, *Clostridium botulinum* releases a potent endotoxin, which is lethal to birds, horses, and dogs, among other animals). Unlike clinically useful antibiotics, these potent endotoxins cannot be used, because of their lethal activity in extremely low concentrations.

In addition to its use in small animals (dogs and cats) as a therapeutic and prophylactic medication, penicillin G is widely used in large, production animals. In these animals, perhaps the most important disease for which penicillin is indicated is streptococcal bovine mastitis. Other diseases involving livestock for which penicillin is indicated are anthrax in all species, erysipelas in sheep and pigs, strangles in horses, and certain clostridial diseases in cattle and sheep.[2]

Table 5-2 lists routes of administration and dosage ranges for penicillin G and semisynthetic penicillins.

TABLE 5-2
Routes of administration and dosage ranges for penicillin G and some semisynthetic penicillins

Drug	Administration route and available dosage forms	Dosages for dogs, cats, and most small domestic animals (adults)
Amoxicillin sodium	Oral (capsule and liquid)	5-40 mg/kg every 4-6 hours
Ampicillin sodium	Oral (capsule and liquid)	10-20 mg/kg every 6 hours
	IM, IV, SC	5-10 mg/kg every 6 hours
Carbenicillin disodium	IV	15 mg/kg every 8 hours
Carbenicillin indanyl sodium	Oral (capsule and liquid)	30-40 mg/kg every 8 hours
Cloxacillin sodium	Oral (capsule and liquid)	10-40 mg/kg every 4-6 hours
Dicloxacillin sodium	Oral (capsule and liquid)	11-55 mg/kg every 8 hours
Methicillin sodium	IM, IV	20 mg/kg every 6 hours
Nafcillin sodium	Oral (capsule and liquid)	30-80 mg/kg every 4-6 hours
	IM, IV	10-40 mg/kg every 4-6 hours
Oxacillin sodium	Oral (capsule and liquid), IM, IV	10-40 mg/kg every 6 hours
Penicillin G benzathine	IM	25 mg/kg every 5 days
Penicillin G (sodium and potassium)	Oral	25 mg/kg every 6 hours
	IM, IV, SC	12.5 mg/kg every 4 hours
Penicillin G procaine	IM, SC	12.5 mg/kg every 12-24 hours
Penicillin V potassium	Oral (tablet and liquid)	10 mg/kg every 8 hours
Phenethicillin sodium	Oral (tablet)	10 mg/kg every 8 hours

Data from Kirk, R.W.: Current veterinary therapy, Philadelphia, 1980, W.B. Saunders Co., vol. 7, Small animal practice; Spinelli, J.S., and Enos, L.R.: Drugs in veterinary practice, St. Louis, 1978, The C.V. Mosby Co.

Semisynthetic penicillins

From the preceding discussions it is apparent that the names of the penicillin-type antibiotics contain the suffix "-cillin"; the prefix usually refers to the organic portion attached to the 6-amino position.

As was mentioned earlier, the semisynthetic penicillins were produced to extend the stability and spectrum of penicillin G. Experimentation with substitutions on the 6-amino position resulted in penicillins that were more resistant to gastric acid. The spectrum of activity was increased to include many gram-negative bacteria that had a natural resistance to penicillin G. The problem of the rapid excretion of penicillin G, which necessitates frequent doses, was largely solved by the development of the benzathine and procaine salts of penicillin. In addition, increasing the half-life seems to have had a generally favorable impact on the spectrum of activity. Ampicillin, and carbenicillin have half-lives from two to three and one-half times as long as penicillin G. Consequently, these two antibiotics exhibit expanded spectrums in comparison to the other penicillins.[1] Hetacillin, which is also in the semisynthetic penicillin group, can be considered equivalent to ampicillin, since it must first be converted to ampicillin before it exhibits antibacterial activity.

Cephalosporins

The cephalosporin antibiotics are semisynthetic derivatives of cephalosporin C, a substance produced by the fungus *Cephalosporium cremonium*. These drugs are structurally and pharmacologically related to the penicillins. Like the penicillins, all have a central nucleus that consists of an organic acid. In the case of commercially available cephalosporins, this organic acid is 7-aminocephalosporanic acid (7-ACA). Like penicillin, 7-ACA contains a beta lactam ring. However, this beta lactam ring is fused to a six-sided dihydrothiazine ring instead of the 5-sided thiazolidine ring of penicillin (Fig. 5-1). Breaking the beta lactam ring system at any point results in total loss of antibacterial activity. In the dry state, cephalosporins are stable for several years at room temperature. In solution, however, most are stable for approximately 4 days under refrigeration and usually at least 1 month when frozen. (Be sure to consult Appendix A for information about the compatibility of cephalosporins with other drugs in intravenous solutions.)

Pharmacological activity

Cephalosporins act primarily in a bacteriocidal fashion; that is, bacteria are killed relatively quickly. Like the penicillins, the cephalosporins interfere with cell wall synthesis. The exact mechanism centers on inhibition of enzymes that produce dipeptidoglycan, a chemical needed for cell wall strength and rigidity. Lacking this strength, the microorganism wall disintegrates as a result of osmotic pressure differences between the protoplasm of the cell and its outside environment. Cephalosporins are more effective against young, rapidly dividing organisms than against mature, nonmitotic cells.[1]

As with most other antibiotics, the bacteriocidal action of the cephalosporins is dose related. If dosages are decreased by two and one-half times, the activity becomes bacteriostatic and the ability to effect "quick" kills of organisms is lost.[6]

Antibacterial spectrum and resistance

Generally cephalosporins are considered "broad-spectrum" antibiotics; that is, they are effective against most gram-positive and some gram-negative organisms. One possible explanation for the resistance of many gram-negative microbes is that they contain fewer mucopeptides, such as dipeptidoglycan, and consequently their cell wall synthesis mechanisms are less vulnerable to the action of cephalosporins.[1]

Most cephalosporins are very resistant to the action of penicillinase per se. Some investigators believe that the resistance exhibited by some species of *Pseudomonas, Enterobacter,* and *Aerobacter,* as well as such bacteria as *Bacillus cereus* and *Escherichia coli,* may be due to their producing an enzyme that breaks the beta lactam ring of the 7-ACA structure. Isolates of organisms known to produce this enzyme have been tested against penicillins, and little, if any, resistance has been demonstrated; thus the enzyme affecting the cephalosporins is not true penicillinase. Consequently the enzymes that break the beta lactam ring portion of 7-ACA have been called beta lactamases and collectively are referred to as cephalosporinases. Of the currently available cephalosporins, cefazolin and cephaloridine are the least resistant and cephalothin the most resistant to cephalosporinases.

Pharmacokinetics

Cephalosporins that can be administered orally are very efficiently absorbed from the gastrointestinal tract. Absorption is delayed by food, with the consequence being lower and postponed peak serum levels, although the total amount of drug absorbed does not seem to be affected. Table 5-3 lists routes of administration for most of the cephalosporins used in veterinary medicine.

TABLE 5-3
Routes of administration and dosage ranges for some cephalosporins

Drug	Administration route and available dosage forms	Dosage for most adult domestic animals
Cephalexin	Oral (capsule and liquid)	30 mg/kg every 12 hours
Cephaloridine	IM, SC	10 mg/kg every 8-12 hours
Cephalothin sodium	IM, SC	35 mg/kg every 8 hours
Cephapirin sodium	IM, SC	35 mg/kg every 8 hours
Cephaloglycin	Oral (capsule)	30 mg/kg every 12 hours

Data from Kirk, R.W.: Current veterinary therapy, Philadelphia, 1980, W.B. Saunders Co., vol. 7, Small animal practice; Spinelli, J.S., and Enos, L.R.: Drugs in veterinary practice, St. Louis, 1978, The C.V. Mosby Co.

Following absorption from the gastrointestinal tract or injection site, cephalosporins are distributed to most tissues and fluids. Being ionic in the bloodstream, they do not pass the blood-brain barrier or the meninges to any significant amount, even when the meninges are inflamed. As would be expected, cephalosporins are not significantly bound to plasma proteins. They do, however, readily cross the placenta; fetal blood levels can be 10% or more of maternal serum concentrations. In addition, low concentrations can be found in the milk of nursing animals. Not all cephalosporins are detoxified in the liver, yet all are rapidly excreted via the kidneys. As a result it can be expected that impaired kidney function will lead to higher serum levels for all cephalosporins and to extended half lives for some.

Indications for use and individual agents

Generally, cephalosporins should not be considered "first-line" antibiotics (those used first) for treatment of an infection; they are used when other antibiotics are unsuitable because of toxicity or spectrum. However, in *Klebsiella* infections, cephalosporins are more effective than penicillins and therefore can be considered first-choice drugs.

Penicillins are generally the drugs of choice for use against susceptible staphylococci and streptococci, while ampicillin should be used for infections caused by susceptible strains of *E. coli*.[1]

The addition of organic molecules at positions R_1 and R_2 (see Fig. 5-1) broadens the spectrum of the cephalosporins without significantly reducing their resistance to gastric acids. As their spectrum broadens, cephalosporins becomes more potent, and consequently their use should be restricted to organisms that do not respond to more traditional medications. Bacterial strains that are resistant to first-generation cephalosporins are already on the rise, a situation that has necessitated altering their spectrums to the extent that second and third-generations of cephalosporins have been created. If the use of these newer cephalosporins is not restricted, we will be caught in an unending cycle of creating more potent, and thus more toxic, cephalosporins to kill increasing populations of organisms that have emerged because of excessive use of a previous generation of these drugs. The ultimate absurdity of this cycle is that we would eventually create a generation of antibiotics potent enough to kill existing bacteria but too toxic for clinical use.

Classification of cephalosporins into generations is currently arbitrary, based largely on manufacturers' advertising. The cephalosporin-type antibiotics most often used in veterinary medicine, however, are generally agreed to be first generation.

Cephalothin, cephaloridine. Both these drugs are available as parenteral products for intravenous or intramuscular use. It is strongly recommended, however, that cephalothin be administered only by intravenous injection, since intramuscular injection is very painful. Cephalothin is likewise irritating to veins; the concentration of the intravenous solution and the infusion rate should be such that drug-induced phlebitis starting at the injection site is avoided or at least minimized.

Frozen solutions of cephalothin in glass vials or syringes are stable for up to 6 weeks. Care should be taken if the frozen drug is warmed to facilitate thawing. Once thawing is completed, no heat should be used. Once thawed, solutions should not be reheated.[1] The intravenous dosage of cephalothin for smaller animals (dogs and cats) is usually 35 mg/kg every 8 to 12 hours.[7]

Cephaloridine exhibits essentially the same spectrum as cephalothin but was designed to be less painful upon intramuscular injection. It is not used widely in veterinary practice, since it has demonstrated kidney toxicity in rats, mice, and rabbits and there is no reason to assume that a similar effect would not occur with other species.[9] The dosage for both dogs and cats is 10 mg/kg every 8 to 12 hours, with adequate kidney function being a prerequisite to therapy.[7]

Cephapirin, cephaloglycin. These drugs are of limited use in veterinary practice. Cephapirin is given only parenterally, and cephaloglycin is administered only orally. Parenteral solutions of cephapirin can be frozen (for at least 60 days), thawed, and administered. The spectrum of both drugs approximates that of most cephalosporins, and their excretion is rapid. Since high concentrations of cephapirin are found in the urine, as opposed to generally inadequate serum levels, cephapirin is recommended for urinary tract infections, with dosages being in the range of 5 to 15 mg/kg, three or four times daily.[9]

Tetracyclines

In contrast to the serendipidous discovery of penicillin, the development of tetracycline-type antibiotics was the result of the first systematic screening of soil samples for antibiotic producing microorganisms. In 1947, after screening approximately 100,000 samples from all over the world, Duggan discovered an organism of the genus *Streptomyces* that inhibited the growth of adjacent microbes on a Petri dish. After 5 more years of work, it was discovered that the antibiotic produced by this organism had a unique structural formula—4 fused, 6-sided rings. Thus all antibiotics with this structure are called tetracyclines (tetra = 4; cycle = circle).[2,8]

Chemically the tetracycline antibiotics differ from each other as a result of differing molecules or atoms being attached to the R_1, R_2, and R_3 positions, as noted in Fig. 5-1. However, relatively few modifications can be made to the structure without loss of antibacterial activity. Chlortetracycline, a typical tetracycline-type antibiotic, has a chlorine atom, a methyl group, and a hydrogen atom on positions R_1, R_2, and R_3, respectively:

Changing any of the other groups or atoms attached to the four joined rings results in significant or total loss of antibacterial activity.

Because of their relatively low toxicity, tetracyclines have been used extensively in production animals. As a result of their stability in dry form, these drugs can be mixed with feeds and given to herds or flocks of animals. Although less stable in aqueous solutions, tetracyclines retain enough activity to be added to a water supply for mass distribution to animals for treatment or prevention of certain infectious diseases.

Unlike the situation with regard to penicillins or cephalosporins, the degradation products of tetracyclines (degradation can result from improper storage), namely epianhydrotetracycline and anhydrotetracycline, are toxic. In animals they have been reported to produce vomiting and symptoms of acute proteinuria, glycosuria, and acidosis. The toxicity develops rapidly, usually within 2 or 3 days, after ingestion of the degraded or partially degraded drug. High heat and humidity are the environmental conditions that promote the degradation of tetracycline-containing feed mixes. The inclusion of lactose in oral tetracycline capsules prevents this decomposition.[8]

Pharmacological activity

The pharmacological mechanism by which tetracyclines inhibit microbial growth is not entirely understood. However, certain chemical properties of the tetracyclines offer circumstantial evidence as to how this inhibition may occur. The fundamental tetracycline structure is a good *chelating* agent. Chelating agents combine with metallic cations, such as calcium (Ca^{++}), magnesium (Mg^{++}), iron (Fe^{++}), copper (Cu^{++}), and others that have two positive charges, and effectively stop them from reacting with any other biological agents (such as the protoplasm of microbes). Although present in only trace amounts, metallic cations are necessary for proper functioning of enzymatic systems that are vital to all cellular life. It has been postulated that tetracyclines irreversibly bind with physiologically important metallic cations in a cell, thereby making them unavailable for enzymatic use. The biological effect of this chelation process is inhibition of enzyme systems that are necessary for the production of protein. Protein is required for the continued survival of microbes as well as the cells of higher animals. Its decreased production, or its absence, does not cause sudden cell death, but eventually, after preexisting protein stores have been exhausted, cellular dysfunction and destruction will result.

Since tetracyclines chelate with divalent cations (cations with two positive charges) to form insoluble, nonabsorbable complexes, their concurrent administration with other drugs or feeds containing these cations (especially calcium and iron) is not recommended. Chelation could result in precipitation of the drug–metallic cation complex in the stomach, with resultant elimination via the intestines.

Antibacterial spectrum and resistance

Tetracyclines are broad-spectrum antibiotics; they exhibit antimicrobial activity against many gram-negative and gram-positive bacteria. Their coverage overlaps the coverages of penicillin and the cephalosporins. In most cases of mutual coverage, penicillin should be the first-line drug. Because of their effect on protein synthesis, tetracyclines are bacteriostatic rather than bacteriocidal; thus susceptible microbes are not killed as fast as they are by pencillins or cephalosporins. In some situations, however, rapid killing of pathogens is not beneficial. If an animal's disease has progressed to a life-threatening situation, rapid lysis of an infectious organism (as done by bacteriocidal drugs) can liberate a large amount of endotoxin into the system within a short period of time. Thus a critical situation could be made worse. Indeed, even in less serious situations it is not uncommon to notice a transient worsening of an animal's condition after administration of the first few doses of a bacteriocidal drug, because of the sudden release of pathogenic bacterial endotoxins.

In general, gram-positive bacteria are affected by lower doses than gram-negative bacteria are. In vitro testing indicates that some strains of staphylococci and streptococci are sensitive to the tetracyclines, as are certain strains of *Clostridium*, *Klebsiella*, *Haemophilis*, *Corynebacterium*, *Aerobacter*, *Escherichia*, *Salmonella*, *Shigella*, *Bacillus*, *Bacteroides*, *Chlamydia*, and *Mycobacterium*. Tetracyclines are also of value in the treatment of brucellosis in animals and chick embryos.[6,9]

Although bacterial resistance to tetracyclines has been demonstrated, it is not conclusive whether this resistance results from genetic changes in the bacteria or from the emergence of a similar strain (brought about by destruction of the competitive, sensitive strain) that is resistant to the tetracyclines. As would be expected, microbes that display apparent insensitivity to one tetracycline usually are "cross-resistant" to the others. The term "cross-resistant" is used to describe an organism that is resistant to drugs of the same antibiotic class as well as to more than one antibiotic class. For example, a microorganism can be resistant to all tetracyclines as well as to some penicillins. Conversely, the term "cross-sensitive" is applied to microbes that are killed by all drugs in a particular antibiotic class as well as to some drugs in different antibiotic classes.

The use of tetracyclines in combination with other antimicrobial drugs has been tried, with limited success. As was mentioned earlier, concurrent use of bacteriocidal and bacteriostatic drugs—such as the penicillins and the tetracyclines, respectively—is not advocated, since bacteriostatic activity inhibits mitosis, which is the optimal condition for bacteriocidal activity. Ample documentation in the literature attests to the fact that the penicillin and tetracycline combination is not effective. In practice actual therapeutic antagonism between penicillin and tetracycline has been observed.[6]

Occasionally, however, when tetracycline is administered concurrently with another bacteriostatic antibiotic, the clinical result can be greater than that produced by either drug alone (an effect called "synergism"), as demonstrated by the routine practice of treating brucellosis in animals with concurrently administered tetracycline and streptomycin.

Pharmacokinetics

All tetracyclines are incompletely absorbed from the gastrointestinal tract; however, for most animals adequate blood levels can be reached. The tetracyclines have acidic pH values (approximately pH 2), and therefore a significant amount of the drug remains nonionized in the stomach. Consequently, in animals with single-chambered stomachs, most absorption occurs from the stomach and from the upper portions of the small intestines. Although tetracyclines are tolerated well by most animals, the innately irritating nature of these drugs can be associated with gastrointestinal disturbances such as nausea, vomiting, loose stools, and diarrhea when they are given to pigs, cats, and dogs. Phlebitis and pain are usually associated with intravenous administration, especially if the same vein is used repeatedly. Peripheral blood dyscrasias such as leukocytosis and atypical lymphocytes have been reported and are presumed to result from the irritability of the tetracyclines on blood elements.[2,6]

After absorption tetracyclines are distributed in most tissues and fluids, with the highest concentrations usually appearing in bone marrow, spleen, lymph nodes, liver, lungs, and kidneys. Lesser concentrations are found in saliva, milk of nursing animals, and various portions of the eye. The concentration in milk is relatively high in comparison to the concentrations of other medications. Tetracyclines therefore should not be administered to nursing animals; their chelating activity causes them to bind to the dentine and enamel of unerupted teeth, resulting in marked discoloration (mottling) upon emergence. It is also unwise to administer tetracyclines to pregnant animals, since they cross the placental barrier and are deposited in developing teeth and skeletal bones. From 20% to 70% of an administered dose depending upon the particular tetracycline used it can be bound to plasma; chlortetracycline is bound the most and oxytetracycline the least. Tetracyclines also diffuse into brain, prostatic fluid, and semen. It is unclear whether their presence in semen predisposes offspring to congenital abnormalities; however, their administration to animals intended for breeding purposes cannot be recommended at this time.

All tetracyclines are detoxified in the liver and excreted primarily in urine. In addition, as is true of penicillin, a portion of the dose is excreted by way of bile into the intestines, from which the drug can be reabsorbed. Because of this enterohepatic cycle, tetracyclines may remain in the bloodstream (traveling between kidneys, intestine, and systemic blood) for extended periods of time after administration has stopped. Impaired kidney or liver function results in prolonged and/or inordinately high blood levels.

Indications for use and individual agents

Specific diseases that respond to most tetracyclines include pasteurellosis, strangles, leptospirosis, calf diphtheria, vibriosis in cattle, and infectious feline influenza. Nonspecific diseases that can be treated with tetracycline-type antibiotics include mastitis, metritis, gastroenteritis (including pig and calf scours), and bacterial infections that accompany viral diseases.[2]

As was mentioned earlier, the bacterial spectrum of the tetracyclines overlaps that of the penicillins. In any of the diseases just mentioned, tetracycline should be used only if previous therapy with a penicillin or semisynthetic penicillin has proved unsuccessful or if laboratory data indicate that the organism is resistant to the penicillins.

Recommended doses for the tetracyclines are noted in Table 5-4. It was mentioned earlier that products containing calcium, iron, and other divalent cations (especially dairy products, which are rich in calcium) should not be given with tetracyclines. Indeed, it is best to administer these drugs on an empty stomach, since other food groups may be chelated by tetracyclines. If tetracycline-induced stomach irritability makes administration on an empty stomach impractical, then the medication may be given with nondairy products that are low in mineral content. Antacids should not be given to allay stomach distress, since they traditionally are high in divalent cations such as calcium and magnesium.

Tetracycline, chlortetracycline, and oxytetracycline can be given orally, intramuscularly; or intravenously, but absorption is best from the gastrointestinal tract. Tetracycline blood levels are usually higher and are maintained longer than oxytet-

TABLE 5-4

Routes of administration and dosage ranges for commonly used tetracyclines

Drug	Administration route and available dosage forms	Dosage	
		Large animals	*Small animals*
Chloretetracycline	Oral (feed mix)	10 mg/kg every 24 hours	Not used
Doxycycline hyclate	Oral (tablet)	Not used	5 mg/kg twice a day
Minocycline HCl	Oral (capsule)	Not used	2-4 mg/kg twice a day
Oxytetracycline HCl	Oral (capsule)	Not used	10-20 mg/kg three times daily
	IM, IV	2.5-10 mg/kg every 24 hours	Not used
Tetracycline HCl	Oral (capsule and liquid)	Not used	20 mg/kg every 8 hours
	IM, IV	Not used	7 mg/kg every 12 hours

Data from Kirk, R.W.: Current veterinary therapy, Philadelphia, 1980, W.B. Saunders Co., vol. 7, Small animal practice; Spinelli, J.S., and Enos, L.R.: Drugs in veterinary practice, St. Louis, 1978, The C.V. Mosby Co.

racycline or chlortetracycline blood levels. If resistance to oxytetracycline and chlortetracycline develops, tetracycline occasionally gives good results. Whether this phenomenon is related to tetracycline's higher and more persistent blood levels has not yet been determined.

There is little difference between the bacterial spectrums of chlortetracycline and oxytetracycline, although the latter is more effective for urinary infections and the former, because of its higher concentrations in lung and spleen, is usually used for diffuse septicemias.[2] Since a large amount of chlortetracycline enters the entero-hepatic circulation, this drug is more apt to disrupt the bacterial balance of the gastrointestinal tract than is oxytetracycline or tetracycline. It is recommended that chlortetracycline, because of its irritability, not be administered by the intramuscular route. Like the other tetracyclines, chlortetracycline is available in many dosage forms, including capsules and powders for mixing with water and foods.[9]

Oxytetracycline is usually considered the most important and widely used tetracyline in veterinary medicine. Its wide use may be related to its greater stability as compared to chlortetracycline or penicillin. Like the other tetracyclines, it is a broad-spectrum antibiotic. It is readily absorbed from the intestines of all mammals, but intestinal absorption in poultry is unpredictable and usually occurs less readily than in other animals. After intravenous injection maximum blood levels are reached within 30 minutes for most animals. Following intramuscular injection blood levels peak after 2½ hours, and resultant blood levels are not as high, although they are maintained for longer periods of time than are the blood levels produced by intravenous doses. Oxytetracycline is also suitable for topical administration (in a cream or ointment base) and for ophthalmic instillation (in an ointment base). The drug is very effective when used in either of these ways.

Doxycycline and minocycline are newer tetracyclines; they exhibit wider spectrums of bacteriostatic activity and require less frequent administration—usually one or two doses daily, depending upon the disease. Unlike the older tetracyclines (oxytetracycline, chlortetracycline, and tetracycline), they are intended only for oral administration and are not available for mixing with foods or water. They are considerably more expensive than the older tetracyclines, even though they require less frequent administration. In order to discourage the rise of resistant microbes, and for reasons of economy, these newer drugs should be reserved for specific pathogens that are not sensitive to the other tetracyclines or to bacteriocidal antibiotics.

Macrolides

The macrolide antibiotics most commonly used for veterinary purposes are erythromycin and tylosin. Another member of this group, oleandomycin, will be mentioned; however, it does not enjoy the popularity of the other two. Like the tetracyclines, macrolide antibiotics were isolated from organisms belonging to the genus *Streptomyces*. Soil samples containing the organisms from which the antibiotics are obtained were gathered in the Philippines and Thailand during the 1950s.

All the macrolide antibiotics have high molecular weights (exceeding 750) and contain a large lactone ring. Lactones are cyclic structures composed of carbon atoms, two of which are attached to an oxygen atom. Sugar molecules are attached to two of the carbon atoms, while other, smaller organic molecules may be bonded to other carbon atoms. Some sugar molecules contain nitrogen (amino sugar), while others do not. Because of this large lactone ring, these antibiotics are also referred to as macrocyclic lactone antibiotics; however, the designation "macrolide" (large lactone salts) is equally descriptive.[7] The provisional structure of tylosin is typical of this class of antibiotics:

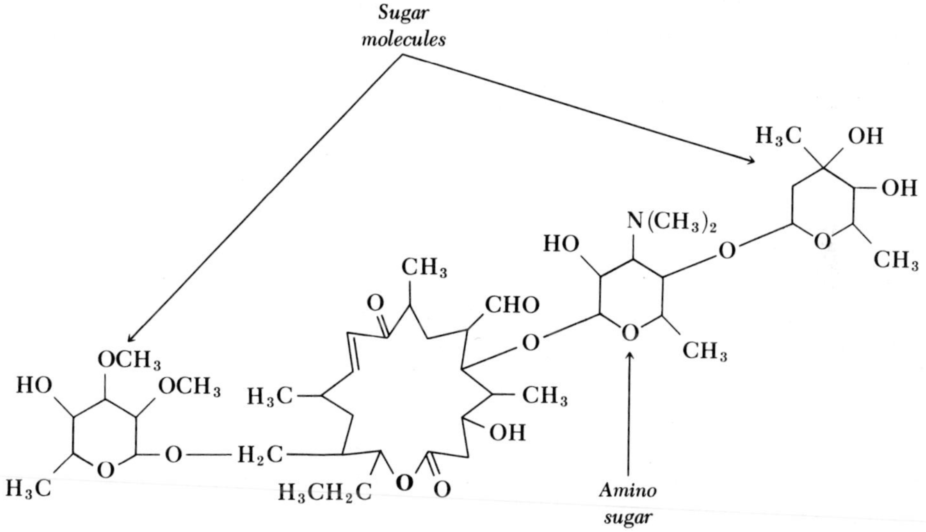

The darker oxygen atom at the bottom of the 16-sided starburst structure is responsible for forming the lactone structure typical of the macrolide class of antibiotics.

Macrolides can be given orally or parenterally, and some (such as erythromycin) are effective when applied topically. These drugs are relatively stable and can be mixed with food or water for administration to large numbers of animals.

Pharmacological activity

By a mechanism that is yet to be precisely determined, the macrolide antibiotics appear to inhibit the formation of protein. This inhibition may be partially a result of chelation (as is true of the tetracyclines), but more probably it is due to competition between the drug and certain amino acids that are intended for incorporation into the protein molecule. As shown in Fig. 5-3, genetic information required to synthesize protein in bacteria flows from the deoxyribonucleic acid (DNA) helix to messenger ribonucleic acid (mRNA) and then to the protein molecule, which is composed of amino acids. A "coding" strand (segment of the DNA chain) is first transcribed into a complementary strand of mRNA. DNA contains four different amino acids: adenine (*A*), guanine (*G*), thymine (*T*), and cytosine (*C*). When mRNA is formed, it has the same amino acids as DNA, except that uracil (*U*) is substituted for thymine.[3] Messenger RNA uses the DNA coding strand as a pattern by which to synthesize itself. For any bacterial mRNA synthesized, the pattern is unchanging: an RNA cytosine is always paired with a DNA guanine, an RNA adenine is paired with a DNA thymine, and uracil (found only on mRNA) is always paired with a DNA adenine.

Each three mRNA amino acids form a "codon," which calls for the incorporation of a particular amino acid into the protein molecule at a specific location. It is

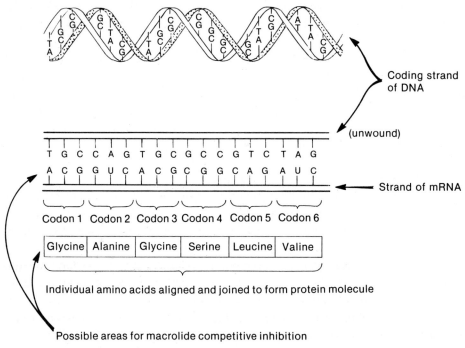

Fig. 5-3. Macrolide inhibition of protein formation. Protein formation is preceded by the unwinding of a portion (gene) of the DNA strand and by its duplication into a "coding strand," which is responsible for transcription of the complentary strand of mRNA. In turn, mRNA directs the assembly of amino acids into protein. Thus bacterial genetic information present in DNA is carried to mRNA, which utilizes it to form a protein molecule. Macrolide and other antibiotics may function by replacing or modifying amino acids in mRNA and/or protein molecules. Ultimately no protein or a false protein is synthesized, which is of no value to the microbe. Lack of the proper protein eventually results in the death of the microbe. (Modified from Chambon, P.: Split genes, Sci. Am., **244:**60-71, May 1981.)

theorized that macrolides may be substituted for any of the amino acids in mRNA or for any one (or more) of the amino acids "called for" by the codon unit. In either case the outcome is similar: either no protein molecule is formed or an incomplete (false) protein is created. Replacement of mRNA amino acids with a macrolide antibiotic molecule disrupts the codon unit, and therefore it cannot "call" for the proper amino acid to be inserted into the protein. Consequently, no protein is formed, or a false protein is formed, which cannot carry out its intended function (that is, repair of cellular walls).

One possible explanation for the incorporation of a macrolide into mRNA is that the antibiotic's structure (or part of it) resembles guanine, thymine, uracil, or adenine and thus it competes with the intended amino acid for the proper position opposite the DNA coding strand. In a similar manner, a macrolide molecule may compete with the amino acid called for by a particular codon unit, thereby either being incorporated into the protein structure or causing synthesis of the protein to stop.

When drugs, presumably because of their molecular structure, compete for biological locations with natural molecules and inhibit the formation of intended products, "competitive inhibition" is said to be taking place. Current data indicate that macrolide antibiotics, acting by the competitive inhibition process, inhibit bacterial protein synthesis, causing the dysfunction and eventual destruction of the bacteria cells.

Antibacterial spectrum and resistance

In normal dosage ranges macrolides are bacteriostatic to mature organisms; however, if doses are increased (as in the case of erythromycin), these drugs can exhibit bacteriocidal activity. The bacteriocidal properties are associated with the destruction of the microbial cell wall.[1]

Generally, the macrolides' spectrum of antibacterial activity is narrow, covering most gram positive organisms and a few gram-negative ones. Macrolides are not affected by penicillinase and therefore can be used for infections caused by penicillinase-producing staphylococci. Cross resistance between macrolides generally does not occur, although prolonged therapy with oleandomycin can cause the emergence of staphylococcus strains that are resistant to other macrolides.[1,8] Laboratory tests have indicated partial cross-resistance between erythromycin and tylosin, but it remains to be seen whether this has any clinical significance. No cross-resistance between tylosin and penicillin or the tetracyclines has been demonstrated.[1,2]

Macrolides are used extensively for simultaneously treating large numbers of animals; however, for the treatment of individual animals most practioners prefer the newer semisynthetic penicillins, which have spectrums similar to those of the macrolides.[9]

Pharmacokinetics

All macrolides are absorbed well from upper portions of the gastrointestinal tract, although erythromycin is partially degraded by gastric secretions. In nonruminants peak blood levels following oral administration are reached in approximately 2 hours, with therapeutic concentrations lasting for 6 hours.

For the most part macrolides diffuse into body tissues and amniotic fluid, and they can be detected in saliva. They cross placental barriers and appear in milk. Small amounts cross into cerebrospinal fluid, but they do not readily cross the blood-brain barrier. Highest concentrations are found in the liver and bile. Detoxification occurs in the liver, with significant amounts being excreted in bile (approximately 30% in most animals), urine (about 15%), milk, and feces.[1,8]

Macrolides are not known to predispose animals to superinfections; however, prolonged therapy should be accompanied by liver function tests, since hepatotoxicity has been linked to their use.

Indications for use and individual agents

Macrolides can be used when penicillins have proved ineffective, possibly because of the presence of penicillinase-producing organisms. Macrolides are useful in pathological conditions of poultry and turkeys (such as sinusitis and synovitis). In pigs they can be administered in the food or water supply to treat or prevent *Vibrio coli*–induced enteritis or scours. For cattle and calves intramuscular injections are beneficial for the treatment of pneumonia, foot rot, and metritis. Likewise, intramuscular injection in dogs and cats is indicated for upper-respiratory-tract infections, cellulitis, otitis externa, metritis, leptospirosis, and bacterial infections accompanying viral diseases.[2] Macrolides have no effect against viruses.

Erthyromycin. In the dry state, injectable erythromycin remains stable for years; however reconstituted solutions should be kept in a refrigerator. Since stability under refrigeration may differ from manufacturer to manufacturer, literature accompanying each brand of erythromycin should be consulted.

Parenteral administration of erythromycin should be limited to the intravenous route, and the rate of administration should be closely monitored to avoid phlebitis. The intramuscular route should never be used, because of resultant tissue necrosis at the injection site. Parenteral erythromycin should be constituted only with sterile water for injection (USP) (which does not contain any preservatives). Use of a reconstituting solution containing preservatives (antimicrobial agents), such as methylparaben, propylparaben, or benzyl alcohol, will result in the formation of a gel rather than a clear aqueous solution.

Since the activity of erythromycin is decreased in acidic media, enteric-coated tablets are recommended when the drug is administered orally. Erythromycin estolate is not affected by stomach acid and is rapidly absorbed. Unfortunately, this compound is associated with liver toxicities and is currently being reviewed by the Food and Drug Administration to determine whether it should be withdrawn from the market.

Another advantage of using enteric-coated tablets is that stomach irritation resulting from erythromycin is largely avoided, without having to administer the drug with food (which enhances degradation by stimulating acid secretion into the stomach).

Erythromycin is also used topically, most often as an ophthalmic ointment for conjunctivitis and other ocular infections.

Oleandomycin. Although oleandomycin produces higher peak blood levels than erythromycin, they are short lived, and consequently this drug's antibacterial activity is generally considered to be less than that of erythromycin. Oleandomycin's most serious side effect is hepatotoxicity following prolonged administration. Consequently its use in the treatment or prophylaxis of infections is not recommended for more than 10 days. Oleandomycin should not be used unless treatment with other macrolides has proved unsuccessful.[2]

As is true of other antibiotics, the possibility of superinfection by fungal organisms exist; however, it is less likely with oleandomycin than with wide-spectrum antibiotics.[8]

Tylosin. Tylosin should not be used in poultry that produce eggs for human use. Chickens must not be slaughtered for human consumption for 3 days after injection of tylosin or for 24 hours after oral administration, whether for treatment or prophylaxis. Turkeys must not be slaughtered for food within 5 days after being given tylosin, and for pigs the waiting time must exceed 21 days. At least a 96-hour wait is recommended before milk is obtained from cows treated with tylosin. Unlike the other antibiotics discussed thus far, tylosin is sold only for veterinary purposes, with most of the drug being used in agribusiness.[2]

• • •

Table 5-5 summarizes doses of the macrolides discussed in this chapter. As is true of tylosin, administration of the other macrolides to animals intended for human consumption is closely monitored by the federal government and by state governments. The detoxification and elimination rates for the individual drugs dictate how long an animal must be free from drug exposure before processing.

The reason for reducing drug residuals to undetectable amounts is to prevent the contamination of food consumed by humans. Foods containing even trace amounts of macrolides, or other drugs, can predispose consumers to anaphylactic reactions. Some antibiotics, such as the tetracyclines, can be converted in the cooking process to toxic substances that can produce significant clinical reactions in persons who ingest them. Drug concentrations may accumulate in developing bones, teeth, and other organs of younger individuals, since their detoxification enzyme systems are not fully developed. Adequate documentation exists as to the adverse affects of the accumulation of tetracyclines in developing teeth; however the potential for damage when tetracyclines accumulate in other tissues of developing youngsters remains unclear. It should not be assumed that food processing destroys residual drug concentrations in food, since some antibiotics and most steroids (which are used to hasten the development of animals and poultry) are stable in high temperatures and over a wide pH range.

It is also necessary to monitor drug intakes in animals whose by-products (such as milk and eggs) are intended for human use.

TABLE 5-5
Administration routes and dosages for commonly used macrolide antibiotics

Drug*	Administration route and available dosage forms	Dosage	
		Small animals (dogs, cats)	Large animals
Erythromycin (as free base and most salts)	Oral (tablets and liquid)	11 mg/kg once or twice daily (dog) 11-22 mg/kg once or twice daily (cat)	Not used
	IM (when IV route is not practical)	4.4 mg/kg every 24-48 hours	2.2-4.4 mg/kg every 24 hours (cattle, horses, sheep) 2.2-6.6 mg/kg every 24 hours (swine)
Tylosin	Oral	7-15 mg/kg three times daily	Not used
	IM	6.6-11 mg/kg every 24 hours	2.2-4.4 mg base/kg each 24 hours (cattle) Swine: same dose as cattle but do not give more than 3 doses Not used in horses or sheep

Data from Spinelli, J.S., and Enos, L.R.: Drugs in veterinary practice, St. Louis, 1978, The C.V. Mosby Co.

*Oleandomycin is not commonly used, because of its expense and its antibacterial spectrum, which is similar to that of the penicillins.

Aminoglycosides

The commonly used aminoglycoside antibiotics (amikacin, gentamicin, kanamycin, neomycin, streptomycin, and tobramycin) are broad-spectrum anti-infectives; however, they should be reserved primarily for treatment of infections caused by gram-negative organisms. These antibiotics, which have high molecular weights, consist of a cyclic nucleus to which one or two amino sugars (hexosamines) are attached by glycoside-type bonding; hence the name aminoglycosides. Gentamicin sulfate illustrates the typical structural formula for these anti-infectives:

$$H_3C-HN-CH(CH_3)- \\ H_2N-CH(CH_3)- \\ H_2NCH_2-$$ R groups

Any commercial gentamicin sulfate product is a mixture of three forms of gentamicin sulfate, which differ only in the composition of the R group (as noted to the right of the core structure). The number of H_2SO_4 molecules depends upon the mix of the R groups. Gentamicin sulfate may vary in composition, depending upon the manufacturer, but all products should exhibit the same clinical activity. Like all other aminoglycosides, gentamicin has two amino-containing sugar molecules (hexosamines) attached to a central deoxystreptamine molecule by ether bonds (—O—). The ether linkages are referred to as "glycoside" bonds; hence the name "aminoglycosides" ("amino-" from the sugar molecules and "-glycoside" from the ether bonding). While the compositions of the hexosamines vary depending upon the particular aminoglycoside, it appears that the deoxystreptamine portion is required for optimal antibacterial activity.

Aminoglycoside absorption from the gastrointestinal tract is generally minimal (with kanamycin being the exception). As a result these drugs are administered orally for enteral infections, while systemic infections require parenteral administration. Aminoglycosides are distributed from the bloodstream into extracellular fluid, since their low partition coefficients prevent them from entering most cells. Likewise, they do not penetrate the central nervous system or ocular tissue. As would be expected because of their low fat solubility, they are only minimally bound to serum proteins. Aminoglycosides have a marked affinity for renal cortical tissue, where they can accumulate in concentrations up to 50 times those achieved in blood. Consequently the most significant side effect of these drugs is nephrotoxicity. Adequate renal function thus is mandatory prior to administration; the aminoglycosides are eliminated via glomerular filtration, and inadequate renal function will only increase the amount concentrated in the kidneys. Ototoxicity is another side effect attributed to these drugs; there is evidence to indicate that the degree of impairment of renal function is directly proportional to the rate of development of ototoxicity (the greater the renal dysfunction, the quicker ototoxicity may occur).[4]

Since aminoglycosides can cause neurological toxicities (such as ototoxicity), it is not surprising that large doses can potentiate the effects of neuromuscular blocking drugs such as d-tubocurarine and succinylcholine.[9] Since neuromuscular blocking drugs are used in conjunction with surgical procedures, it is best to determine aminoglycoside blood levels prior to surgery, to avoid muscular collapse. (Refer to *Small Animal Anesthesia*, the first volume of this series, for a more detailed discussion of neuromuscular blocking agents.)

With the exception of streptomycin, aminoglycosides are stable in temperatures used to cook food. In addition, most are stable in pH ranges from 2 to 11, and although their aqueous solutions can darken as a result of oxidation, potency does not appear to be affected. Specific incompatibilities depend upon the specific drugs with which aminoglycosides are mixed, as well as concentrations, pH, and temperature. However, it is prudent to consider the aminoglycosides incompatible with penicillins and cephalosporins.[1] Accordingly these drugs should not be mixed in the same syringe or intravenous-administration container.

Pharmacological activity

Although the exact mechanism by which aminoglycosides exert their antibacterial effect is uncertain, it appears that they inhibit protein synthesis in susceptible bacteria, with the mode of inhibition possibly being similar to that discussed for the macrolides.

Antibacterial spectrum and resistance

In therapeutic doses aminoglycosides are bactericidal. They are active against many aerobic gram-positive and gram-negative bacteria. They are inactive against fungi, viruses, and most anaerobic bacteria. Organisms of the genera *Actinobacillus, Citrobacter, Enterobacter, Klebsiella, Proteus, Providencia, Pseudomonas, Salmonella, Serratia,* and *Shigella,* as well as *E. coli,* are generally sensitive to aminoglycosides (except kanamycin, the drug in this class to which they mostly commonly show resistance). *Pseudomonas aeruginosa,* seems most sensitive to amikacin, gentamicin, and tobramycin. Aminoglycosides are also active against most strains of straphylococci. Resistance to a particular aminoglycoside can be due to decreased bacterial wall permeability or to the ability to enzymatically modify the drug, the latter method occurring least frequently with amikacin. Amikacin is the newest addition to the aminoglycoside group; it exhibits not only an expanded antibacterial spectrum but an increased potential for discouraging resistance as compared to the other antibiotics of this class. Some bacterial cross-resistance (usually between kanamycin and neomycin) occurs among the aminoglycosides.

Pharmacokinetics

It was mentioned earlier that systemic distribution of aminoglycosides results in their concentrating in the kidney. Another area of concentration is the inner ear. During a course of therapy with an aminoglycoside the inner ear will usually become saturated with the drug, which will be slowly released after therapy has been discontinued. Since high concentrations in the kidney result in nephrotoxicity, it seems reasonable to assume that accumulation in the ear accounts for the reports of ototoxicity associated with aminoglycoside use.

Since drug distribution patterns are similar for all animals, the major contributing factor to the development of these toxicities is dosage. It appears that there is a need for periods of lower blood drug concentrations ("valleys") during treatment in order to prevent ototoxicity and nephrotoxicity. Thus an administration pattern should be used that will produce sustained periods of effective blood concentrations, but with peaks and valleys rather than consistently high levels. Either of two dosage schemes (both of which require the monitoring of blood levels) can be used to accomplish this (see Fig. 5-4):

Scheme 1: *Administer half the dose every half-life of the drug.* Half the original dose is given when the blood concentration falls to half of that produced by the initial dose.

Scheme 2: *Administer the full dose every two to three half-lives of the drug.* Twice as much of the drug is given half as often (as compared to scheme 1); thus the total daily amount administered is the same as in scheme 1 (if the drug is administered every two half-lives). One disadvantage of this pattern is that valley concentrations can fall below effective blood levels before the next dose is given, as noted in Fig. 5-4.

Both dosage schemes have been used effectively with gentamicin.

A less formal, but perhaps more practical, approach for nonhospitalized animals is to periodically monitor urine creatinine levels, since nephrotoxicity will result in

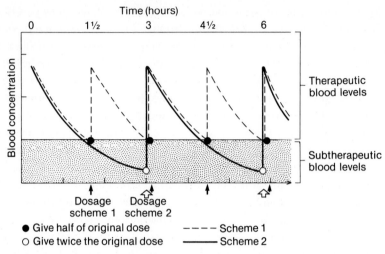

Fig. 5-4. Dosage patterns for aminoglycosides in dogs. Scheme 1 requires more doses to be administered than scheme 2 over the same time period, but ensures higher blood levels. Scheme 2, however, provides the better method to avoid ototoxicity and/or nephrotoxicity. The half-life of gentamicin, for example, in dogs is 1½ hours.[9] If scheme 1 were used, a dose of 2 mg/kg would be given, followed by doses of 1 mg/kg given 1½, 3, 4½, and 6 hours after the first dose. If scheme 2 were used, 2 mg/kg would be given, followed by 2 mg/kg after 3 and 6 hours (if the drug were being given every two half-lives).

their elevation. For most animals nephrotoxicity is irreversible, while ototoxicity is reversible in many cases.[4]

Indications for use and individual agents

Amikacin, gentamicin, kanamycin, tobramycin. These drugs are administered parenterally for short-term treatment of infections caused by certain gram-negative bacteria; these conditions include septicemias, bone and joint infections, skin and soft-tissue infections, respiratory tract infections, and posteroperative infections. These drugs are also indicated for serious infections caused by susceptible gram-positive bacteria, but only after less toxic antibiotics have proved unsuccessful. Although gentamicin is the most frequently used drug in this group, recent data indicate that tobramycin is therapeutically equivalent and that it has less propensity to cause nephrotoxicity and ototoxicity. All four drugs are available as ready-to-use injectable solutions. Kanamycin is also available in oral capsules; it is the only aminoglycoside that can achieve therapeutic blood levels after oral administration.

Streptomycin, dihydrostreptomycin. Clinically dihydrostreptomycin can be considered equivalent to streptomycin. Generally a streptomycin blood level of 5 micrograms (μg) per milliliter of serum is considered a minimum therapeutic amount.

Like other aminoglycosides, streptomycin diffuses very slowly into cerebrospinal fluid, with effective concentrations rarely being achieved. Streptomycin passes the placental barrier relatively easily, with no neurotoxic effects on the fetus having been reported. Approximately 10% of the drug is absorbed after oral administration to dogs and cats, with no appreciable blood levels of drug being detected. As a result streptomycin is useful for susceptible enteral pathogens. Streptomycin is recoverable in milk in significant amounts and thus can be used to treat staphylococcal mastitis. It is essential that milk obtained from cows undergoing streptomycin therapy not be marketed.[2] Even though the temperature reached in the pasteurization process (68°C) is high enough to slowly degrade the drug, it is not maintained long enough to ensure that all the drug is destroyed. In addition, the by-products of streptomycin degradation may have adverse effects in humans.

Streptomycin can cause three types of toxic reactions in animals: (1) a contact dermatitis, which can also occur to practioners who handle streptomycin powders or solutions; (2) a chronic toxicity; and (3) an acute systemic reaction. The chronic toxicity involves the ear and is a result of damage to the eighth cranial nerve. The clinical manifestations are vertigo (dizziness, loss of balance) and/or degrees of hearing loss. Both symptoms can occur within 4 to 5 days if large doses are administered. (With dihydrostreptomycin the ototoxicity usually results in hearing dysfunction rather than vertigo.)

Acute toxicity results in anaphylactoid symptoms—nausea, vomiting, and rapid loss of consciousness. Standard treatment for shock, as well as injectable antihistamines, will usually prove effective. It has been reported that didhydrostreptomycin is less likely to cause this type reaction than is streptomycin.[2]

As is true when any aminoglycoside is used, adequate renal function must be assured before streptomycin or dihydrostreptomycin is administered. In animals with normal kidney function the half-life of streptomycin is relatively short (for example, 1½ hours in dogs).[9]

Neomycin. Neomycin was isolated from *Streptomyces fradiae* found in a soil sample taken from the farmyard of the New Jersey Agricultural College. It was in this same farmyard that the organism producing streptomycin was also discovered. Besides being ototoxic, neomycin is the most nephrotoxic of the aminoglycosides and therefore should be used parenterally only as a last resort. It does not enter systemic circulation after topical application; consequently most of its use is by this route. Neomycin is available as 0.5% and 1% ointments for application to wounds, often in combination with other antibiotics. The drug can be administered orally in all species for use against enteral infections (such as coliform enteritis), since, like most aminoglycosides, it is not appreciably absorbed from the gastrointestinal tract. Oral doses in cows and piglets are effective in the treatment of scours. Neomycin is also used to "sterilize" the intestinal tract prior to enteral surgery.

•   •   •

TABLE 5-6

Routes of administration and dosage for some aminoglycoside antibiotics

Drug	Administration route and available dosage forms	Dosage*
Gentamicin sulfate and tobramycin sulfate	IM, IV, SC	4 mg/kg every 12 hours for 1 day, then 4 mg/kg every 24 hours (also see Fig. 5-4)
Kanamycin sulfate	Oral (capsules), IM, IV	10-55 mg/kg every 6 hours
Neomycin sulfate	Topical (solution or ointment in strengths from 0.5% to 1%)	Since neomycin is the most toxic of all aminoglycosides and has the same spectrum of antibacterial activity as kanamycin, it is not recommended for parenteral use.
Dihydrostreptomycin sulfate and streptomycin sulfate	IM, SC	10 mg/kg every 6-8 hours

Data from Kirk, R.W.: Current veterinary therapy, Philadelphia, 1980, W.B. Saunders Co., vol. 7, Small animal practice; Spinelli, J.S., and Enos, L.R.: Drugs in veterinary practice, St. Louis, 1978, The C.V. Mosby Co.

*Since all aminoglycosides should be considered nephrotoxic and/or ototoxic, safe dosages can be significantly lower than those noted, especially if renal function is not optimal.

Table 5-6 lists suggested dosages for some of the aminoglycosides discussed in this section.

Polypeptides

The two most significant and useful polypeptide antibiotics are polymyxin B sulfate and bacitracin. Both "polymyxin" and "bacitracin" are collective names; each is used to describe a number of very similar antibiotics. The name "polymyxin" is used to refer to polymyxin A, B, C, D, or E (B being the most clinically effective and the least toxic). "Bacitracin" is used to refer to any of at least three different forms of the drug—bacitracin A, B, and C (A being used most often). The polymyxins are produced by *Bacillus polymyxa,* which was isolated from soil samples in 1947. The discovery of the bacitracins makes a slightly more interesting story. They are now produced from the Tracy I strain of *Bacillus subtilis,* which is an aerobic gram-positive organism. In 1943 this particular strain was isolated from debrided wound tissue obtained from a young girl named Tracy. Hence the name: "baci-" from *baci*llus, "trac" from *Tracy,* and "in" from stra*in.*

Structurally the two groups of antibiotics have little in common except that both consist of simple, high-molecular-weight compounds (exceeding 1000) that are composed of amino acids linked to each other to form a cyclic configuration. In each of the polymyxins one of the amino acids is bound to isopelargonic acid (a nonamino acid). In the bacitracins one of the amino acids is bound to a thiazolidine molecule. In addition, the polymyxins and the bacitracins differ from each other in amino acid content.

Polymyxin B sulfate

Polymyxin B sulfate is the most commonly used polymyxin compound. In fact, in practice the terms "polymyxin" and "polymyxin B" generally mean polymyxin B sulfate.

Polymyxin B exhibits surfactant activity. Surfactants are chemicals that have the ability to "wet" surfaces, oftentimes disrupting molecular arrangements. They are commonly used in detergents and are responsible for penetrating and breaking up soiled areas. The ability of surfactants to "wet" surfaces is a function of their capacity to foam. The foaming capacity of polymyxin is evident when a vial of it is reconstituted and shaken.

Polymyxin immediately wets outer cellular layers of a microbe's wall, causing a disruption in its integrity. Since the wall can no longer act as an effective osmotic barrier, cell protoplasm escapes, causing the death of the organism. As a result polymyxin B is rapidly bacteriocidal in vitro. It has a narrow spectrum of antibacterial action, being effective against gram-negative bacteria such as *Aerobacter*, *Escherichia*, *Haemophilus*, *Klebsiella*, *Pasteurella*, *Salmonella*, and *Shigella*. It remains the first drug of choice for treatment of *Pseudomonas aeruginosa*. Polymyxin B sulfate is not significantly effective against gram-positive pathogens.

Even in large doses polymyxin is not absorbed significantly after oral administration. Neither is it absorbed when applied topically, even if the integrity of the skin is broken. Consequently application as an ointment or a wet dressing is useful for local treatment and does not carry the risk of systemic drug absorption.[6] It has been reported, however, that ointments or solutions exceeding 1% polymyxin have irritated even intact skin.[2] Polymyxin is often combined with neomycin and/or bacitracin in topical medications; this combination of ingredients provides a wide antibacterial spectrum. Oral administration of polymyxin B sulfate is useful for eradicating gram-negative pathogens from the gastrointestinal tract.

After intramuscular injection little polymyxin is eliminated within the first 12 hours. Thereafter elimination is rapid, and it becomes difficult to maintain adequate tissue levels.[6,9] Localized pain and swelling can be expected at the injection site. The intensity of these side effects can be reduced, or sometimes the side effects can be eliminated, if injections of procaine are given with the polymyxin B sulfate.[2]

Like the aminoglycosides, polymyxin can have neurotoxic effects, including vertigo and loss of sensation in the head and extremities; the severity of the latter side effect is increased if neuromuscular blocking agents are concurrently administered. The intensified neurological side effects caused by the combination of polymyxin and blocking agents are not reversed by administration of neostigmine, as they are when these effects result from concurrent administration of aminoglycosides and blocking agents.[9] Nephrotoxic effects (for example, albuminuria, renal casts, hematuria) in dogs have been reported after a single intravenous dose of as little as 2.5 mg/kg.[1] Recommended doses for dogs and cats are 2 mg/kg every 12 hours if given by the IM route, and 1.2 mg/kg every 12 hours if given orally.[6]

In order to avoid systemic toxicities, the use of polymyxin is largely confined to topical preparations for the skin, eyes, or ears.

Bacitracin

Bacitracin is effective primarily against gram-positive organisms, in a pattern very similar to that of penicillin. Like penicillin, bacitracin contains a thiazolidine molecule, and, as is true of penicillin, bacitracin's antibacterial activity seems to result from interference with cell wall formation. Unlike penicillin, however, bacitracin is bacteriostatic rather than bacteriocidal.[2] Almost all strains of aerobic and anaerobic hemolytic streptococci are sensitive to bacitracin. In addition, *Actinomyces, Fusobacterium, Corynebacterium, Clostridium, Neisseria,* various strains of staphylococci, and enterococci are sensitive to the drug. No bacterial resistance of any significance has been reported in animals. Likewise no cross-resistance between bacitracin and other antibiotics has been demonstrated; thus bacitracin may be used when others have failed, and vice versa.

In the dry state bacitracin is stable for years, but once reconstituted it loses one third to one half of its potency within 2 weeks when stored at room temperature. Refrigerated solutions retain their original potency for 1 week.

As is true of polymyxin, bacitracin's absorption after oral administration is negligible, partly because of its destruction by gastric acid. Injections should be given only by the intramuscular route. After injection bacitracin penetrates most tissues; however, it does not penetrate the brain, since it does not cross the blood-brain barrier. It may require up to 2 hours to reach maximum blood levels; therapeutic levels may persist for 6 to 8 hours, depending on the dose.[2]

Like polymyxin, bacitracin is primarily used as a topical medication for skin, mucous membranes, and ocular tissue.

Antifungal antibiotics

Just as the antibacterial drugs are classified according to the way they affect bacteria, antifungal (antimycotic) antibiotics can be classified according to the way they affect fungi. Fungistatic drugs prevent growth and multiplication of fungi, while fungicidal drugs destroy fungi relatively rapidly.

Fungi are responsible for external animal and bird diseases—most notably ringworm, which can be caused by organisms of the genera the *Trichophyton* and *Mi-*

crosporum. Fungi are also responsible for systemic diseases such as "brooder pneumonia" in chickens and mycotic "abortion" in cattle.[2]

The modes of action of antifungal antibiotics are similar to those discussed for antibacterial antibiotics; they include inhibition of cell wall formation and disruption of protein synthesis.

Amphotericin B

Amphotericin B, a fungistatic antibiotic, is obtained from *Streptomyces nodosa*. It is a relatively insoluble drug, but its solubility increases as the pH rises. Sodium desoxycholate is added to the injectable product to ensure that the pH of the reconstituted solution remains in the vicinity of 7. Because desoxycholate is a very irritating chemical, injections of the amphotericin product should be given only by the intravenous route. Intense pain and tissue sloughing have been reported when this product is given intramuscularly. The injection site should be continually monitored for signs of phlebitis or infiltration, and the intravenous infusion rate should be adjusted to compensate for the irritating nature of the medication.

Like erythromycin, amphotericin B should be reconstituted only with sterile water for injection (USP), since use of water containing any preservatives (such as benzyl alcohol, methylparaben, or propylparaben) or even unpreserved sodium chloride solutions can cause precipitation upon initial dilution of the product. Unlike the case with erythromycin, a solution of amphotericin B, although perfectly clear, is actually a suspension composed of particles (1 to 50 μ in diameter) that are too small to be seen by the unaided eye. Suspensions that are composed of such particles and that appear to be solutions are referred to as "colloids" or "colloidal dispersions." Since the drug is not dissolved, amphotericin B should not be infused by an intravenous-administration setup that utilizes an antibacterial filter. The porosities of antibacterial filters range from 0.22 to 0.45 μ and consequently will filter out the drug from the solution so that the animal does not receive any medicine.

Amphotericin B acts by binding steroids in fungal walls, causing the walls to become more permeable as a result of a loss of integrity. Cellular protoplasm is lost by passage through the wall, leading to cessation of many cellular functions.

Amphotericin B is nephrotoxic; its use requires the monitoring of blood urea nitrogen (BUN) and blood creatinine levels.[9]

Griseofulvin

The fungistatic antibiotic griseofulvin exerts its action largely by interupting microbial division during the metaphase stage. The exact mechanism seems to be the disruption of mitotic spindle structures. In addition the drug is believed to cause the formation of defective DNA. Since defective DNA is not able to direct microbial activity, growth and reproductive functions are inhibited.

In the oral form (capsules, tablets, or suspensions) the best absorption occurs when the diameters of the drug particles are 4 μ (microsize) or less (ultramicrosize). Unless the trade or generic name includes the term "microsize" or "ultramicrosize" or otherwise indicates that the largest drug particle diameter is in the area of 4 μ, absorption will be minimal, resulting in longer courses of therapy.

Following oral administration, griseofulvin is absorbed from the duodenum; the degree of absorption is inversely proportional to the size of the particles (the smaller the particles the more drug absorbed). Upon absorption the drug concentrates primarily in skin (keratin precursor cells), hair, and nails. As a result, griseofulvin is beneficial in treating mycotic infections in these areas, providing the pathogen is a susceptible species of *Trichophyton, Microsporum,* or *Epidermophyton.* Since griseofulvin is not effective against other fungal pathogens, the infectious agent should be identified before therapy is started.

Because of griseofulvin's high partition coefficient, detoxification in the liver occurs slowly in mammals, with the drug requiring several days to be totally excreted, even after a single dose. The drug crosses placental membranes in dogs and is suspected of being toxic to the embryo and teratogenic.

Only oral dosage forms are available (capsules, tablets, or suspensions). The duration of treatment depends upon the length of time required to replace infected skin, hair, or nails. Treatment of mycotic nail infections in smaller animals (such as dogs) with doses of 50 mg/kg given once daily can require up to 12 weeks. Large animals should be treated for at least 10 days and preferably 14 days.[2]

Miconazole

Miconazole, a synthetic drug, is the newest of the antifungals. It exerts its activity by interfering with intracellular enzymatic activity. As the dose increases, the drug is initially fungistatic and then fungicidal, causing an alteration in cell wall permeability in the higher dosage ranges. In addition to its antifungal activity, miconazole is also effective against all gram-positive bacteria.

After intravenous or oral administration, the drug is distributed in most tissue masses and fluids. It crosses the blood-brain barrier, but only in small amounts, and apparently does not cross placental tissue in animals. It is not known whether miconazole is excreted in milk. Although tablets are available, the intravenous route is preferred because absorption is erratic when the drug is given by mouth. Intravenous solutions of miconazole are not as irritating as those of amphotericin B.

Miconazole has proved effective in fungal infections that do not respond to amphotericin B therapy. Concurrent use of miconazole and amphotericin B, however, cannot be recommended at this time, since preliminary in vitro tests suggest an antagonism may occur between these drugs.

Nystatin

Nystatin was discovered by soil survey personnel of the New York State Department of Health (hence the name: "ny" from *New York*, "stat" from *State*). Nystatin's mode of antifungal activity is similar to that of amphotericin B. Consequently cell wall integrity is compromised, leading to cellular dysfunction and destruction by the host's biological mechanisms. Although nystatin has fungistatic and fungi-cidal activity against a number of pathogens, it is usually used for *Candida (Monilia)* organisms, since they rarely develop resistance to it.

Oral administration is usually intended for *C. albicans* infection of the gastrointestinal tract, which in some cases is a result of antibacterial drug therapy. Nystatin is poorly absorbed from the gastrointestinal tract and is excreted almost entirely in the feces.

Nystatin is available in ointment form for topical application. Negligible amounts of the drug are absorbed by this route, even if the skin is broken. Other dosage forms include an oral suspension, which can be either applied to the mouth or swallowed, and an injectable form.

The recommended oral dosage is 100,000 units every 6 hours, whether the drug is intended for the oral cavity or for gastrointestinal use.[2,7]

* * *

This discussion has included only antibiotic antifungal drugs. Efficacious non-antibiotic (mostly topical) antifungal preparations, such as gentian violet, undecylenic acid and its zinc salt, and salicylic acid, are available and should not be discounted as first-line preparations or as last resorts if antifungal antibiotics prove unsatisfactory.

Other antibiotics

Chloramphenicol

Chloramphenicol is different from the other antibiotics thus far studied in that it has a very simple structure, as shown in Fig. 5-1, and it is the only antibiotic that is manufactured totally synthetically.

Chloramphenicol was isolated from a *Streptomyces* organism found in Venezuelan soil samples. The antibiotic is very stable, demonstrating no clinical decrease in activity after being boiled in water for 5 hours.[2] Because it is so stable it should not be used in food-producing animals, since it is likely that food processing temperatures would not destroy residual amounts of the drug.[9]

Pharmacological activity and pharmacokinetics. Chloramphenicol is considered bacteriostatic; however, it can be bacteriocidal if doses are increased.[2] Despite years of intensive study, chloramphenicol's exact antibacterial mechanism of action is not understood. Although the drug is known to interfere with protein synthesis (as aminoglycoside and polypeptide antibiotics do), it is unclear whether it competitively displaces the mRNA amino acids (cytosine, adenine, uracil, guanine), to form false mess-RNA, or competes with other amino acids for positions on mess-RNA codons.[8]

Oral administration results in rapid and almost complete absorption of the drug, uptake being so efficient that oral and parenteral doses can be the same in mammals with single-chambered stomachs.[9] Blood levels and their duration are proportional to dose. Peak blood concentrations are usually reached in 2 to 4 hours, with up to 45% of the drug being bound to plasma.

The extent of distribution of chloramphenicol exceeds that of the tetracyclines; however, the rate of distribution is the same as that of the tetracyclines. Chloramphenicol diffuses easily across the blood-brain barrier and into cerebrospinal fluid. Likewise it effectively crosses placental barriers; fetal blood concentrations can reach up to 75% of the concentration of the mother. Significant amounts of chloramphenicol are excreted in milk, a situation that in humans has been linked to infant deaths.

In most animals chloramphenicol is conjugated in the liver. (Cats, however, like newborn human infants, appear to have another hepatic detoxification mechanism, which causes an amide salt of the drug to be formed.) Elimination of chloramphenicol depends upon adequate hepatic and renal function and therefore these parameters should be monitored and evaluated before and during therapy.[9]

It appears that only chloramphenicol *base* is capable of being absorbed and is microbiologically active. For this reason oral dosage forms are most often composed of the free base, in order to hasten absorption. Parenteral forms of chloramphenicol most often consist of the sodium succinate salt (which facilitates dissolution) and thus require hydrolyzation by plasma enzymes so that the sodium succinate portion is removed from the chloramphenicol molecule. Once that portion has been removed, the molecule becomes biologically active, demonstrating antibacterial activity.

Chloramphenicol can also be given by the intramuscular, intravenous, or subcutaneous routes, without irritation at the injection site. It is also available for ophthalmic use, either as a solution or as an ointment. When the drug is applied in either of the latter two forms, it is necessary to use only chloramphenicol base, since enzymes necessary for conversion of any chloramphenicol salt to the base are probably not present in ocular tissue.

Antibacterial spectrum and resistance. Another unique aspect of chloramphenicol is that not only is it effective against gram-negative and gram-positive bacteria, but it exhibits activity against certain viruses and rickettsiae. A broad-spectrum antibiotic, it exhibits bacteriostatic action against *B. anthracis*, the *E. coli–Salmonella* group, and *Brucella, Corynebacteria, Erysipelothrix,* and *Pasteurella* species. In addition it is effective against *Proteus vulgaris, Psuedomonas aeruginosa,* and most staphylococci and streptococci.

Unlike the situation with regard to some other antibiotics, resistance to chloramphenicol develops slowly, in a stepwise fashion, rather than in one step as is the case with streptomycin.[8] Thus far resistance to chloramphenicol does not seem to be a clinical problem. In one study 88 strains of bacteria were isolated from diseased animals and birds (representing 15 species), and not one demonstrated resistance.[2] The fact that a microbe is resistant to other wide-spectrum antibiotics (such as the tetracyclines) does not necessarily mean the organism will be resistant to chloramphenicol.

Indications for use and dosage. Suppression of blood cell formation because of bone marrow depression has been reported after the administration of chloramphenicol, although the frequency is extremely low. This phenomenon usually occurs as a result of high doses being given over long periods of time, and it usually subsides when the drug is discontinued. Accordingly, since the antibacterial spectrum of chloramphenicol is similar to that of the tetracyclines, it would seem prudent to use tetracyclines initially. If results are unsatisfactory, the use of chloramphenicol may be justified.

Chloramphenicol has been effective in treating calf and pig scours, kennel cough, infectious bovine keratitis (when the drug is applied as an ophthalmic solution or ointment), foot rot in sheep, viral pneumonia, and calf diphtheria.[2]

Recommended oral and parenteral doses are as follows:

Horse	25-50 mg/kg every 6 to 8 hours[9]
Cat	50 mg/kg every 12 hours
Dog	50 mg/kg every 8 hours[6]

Clindamycin and lincomycin

Clindamycin and lincomycin are structurally unrelated to the antibiotics discussed thus far, but these two drugs are very similar to each other:

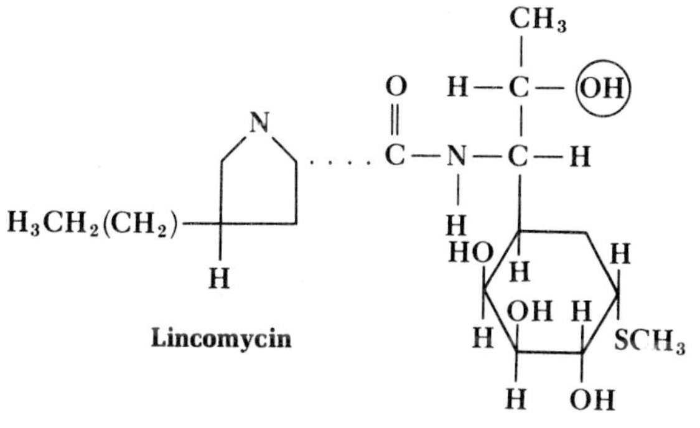

Lincomycin

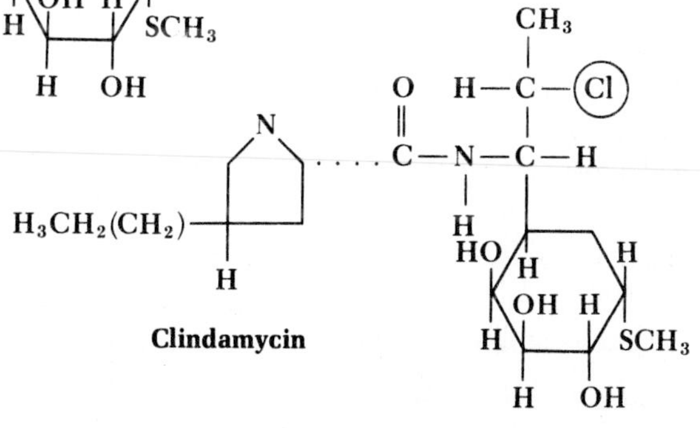

Clindamycin

Replacement of only lincomycin's hydroxyl group (circled) with a chlorine atom (circled) forms clindamycin. Although this minor change does not significantly affect the antimicrobial spectrum, it does substantially increase absorption, thereby decreasing the intestinal side effects associated with lincomycin. The only structural feature these drugs share with the aminoglycosides and some macrolide antibiotics is the presence of amino sugars.

Clindamycin and lincomycin are bacteriostatic. They are effective primarily against gram-positive organisms that are sensitive to erythromycin. Their mode of action is to interfere with cell wall integrity, presumably by inhibiting protein formation. The exact mode of protein inhibition appears to be interference with allignment of amino acids with specific codon units on mRNA.

Lincomycin was marketed first. Frequent and severe gastrointestinal disturbances, such as diarrhea and vomiting, related to significant changes in intestinal flora led to the development of clindamycin. Although it exhibits fewer of these symptoms, clindamycin is not devoid of such side effects. It is recommended that, like the use of lincomycin, the use of clindamycin in cats and horses be considered a last resort, because of reports of severe gastrointestinal disturbances related to lincomycin use in these animals.[9]

Naturally occurring resistance to clindamycin is being reported in certain strains of *Staphylococcus aureus*. In addition, some organisms that are resistant to lincomycin have shown cross-resistance to clindamycin. Clinically an increasing number of organisms that are resistant to erythromycin are also exhibiting insensitivity to clindamycin. It is recommended that clindamycin and erythromycin not be used concurrently, since the clinical effects of clindamycin appear to be reduced in the presence of erythromycin. This situation may be due to their competing for the same mRNA codon unit(s).

In view of the side effects associated with these drugs as compared to their potential benefits, conservative antibiotic use dictates that erythromycin be the first choice for organisms that are sensitive to these drugs. If the results are unsatisfactory, clindamycin and lincomycin (in that order) may be considered. They are both available in oral and parenteral dosage forms.

• • •

This review of antibiotics has centered on "traditional" drugs—in other words, drugs that have demonstrated significant clinical value over a number of years. As new antibiotics become available, their extent of use should be based on the advantages they exhibit as compared to the "traditionals," especially in terms of side effects, antibacterial spectrums, and propensity for the development of resistant microbes.

Side effects of antibiotic therapy

Any antibacterial drug that exhibits bacteriocidal activity as a result of cell wall disruption (for example, penicillins and cephalosporins) can be expected to demonstrate, or at least to have the potential for, acute blood toxicities. Biological reactions, structures, and chemicals responsible for cell wall formation in bacteria are similar to those needed for cell wall synthesis in blood cells. Antibacterials, such as antibiotics, that affect cell wall integrity cannot differentiate between pathogens and blood cells, and consequently their pharmacological actions are responsible for lysis of blood cells as well as pathogenic bacteria. Hematological side effects of cephalosporins and penicillins can include hemolytic anemia, mild and transient neutropenia, thrombocythemia or thrombocytopenia, and reversible leukopenia. In addition, in rare cases aplastic anemia and agranulocytosis have resulted from the use of some cephalosporins. The severity of these hematological effects is dose and drug related, and the effects usually disappear upon discontinuation of the drug.

With the exception of anaphylactic reactions, hematological side effects represent the most serious aspect of antibacterial therapy. They occur quicker and more often with antibiotics, since these drugs are more potent and act quicker than other antibacterials, such as the sulfonamides (discussed in the following section). In addition, adverse effects on the blood are more acute if an antibiotic is bacteriocidal in normal doses. Unlike bacteriostatic antibiotics, bacteriocidal antibiotics are specific antagonists of cell wall formation and integrity; hence the cell is destroyed quicker. Bacteriostatic antibiotics generally affect biological processes associated with mitosis and thus do not generally kill bacteria but prevent their multiplication, the rationale being that the host's defenses will ultimately destroy the pathogens if their numbers are kept from increasing. In most infections the number of pathogens is far less than the number of blood cells. Thus even if blood cells and bacteria are destroyed on a one-to-one basis, the pathogens will be obliterated long before the blood picture is significantly affected. Conversely, if the number of pathogens is inordinately high, indicating an advanced infectious condition at the time therapy is initiated, the ratio of blood cells to pathogens is smaller and more antibiotic will be required. This increases the potential for hematological side effects resulting from therapy.

The use of any anti-infective, especially antibiotics, should incorporate the following principles:

1. Anti-infective therapy should begin as soon as the need is evident (to inhibit pathogenic multiplication).
2. The choice of drug should be based on microbiological data whenever possible (to ensure that pathogens are susceptible to the drug).
3. The course of therapy should be long enough to ensure that the pathogenic count no longer poses a threat to the animal.

The correct choice of drug, based on laboratory findings, cannot be overemphasized. If a drug is being administered that does not have the proper spectrum, only the destruction of blood cells is occurring. The pathogens are not being adversely affected, and consequently when the correct drug is used, higher doses, which carry the possibility of greater side effects, may be required.

The third principle should not be interpreted so that the course of therapy is overextended. Administering an antibiotic after the possibility of infection has passed is analagous to administering the improper antibiotic. The potential for adverse side effects is increased. In addition, the normal bacterial flora of the gastrointestinal tract can be altered so that the class(es) of microorganisms resistant to the drug begin to dominate, with the result being an abnormal microbial overgrowth. This constitutes a pathological condition called "superinfection," which usually leads to excessive destruction of intestinal bacteria, with resultant overgrowth of endemic fungi. Quite often the superinfection can be more life threatening than the original infection.

A related condition that may occur because of improper use of antibiotics (that is, incorrect drug given or correct drug given for too long) is domination of a bacterial strain that is similar to the pathogen but resistant to the drug.

Development of diarrhea or abnormal stools during antibacterial therapy can be a signal that drug therapy should be reevaluated as to dosage and drug. Antibiotics, like other antibacterials, do not differentiate between beneficial and pathogenic bacteria, and as a result both are destroyed if they are susceptible to a drug. Significant destruction of normal bacterial flora in the intestinal tract alters the absorption process, with resultant changes in excretory habits and products. However, diarrhea or abnormal stools do not necessarily mean that a drug is having an adverse effect, since pathogens, by destroying normal flora, can produce a similar response.

Usually, drug-induced gastrointestinal changes will appear before significant blood disorders, and therefore a practioner should carefully review these symptoms with respect to therapy.

Like any major drug class, anti-infectives, and especially antibiotics, can also produce unanticipated, anaphylactic reactions. Fortunately, even though penicillins and cephalosporins have similar structures, if an animal is allergic to one of these drug classes there is less than a 5% chance that it will be allergic to the other.

Reports of skin toxicity (for example; pruritis, erythemias, nonspecific rashes) are not uncommon during antibiotic therapy. It is the responsibility of the practitioner to judge the degree of the dermatological response and then determine if symptomatic treatment is required. Such treatment may require only the application of a soothing cream or lotion or the administration of systemic drugs such as antihistamines and/or steroidal hormones. In many cases skin eruptions will diminish as therapy continues; however, a practitioner should be prepared to discontinue therapy with a particular drug as a result of debilitating skin problems.

In general, each antibacterial drug class is associated with an inordinately high number of particular side effects (for example, the sulfonamides' propensity to produce skin toxicities). In addition, it should always be remembered that each drug can exhibit not only side effects common to its class, but rare, idiosyncratic reactions peculiar to that drug. Only the most serious and/or more common side effects have been and will be discussed in this book. Specific product information, such as package inserts, should always be consulted for information about the potential side effects of individual drugs in any class.

SULFONAMIDES

The sulfonamides were the first antibacterial drugs to be used clinically in large patient populations; their use predated the extensive use of penicillin by approximately 7 years. The original sulfonamide, Prontosil, was initially used as a red dye in 1932. Unfortunately it was not until 1937 that investigators, in England, prepared a derivative of Prontosil called sulfapyridine and found it to be enormously successful in the treatment of pneumonia. Immediately afterward, a series of sulfonamides was synthesized. More than 3300 have been produced to date, but only a handful have proved clinically useful. The advent of antibiotics has been primarily responsible for the reduction in sulfonamide research and development.

All the clinically useful sulfonamides can be characterized by the general structure illustrated in Fig. 5-1, in which R is an organic group. The most active sulfonamides, such as sulfisoxazole, use cyclic structures as organic substitutions.[1] Although a few sulfonamides have organic groups on one of the two hydrogen atoms attached to N, it appears that two hydrogen atoms are needed for maximal effectiveness.[5] The following profile of selected sulfonamide antibacterials on p. 148 illustrates the conformity in the basic sulfonamide nucleus for many of these drugs as well as the consistency in their nomenclature.

The darker portion in the structural formulas of these drugs represents the sulfonamide core, which is responsible for the antimicrobial effect. The antimicrobial effect is maximized and absorption from the gastrointestinal tract enhanced if the para nitrogen atom (arrow) has two hydrogen atoms attached to it rather than an organic portion. As would be expected because of its structure, salicylazosulfapyridine is not appreciably absorbed from the gastrointestinal tract and therefore is used for intestinal pathogens.

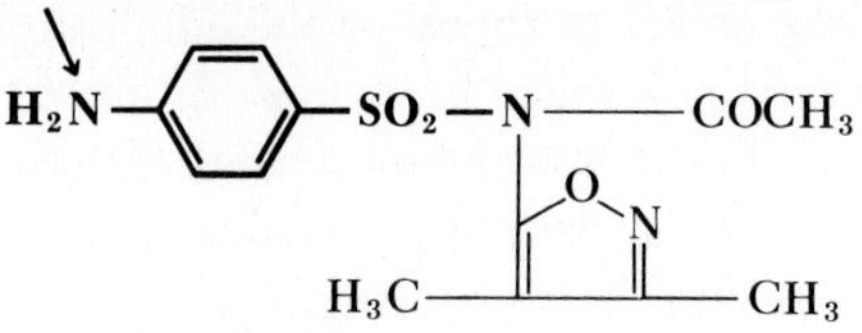

$$H_2N - \bigcirc - SO_2 - N - COCH_3$$

Acetylsulfisoxazole

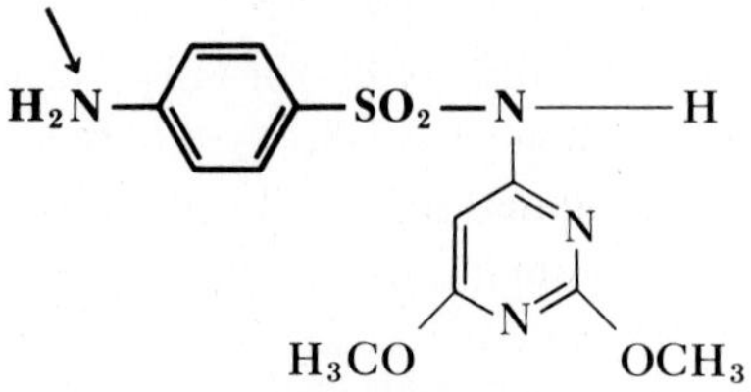

$$H_2N - \bigcirc - SO_2 - N - H$$

Sulfadimethoxine

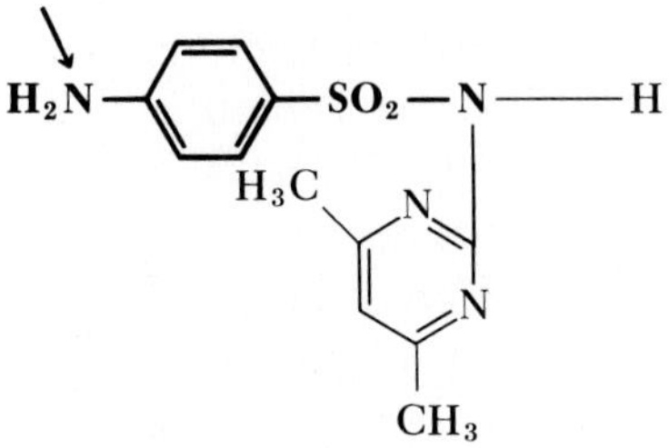

$$H_2N - \bigcirc - SO_2 - N - H$$

Sulfamethazine

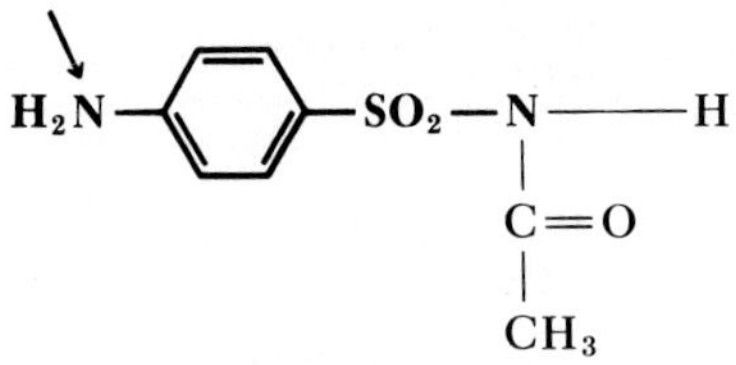

$$H_2N - \bigcirc - SO_2 - N - H$$

$$C = O$$

$$CH_3$$

Sulfacetamide

$$HO - \bigcirc - N = N - \bigcirc - SO_2 - N - H$$

$$COOH$$

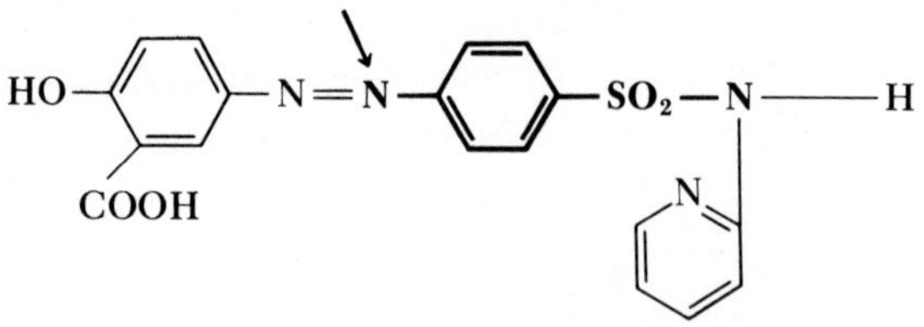

Salicylazosulfapyridine

Pharmacological activity

One way to classify bacteria is to separate those that make their own folic acid from those that must receive it from outside (dietary) sources. Folic acid, an essential nutrient required for most complex and simple life forms is formed as a result of the combination of three distinct organic molecules: (1) Glutamic acid is combined with (2) a dihydropteridine derivative to form dihydropteroic acid. This combines with (3) *p*-aminobenzoic acid (PABA) to form folic acid.

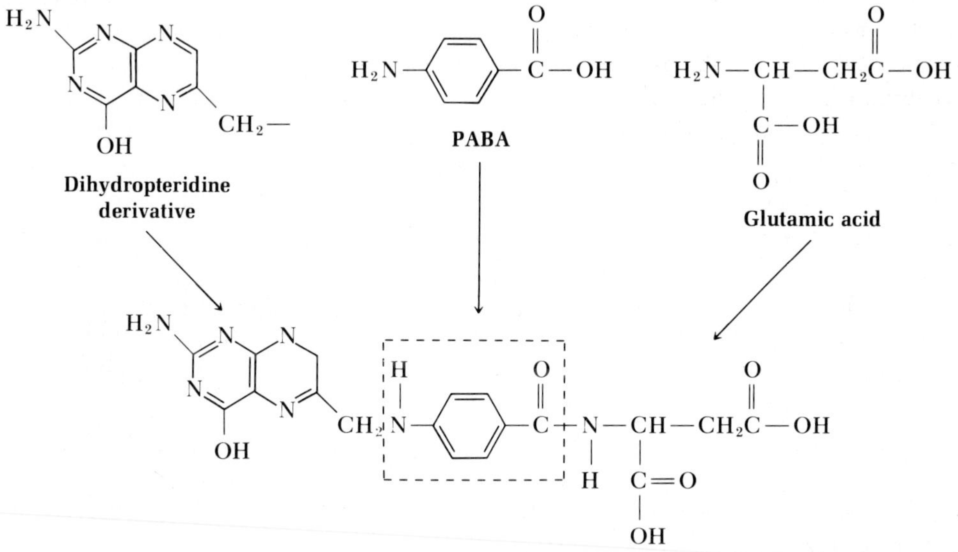

Dihydropteridine derivative

PABA

Glutamic acid

Folic acid

PABA is structually similar to the sulfonamide core, and thus the sulfonamide drugs competitively inhibit PABA from being incorporated into the folic acid molecule. The theory of competitive inhibition by the sulfa drugs is clinically subtantiated, since increasing the concentration of sulfa drugs increase their effect.

The most generally accepted theory about the action of sulfonamides is that these drugs, because of their structural similarity to PABA, compete with it in binding to dihydropteric acid. Attachment of a sulfonamide to dihydropteroic acid stops the formation of folic acid and inhibits cellular functions that depend upon it. In addition, it seems likely that sulfonamides compete with PABA in any other biological mechanism in which PABA is required. Because these drugs' mode of action involves competition in the synthesis of folic acid, *sulfonamides are effective only in microbes that are capable of manufacturing folic acid*. They are not effective in microbes that receive it from exogenous sources.

Antibacterial spectrum and resistance

Since only organisms that must make their own folic acid are sensitive to sulfon-amides, microbes that are able to use preformed folic acid or that do not require this metabolite are not adversely affected by these drugs. Because folic acid inhibition affects cellular reproductive and growth activities rather than causing immediate destruction of the microbe, sulfonamide activity is generally considered bacteriostatic rather than bacteriocidal. The spectrum of their antibacterial action is wide, including many gram-positive and gram-negative bacteria.[9] Sulfonamides are not effective against viruses, fungi, or rickettsiae.

Resistance to sulfonamides is already clinically significant. In an attempt to minimize the development of bacterial resistance and to achieve desired clinical effects, sulfonamides have been used in conjunction with certain antibiotics. In order for these combinations to be effective, the microbes must be sensitive to both drugs. Relatively few such combinations have proved consistently useful. The most notable successes have been the combination of streptomycin and a sulfonamide, for treatment of influenzal meninigitis and brucellosis, and the combination of penicillin and a sulfonamide, for treatment of bacterial endocarditis. It should be emphasized that such combination drug therapy should be initiated after the use of the individual drugs has proved unsatisfactory.

Pharmacokinetics and side effects

Sulfonamides can be administered orally, parenterally, or topically; the latter route is most often used for ophthalmic preparations. The only sulfonamides that show significant activity in the eye are sulfisoxazole and sulfacetamide. The latter drug is available as a 10% ophthalmic ointment and in 10% and 30% ophthalmic solutions. The 30% solution is unquestionably more irritating to the eye, and it is doubtful whether it is significantly more effective than the 10% solution. As is true in regard to other ophthalmics, best results are most often obtained by using the ointment rather than a solution.

Orally administered sulfonamides can be classified as "systemically effective" (absorbed well from the gastrointestinal tract) and "gut active" (not absorbed well from the gastrointestinal tract). In small, single-chambered-stomach animals, up to 90% of a dose of a systemic sulfonamide is absorbed from the gastrointestinal tract. As would be expected, absorption in ruminants is not as predictable, and attainment of therapeutic blood levels requires a longer time.

Sulfonamides have relatively high partition coefficients and consequently are highly bound to plasma; with some sulfonamides, up to 95% of an administered dose will be bound. Only free, unbound sulfonamide has antibacterial action. It has been theorized that only after plasma binding sites have been occupied does a sulfonamide begin to concentrate in the aqueous portion of blood in therapeutic amounts. Once in the aqueous portion of blood, sulfonamides are distributed rather extensively into most fluids and tissues. Sulfonamides whose partition coefficients are high enough cross the blood-brain barrier and reach therapeutic concentrations in cerebrospinal fluid. Most sulfonamides readily pass placental barriers, and most are partially excreted in milk.

Once therapeutic blood levels are reached, oral doses every 8 hours in animals with single-chambered stomachs and every 12 hours in mature ruminants are sufficient to maintain these levels.[2]

Sulfonamide detoxification occurs in the liver and involves conjugation with glucuronic acid and/or the addition of an acetyl group ($-CH_2COOH$) to the para nitrogen atom in place of one of the hydrogen atoms.

Increasing the pH of the urine (alkalinization) increases solubility of free sulfonamide and its acetyl metabolites, thereby enhancing their excretion. Accumulation of free sulfonamide or its acetyl metabolites in the kidney may result in a condition known as crystalluria, which will be discussed shortly. In order to prevent crystalluria in carnivores, it is advisable to alkalinize the urine. This can be done by administering sodium bicarbonate, sodium citrate, or sodium acetate; the last chemical is the most preferred, since it produces the longest-lasting effect. The urine of herbivores is normally on the alkaline side, and further alkalinization is not normally necessary.

Crystalluria has been reported in animals but is more prevalent in humans, since the latter produce a greater percentage of acetylated sulfonamide metabolites (which are less soluble than the glucuronide conjugates) than most animals. Since sulfonamides and their detoxification products have low water solubilities, they can precipitate, forming needle-like crystals in the urine (crystalluria). If this precipate occurs in kidney tubules, these crystals can puncture the lumens, causing proteinuria, hematuria, oliguria, and very possibly kidney failure. To prevent crystalluria, the following measures are advisable:

1. *Alkalinize the urine of carnivores* (which enhances the solubility of sulfonamides and their biological derivatives).
2. *Give large amounts of neutral or nonacidic fluids—preferably water* (provides more urine volume to aid sulfonamide solubility).
3. *Do not exceed recommended dosages for the particular drug.*

Side effects that are more common than crystalluria include skin rashes and blood dyscrasias. Dyscrasias are linked to the general inhibition of folic acid formation, since folic acid plays a role in the formation of blood elements. It should be realized that sulfonamides inhibit folic acid synthesis in the animal as well as in the pathogen.

Side effects associated with long-term sulfonamide administration in ruminants include dehydration as a result of prolonged diarrhea, direct irritation of the gastrointestinal tract, and digestive disturbances resulting from the destruction of intestinal bacteria.

Toxicity in poultry is demonstrated by decreased egg yield and a thinning of the shell.

Acute toxicities can occur after injection; in cattle they include pupil dilation, muscle weakness, and uncoordination. Dogs also exhibit the ocular side effect, as well as uncontrolled running movements, nausea, and, rarely, convulsions (after large parenteral or oral doses).[9]

Most side effects that result from large doses or long-term therapy gradually subside once the drug is discontinued.[2]

Principles of therapy

In view of the pharmacological and pharmacokinetic properties of sulfonamides, the following principles regarding their use have proved beneficial:

1. If a sulfonamide is indicated, begin administration as early in the course of the disease as possible. As the infection progresses, pathogens proliferate and the ability of the drugs to compete with PABA decreases.
2. Administer plenty of water to all animals, and use urinary alkalinizers for carnivores.
3. Discontinue drug administration in the presence of proteinuria, hematuria, or any other sign of abnormal renal function.
4. Reevaluate the appropriateness of sulfonamide therapy if clinical results are not apparent within 3 days.
5. Do not continue therapy for more than 8 consecutive days without evaluating clinical benefits and side effects. This reduces the possibility that resistant bacterial strains will develop. It also minimizes side effects associated with decreased vitamin production by normal intestinal bacteria (especially in herbivores) because of their being inhibited by the sulfonamide.
6. Continue therapy for approximately 48 hours after the disappearance of clinical symptoms. This helps to prevent reemergence of the infection.
7. Give larger doses initially, to reach therapeutic blood levels, followed by regularly repeated smaller doses.[2]

Indications for use

Generally, antibiotics are preferred over sulfonamides because of the reduced potential for side effects. However, if antibiotic therapy has proved unsuccessful or is not indicated, sulfonamides are sometimes effective as second-line drugs for such conditions as strangles, pasteurellosis, foot rot in cattle, pneumonia, metritis, and urinary tract infections.

Because of their tendency to cause skin rashes, sulfonamides are not the drugs of choice for topical application to wounds. In addition, adeqate documentation exists to show that their physical presence may actually retard the healing process.

• • •

The advent of sulfonamides and the subsequent introduction of antibiotics has overwhelmed practioners with chemical means to combat infectious diseases. Many pathological conditions that previously were fatal are now regarded as minor or nuisance infections. The steady emergence of resistant organisms, however, must serve as a warning that carelessness in the nondrug management of infections cannot be compensated for by drugs. The realization that microbes are becoming increasingly resistant to even our mightiest antibacterials has already fostered a search for new drugs. It should also foster renewed interest in and concern for aseptic procedure and proper nondrug management of infectious diseases.

Anthelmintics

Originally the term "anthelmintic" was reserved for drugs that were intended to act against parasites of the intestinal tract, but the term has been expanded to include drugs used to eradicate parasites from blood and tissue as well.

Treatment for parasites presents problems that are not encountered with simpler organisms, such as bacteria or fungi. In most cases parasites are sophisticated, complex animals that are resistant to most of the anti-infective drugs thus far considered.

In order to be maximally effective and minimally-toxic to the host, an anthelmintic should reach only the area where the infestation resides. Drugs used for intestinal parasites, such as tapeworms, flukes, and roundworms, can be formulated to have low partition coefficients, to be ionized in the gastrointestinal tract, and to be refractory to enzymatic activity designed to promote absorption. All these characteristics prevent drug absorption from the gastrointestinal tract.

Relatively potent drugs can be used when the parasite is confined to the gastrointestinal tract. Most anthelmintics are innately irritating to the gastrointestinal tract, and thus nausea, vomiting, and loss of appetite are common symptoms associated with anthelmintic administration. However, the drug should not be more toxic to the mucous membrane lining the gastrointestinal tract than it is to the parasite, or even equally toxic. Excessive irritation of the tract wall can result in overt amounts of the drug migrating from the tract into the bloodstream. If abundant amounts of a drug not intended for systemic circulation enter the bloodstream, most certainly toxicities and possibly death will result, especially if the drug is slowly detoxified or not detoxified at all.

Treatment of systemic parasites such as heartworms requires a drug that is effective but not overly damaging to internal organs or to blood. This has led to use of new drugs that are more toxic to the parasite than the host. It cannot be assumed, however, that these drugs are totally innocuous to the host. Drugs such as dichlorvos are organophosphate derivatives, and the main reason an animal is not overtly affected is its greater mass as compared to the parasite. Thus, large doses of systemic anthelmintics should be avoided to protect the host. Therapy for infected animals has centered on small doses given for long periods of time. In addition, the importance of prophylactic therapy, which requires doses smaller than those used therapeutically, has been stressed. As is true of any drug, the most desirable anthelmintic is the one that has the highest therapeutic index.

The screening of potentially useful anthelmintics poses problems that are not encountered with other anti-infectives. The wide variations between species of helminths, their behavior in the host, symbiotic associations between the host and parasite, and the susceptibility of the host to the parasite and the drug are all difficult to simulate in vitro.

This has been only a short introduction to anthelmintics; before any particular drug is administered, books that deal exclusively with parasitic infections and their treatment should be consulted and product information should be carefully read.

IMMUNOLOGICALS (BIOLOGICALS)

Products derived from living entities and used to immunize animals are traditionally categorized as "biologicals."[9] However, since the term "immunologicals" more accurately describes the action of these products, this term will be used in this discussion. Like some antibiotics, immunologicals can be natural by-products or derivatives of natural by-products. Consequently these products can contain living, modified, or killed organisms. A significant distinction between the previously discussed drugs (as well as those described in later chapters) and immunologicals is the manner in which the desired biological response is achieved. Immunologicals most often stimulate biological systems to produce the therapeutic substances (antibodies) that destroy the invading material (antigen). "Drugs" are the therapeutic substances themselves. The distinction between immunologicals and drugs is not always this clear cut, since immunological products containing antibodies can be considered to be the therapeutic chemicals.

History of immunological practices

Immunologicals are used in veterinary practice to render an animal resistant, or relatively resistant, to an abnormal condition—namely, a disease. This process is referred to as "conferring immunity" on the animal. The word "immunity" is derived from the Latin "immunus," meaning "safe."

For centuries people realized that an infectious disease could sometimes be prevented by exposing healthy individuals to persons that had survived a course of the disease. During the seventeenth century the intelligentsia of Europe sometimes followed the practice of briefly mingling with people who were alleged to have had smallpox and lived. The Chinese carried this concept one step farther by powdering the scabs of smallpox victims and inhaling them. Africans rubbed the exudate from smallpox pustules into surgical wounds in healthy individuals. All these measures represented crude attempts at conferring immunity by "vaccination." Although now commonly done by injection, vaccination can also include introduction of a substance by inhalation or by any other means that places it on an absorbing tissue.

The success of these early attempts was sporadic, owing to the fact that there was no way of accurately determining how much of the pathogenic substance (antigen) was being introduced to the body. If the amount was less than that needed to cause a clinical infection, chances were good that the person would not suffer the full effects of the disease and would become immunized. Conversely, greater amounts of the antigen could result in a normal disease process. Continued research into the phenomenon of the immune response has resulted in standardized vaccines and efficient vaccination procedures.

The immune response

A greater understanding of the immune response has been responsible for the advent of more reliable vaccines. As insight continued to develop, it was realized that a terminology for immune-related processes and resultant medications was needed. As the immune response is reviewed here, the terms involved will be explained to a degree consistent with the introductory nature of this discussion.

The discussions of antibiotics and sulfonamides centered on drugs used to kill or inhibit the growth of pathogenic microbes. Although the infections caused by these organisms can represent life-threatening situations, treatment with antibiotics or sulfonamides does not cause an animal to develop any lasting mechanism to protect itself from future infections of the same organism. Consequently bacteria, fungi, or viruses could reinfect animals an indefinite number of times. Certain microbes and/or the toxins they produce (endotoxins), however, can stimulate hosts to synthesize substances (antibodies) that destroy the pathogenic agents and create a mechanism that offers more protection to the animal against these specific agents than it had prior to its exposure to them. Such microbes or endotoxins are called "antigens," and the mechanism that kills or neutralizes the antigens is called the "immune response."

Although the term "antigen" is usually associated with infectious agents, it also is used to describe substances that can elicit an *idiosyncratic, noninfectious* response in an *individual* animal. Clinically such antigens are referred to as "allergens." Allergens can include such diverse substances as pollen, food, house dust, animal dander, and drugs; they will be discussed more fully in the discussions of steroids and antihistamines, in Chapter 6. Antigens are usually high-molecular-weight substances that contain nitrogen. Most noninfectious antigens are proteins that are not found in an animal's body and thus represent foreign substances.

Once an antigen penetrates an animal's natural defenses and gains access to the blood, it is "recognized" as an antigenic substance, probably by specific blood elements. The exact mode of the recognition process is unclear; however, it is evident that the precise structural configuration and chemical composition of the antigen are determined. Identification of the antigen leads to synthesis of "antibodies," which are modified, high-molecular-weight proteins. Specific antibodies are formed for each antigen although some overlapping of antibody coverage is not uncommon. That is, the same antibody can be effective against more than one antigen. Synthesis of antibodies occurs primarily in lymph tissue, while antibodies are transported primarily in the globulin portion of plasma.

The first synthesis of an antibody specific to an antigen requires a longer period of time than subsequent production of the same antibody, because recognition of the antigen and development of a DNA-mediated code for formation of the antibody must first occur. Therapeutic amounts of antibodies do not circulate in the blood for the life of an animal; however, the code for making specific antibodies is retained, possibly in the lymph cells. Thus the first exposure to an infectious antigen usually results in the animal contracting the full effects of the disease, presum-

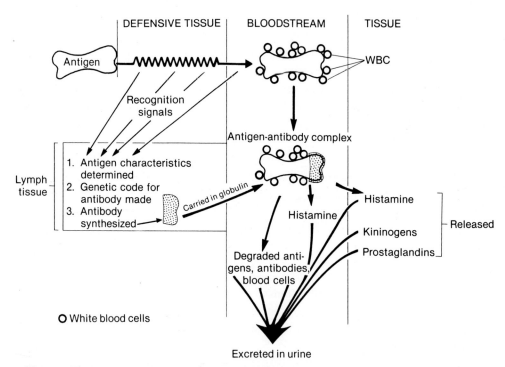

Fig. 5-5. The immune response. After an animal's first exposure to an antigen, identification of the antigen and the initial formation of antibodies require a certain amount of time, hence clinical symptoms of the disease become apparent. However, once the genetic code for synthesizing the specific antibody has been "set," repeated exposure to the antigen usually results in the rapid production of antibody blood levels. Consequently little or no clinical effect of the disease is apparent.

ably because the microbe has enough time to multiply while the recognition and antibody production processes are occurring. The first exposure to the antigen forms the lasting code for its production. Subsequent exposures of the animal to the antigen result in rapid antibody formation, since the code for its formation is remembered. This usally destroys the infectious antigen before it can cause clinical symptoms of the disease.

It is important not to confuse the terms "antibody" and "antibiotic." As just explained, antibodies are produced by an individual animal in response to invasion by an antigen. An antibody is a proteinaceous substance that is usually specific for an antigen and that interacts with it to cause its destruction or neutralization. Antibiotics are produced by microbes and do not have the degree of specificity for particular substances that antibodies do. In addition, antibiotics are not effective against toxins as are some antibodies.

Destruction of an antigen by an antibody seems to be as much a surface phenomenon as it is an internal chemical reaction between antibody and antigen. Apparently the antigen is first identified by the antibody as a result of cell wall "indicators." These same indicators may also serve as receptor areas for the antibody to attach onto the antigen, thereby forming an "antibody-antigen complex." After the antigen is engulfed by antibodies, chemical reactions that probably involve cell wall disruption and inhibition of biological functions (in living antigens) occur to eventually kill or neutralize the antigen. The aftermath of the battle between antigens and antibodies results in remnants of the antibodies and antigens circulating in the blood and finally being excreted in the urine. A more significant consequence of this complex struggle (which will be examined more closely in Chapter 6) is the release of histamine, kininogens, and prostaglandins.

The immune response (which is summarized in Fig. 5-5) results in the animal receiving "active immunity" to a particular disease caused by an infectious antigen. As the name implies, this type of immunity is a result of an active, in vivo process, which results in the formation of antibodies and a code for their more efficient production in the future. Active immunity results in lasting protection for the animal—not always, however, for a lifetime.

Classification of immunologicals

Immunologicals can be clasified according to the type of immunity they confer. Those that are composed of antigenic substances (that is, fully virulent microbes, attenuated microbes, killed microbes, or toxoids) confer active immunity, since they stimulate the immune response. Other immunologicals contain antibodies that were formed by animals exposed to antigens. These preparations confer *passive immunity*, which is temporary and only designed to protect an animal that has been exposed to the fully virulent disease and that is displaying or may display, its clinical symptoms. For life-threatening diseases there is no time to wait for the animal's immune system to produce antibodies, which usually requires 10 to 14 days, or more, after the first exposure. Thus antibodies specific to the disease are injected in an attempt to kill or neutralize the antigen.

Products for active immunization

After determining what provokes active immunity, researchers developed pharmaceuticals that mimic the in vivo activity of antigens. The word "vaccine" was used to describe only the first inoculum of cowpox virus, which was used to prevent smallpox in humans. Over time, however, the term "vaccine" has come to describe any preparation that is capable of producing active immunity. Active immunity can be conferred by four types of immunologicals:

1. Preparations containing the fully virulent organisms but in low enough concentration (subclinical amounts) that the recommended dose will not contain enough organisms to elicit the full effect of the disease but will initiate the immune reaction.

2. Preparations containing "attenuated" (also referred to as "modified live") organisms. Attenuation is a process by which the virulence of organisms is reduced to the point that they do not usually produce full clinical symptoms but do cause the immune response to occur. Attenuation can be accomplished by (a) exposing the organism to temperatures (high or low) that are not suitable to its survival, (b) drying it, (c) altering the nutrients in its growing media, or (d) subjecting it to "serial passages." This last procedure involves injecting organisms into an animal, allowing them to multiply for a while, and then transferring the progeny to another animal, and so on. The greater the number of transfers, the more attenuated (less virulent) the organism becomes. Another method used to attenuate organisms is to grow them in artificial media. Oftentimes kidney tissue is used, since it represents foreign media to most antigens. Invasion routes for many antigens do not involve kidney contact, and therefore they do not develop maximum virulence when forced to survive on kidney tissue. Thus they become attenuated.[9] Usually the method used to attenuate an antigen will be noted on the label of the immunological product (for example, "Rabies vaccine—tissue culture origin").

3. Preparations containing killed organisms. Although the bacterium or virus is killed, it still contains antigens that can induce the immune response. Usually bacteria are killed by excessive heat or by being exposed to antibacterial chemicals such as phenol.

4. Preparations containing toxins that have been modified to reduce their virulence. These products are more correctly referred to as "toxoids" rather than as vaccines.

As was previously mentioned, the term "vaccine" was originally used to refer only to the material used for immunizing against smallpox. However, its meaning has been extended to include all antigenic materials made from viruses, bacteria, and rickettsiae. Another point of confusion can occur with respect to the difference between vaccines and antigens. The term "antigen" is used to describe all antigenic substances, including vaccines. Thus all vaccines are antigens, but not all antigens are vaccines.

Immunologicals made from bacteria can be classified according to whether or not the whole bacterium is present. When the entire bacterium is present, *in suspension,* regardless of whether it is attenuated or killed, the immunological should be classified as a *bacterial vaccine*. When only the *soluble* antigenic material derived from the bacteria is present, the product should be classified as a *bacterial antigen*.

Bacterial vaccines are divided into two major classes according to source:

1. Stock vaccines, which are the more commonly used of the two classes, are made from cultures retained by pharmaceutical manufacturers.
2. *Autogenous vaccines* are prepared from an animal's own infection. The antigen obtained from the blood or any lesions that may result from the disease is used to prepare the vaccine, which is then injected into the animal. Autogenous vaccines are usually used only when an animal shows sensitivity to stock vaccines because of the tissue they were prepared from or when the vaccine specific to an antigen is not available commercially.

Further classification of bacterial vaccines involves how many strains or species of microorganisms are present in a product. A *monovalent* bacterial vaccine is made from a single species, while a *polyvalent* vaccine contains more than one species of bacteria.

In addition, bacterial vaccines can be classified according to on how the antigenic material is treated. As was mentioned earlier, organisms can induce immunity if they are injected as (1) fully virulent but in subclinical concentrations, (2) attenuated, or (3) killed. Consequently we can subdivide monovalent or polyvalent, stock or autogenous bacterial vaccines in terms of how their antigenic material is presented into the animal—fully virulent, attenuated, or killed. The term "bacterin" is used to describe a monovalent or polyvalent vaccine that is composed of killed bacteria as opposed to fully virulent or attenuated bacteria.

Fig. 5-6 summarizes my paricular method of categorizing bacterial immunologicals that are capable of producing active immunity.

Antigens also include exotoxins produced by some pathogenic bacteia. In some instances it is these toxins, rather than the organisms themselves, that cause symptoms of the disease as in the case of tetanus. The soluble toxins are not used as such but are converted into toxoids, which are materials that result from treating toxins with chemicals, such as formaldehyde, and incubating them at 40° C for periods of a month or longer. To produce maximum effectiveness, these soluble toxins are then precipitated or absorbed from solution by being mixed with aluminum salts. When injected as a relatively insoluble aluminum precipitate, the toxoid persists for extended periods before becoming absorbed. This allows a gradual and prolonged release of modified toxin (toxoid) into the animal, thereby lessening the chances that the full effects of the disase will occur. The result is that the toxoid, like a vaccine, can induce the immune response but cause few, if any, clinical signs of the disease. Unlike the situation in regard to vaccines, it is uncommon to use toxoid preparations containing more than one modified toxin.

Vaccines and toxoids are intended for administration to healthy animals to prevent them from contracting specific diseases. It is imperative to ensure that an animal does not have a chance to contract the disease it is being vaccinated against before its antibody titer has increased to a prophylactic concentration as a result of the inoculation. Immunity normally requires 10 to14 days to develop, but in some cases it may be several weeks before full immunity is reached.[2] In addition, if the animal has the disease at the time of vaccination, it will suffer an exaggerated re-

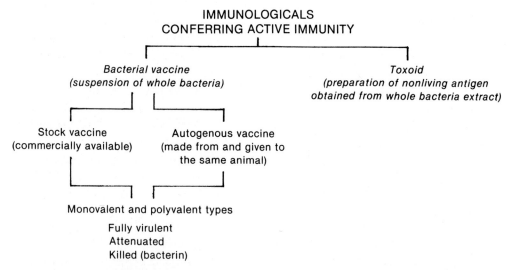

Fig. 5-6. Classification of immunologicals that confer active immunity. Immunologicals conferring active immunity are divided into two major groups those that immunize animals against living organisms and those that immunize animals against toxins. Vaccines are used for immunization against living organisms, while toxoids stimulate in vivo production of antibodies used to destroy toxins. Autogenous vaccines are rarely used, since the need for them seldom justifies the expense of production.

sponse, especially if a fully virulent type of immunological is used. It is important to remember that "vaccines" and "toxoids" are used to confer protection upon healthy animals and not to treat an existing or imminent antigen invasion.

Products for passive immunization

After their production, antibodies circulate in the proteins of the globulin fraction of blood serum. The aqueous portion of blood (in which blood cells and platelets are suspended) is practically devoid of antibodies. Because antibodies are localized in a specific portion of serum, high degrees of purification and concentration are possible when they are extracted to make commercial immunological products.

Antibodies that are to be used therapeutically are usually produced by active immunization of an animal—usually a horse or rabbit, since sensitivity reactions to their proteins by other animals are not common. After collection the serum is processed so that the antibody-containing portion is separated from as many other proteins as possible, to reduce the chance of sensitivity reactions in recipient animals. However, since antibodies are proteins themselves, they can act as noninfectious antigens in other animals. Reactions to foreign antibodies can range from mild, transient skin rashes to anaphylactic shock. If a practitioner believes they are warranted, certain skin and ophthalmic tests can be done to identify animals that will respond adversely to the serum. Unfortunately these tests are neither infallible nor always definitive.

The processed serum, properly assayed, represents a standardized amount of antibodies that can be injected into an animal to temporarily protect it (confer passive immunity) against specific antigens, whether they are living or not. The term "antibody" pertains to a wide variety of substances that are antagonistic to, or capable of neutralizing, the antigens responsible for their production. There are numerous types of antibodies, their classification being based on how they interact with antigens. Clinically, however, antibodies are classified as either antibacterial (or antiviral) or antitoxic. A product that kills living, infectious antigens is known as an "antiserum" or an "immune serum." A preparation that neutralizes nonliving antigens (toxins) produced by microorganisms is called an "antitoxin." The use of antisera or antitoxins should be reserved for animals that are expected to develop a disease within a short period of time (less than 10 days) or for those already demonstrating symptoms of a disease. The purpose of these products is to provide enough antibodies so that the antigenic agent will be destroyed before the full effects of the disease are realized. Protection is transient, usually lasting 10 to 14 days. If prolonged protection is desired, the animal should be administered a vaccine or a toxoid after symptoms of the disease or the possibility of its having contracted the disease have passed.

•   •   •

It is especially important that all persons who are called upon to dispense or administer immunologicals have an absolute understanding of the nomenclature used to describe these products. The terms presented here represent a workable baseline, but product information should always be read, since other, sometimes company-specific, wording can be used to describe the activity of a pharmaceutical. The doses of active or passive immunologicals are often expressed in units of activity rather than in terms of absolute weight (such as grams or milligrams). This is necessary because these agents are essentially impure drugs (they contain other proteins besides the antibodies or antigens) that are obtained from various animal sources. Doses are standardized by determining the magnitude of the biological response that results from a particular dose and comparing it to a standard. For example, the standard for a particular vaccine could be expressed in terms of the antibody titer produced in a particular strain of animal. Different batches of this vaccine would be diluted or concentrated until the same administered volume as the standard produced comparable antibody levels in the same animal strain. This comparison of dose to biological response is called a "bioassay" (short for "biological assay") because a live animal instead of laboratory instruments is used as the end-point indicator.

Obviously, standardization of the doses of a pharmaceutical is essential to the production of adequate immunity, but other factors must also be considered. Proper storage is required to maintain the potency of an immunological. Most immunologicals require refrigeration. Exposure to room conditions could destroy the antigens or antibodies to the extent that immunity would not be achieved. Proper doses are mandatory. Because doses are based on eliciting biological responses, it is commonplace to use the same volume of a product for large and small animals of the same species, if they are mature. Since most immunologicals are administered by injection, proper aseptic technique must be followed so that an animal's condition is not further compromised by introduction of other pathogens. Furthermore, if an animal demonstrates symptoms of infection, which, unknown to the practitioner, are a result of the administration technique, they could be interpreted as being caused by the immunological agent.

REFERENCES

1. American Society of Hospital Pharmacists: Hospital formulary, vol 1, 8:12:02, 8:12:12, 8:12:16, Washington, D.C., 1980, The Society.
2. Brander, G.C., and Pugh, D.M.: Veterinary applied pharmacology and therapeutics, Oradell, 1972, Medical Economics Book Division, Inc.
3. Chambon, P.: Split genes, Sci. Am., **244:**60-71, May 1981.
4. Garand, R.A.: Ototoxicity and nephrotoxicity associated with aminoglycosides, seminar paper toward master's degree in pharmacy, Boston, 1978, Northeastern University.
5. Goldstein, A., Aronow, L., and Kalman, S.M.: Principles of drug action, New York, 1968, Harper & Row, Publishers, Inc.
6. Goodman, L.S., and Gilman, A.: The pharmacological basis of therapeutics, ed. 3, New York, 1968, Macmillan, Inc.
7. Kirk, R.W.: Current veterinary therapy, Philadelphia, 1980, W.B. Saunders Co., vol. 7, Small animal practice.
8. Krantz, J.C., and Carr, C.J.: Pharmacologic principles of medical practice, ed. 6, Baltimore, 1965, The Williams & Wilkins Co.
9. Spinelli, J.S., and Enos, L.R.: Drugs in veterinary practice, St. Louis, 1978, The C.V. Mosby Co.

6

Anti-inflammatory drugs

PERFORMANCE OBJECTIVES

After completion of this chapter the student will:

- Define the inflammatory response
- List and distinguish between the different types of trauma in terms of how they cause the inflammatory response
- Differentiate between the pharmacological effects of epinephrine and the glucocorticosteroids with respect to the inflammatory response
- List four major differences between mineralosteroidal and glucosteroidal activity
- List four dosage concepts relevant to the administraton of glucocorticosteroids
- Name the three most potent glucocorticosteroids
- List two major differences between glucocorticosteroids and nonsteroidal anti-inflammatory drugs in terms of how they combat inflammatory reactions
- Differentiate between the pharmacological actions of antihistamines, glucocorticosteroids, and nonsteroidal anti-inflammatory drugs with respect to suppression of inflammatory processes

TRAUMA AND THE INFLAMMATORY RESPONSE

As their name suggests, anti-inflammatory drugs are used to reverse or inhibit the "inflammatory response." The inflammatory response is the name given to a series of biological reactions that occur in response to a traumatic episode in an animal's body. Before the anti-inflammatory drugs are discussed, it would be helpful to review the types of trauma and the types of inflammatory responses that occur as a result of them.

Essentially there are two types of trauma—nonimmunological and immunological. Nonimmunological trauma results in tissue destruction largely because of physical contact between tissue and the insulting agent. An example of such trauma would be a surgical incision or an injury that causes immediate, oftentimes localized, destruction of tissue. Immunological trauma is chemically mediated; it can result from either exogenous or endogenous chemicals (chemicals that arise from outside the body or chemicals produced by the body, respectively). Chemicals that are responsible for immunological trauma are usually referred to as "toxins," "antigens," or "allergens." Immunological trauma is not always an acute episode; many times such trauma represents a chronic pathological condition, such as arthritis. The response to an acute immunological traumatic episode is called an "anaphylactic reaction"; such a reaction can be caused by a variety of chemicals, ranging from bee venom to penicillin. Fig. 6-1 outlines the types of trauma and gives specific examples of each type.

The inflammatory response is a fundamental pathological process that occurs as a result of an injury or abnormal stimulation caused by a physical, chemical, or

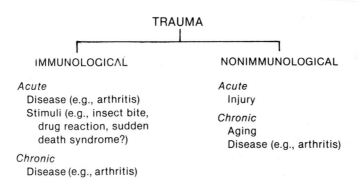

Fig. 6-1. Types of trauma. Trauma can be defined as any injurious episode. If the episode involves activation of the immunological system, the trauma is said to be immunologically mediated. Most sudden trauma experienced by animals is a result of physical injury such as a wound. This type of trauma is classified as nonimmunological trauma. In its broadest interpretation, nonimmunological trauma can include the aging process. Diseases such as arthritis can be classified as either immunological or nonimmunological, depending on their origins.

biological agent. The process involves numerous and complex biological reactions, which can occur in blood as well as tissue. Although the inflammatory process is considered a pathological reaction, it is nature's way of combatting cellular destruction arising from traumatic insults. Cellular destruction arising from nonimmunological trauma is usually immediate and does not progress significantly over time. The inflammatory response to nonimmunological trauma therefore is usually limited to localized reactions that aid in the repair and healing of tissue. Immunological trauma, however, because it can involve many organ systems, can evoke an exaggerated, systemic inflammatory reaction, which affects an animal's entire body.

In both types of trauma, clinical manifestations of the inflammatory response consist of *redness and warmth* and *swelling and pain*. The redness and warmth (localized or systemic) are due to excessive blood being shunted to the affected areas. Damage to tissue causes many endogenous substances to be released from cells. Two of these substances are leukotaxine and necrosin. Leukotaxine attracts blood elements (for example, polymorphonuclear neutrophils) from the bloodstream into the affected area. Necrosin increases the permeability of capillaries in the inflamed area, thus allowing fluid, protein, and white blood cells easy access to the damaged tissue. These blood elements aid in removing organic debris, such as dead tissue, and injurious material (such as toxins) from the area. In addition, white blood cells may be instrumental in neutralizing or killing the causative agent. Necrosin also activates any fibrinogen in fluid leaked from cells, causing it to clot much as blood does. Clotting of leaked cellular fluid prevents the flow of injurious material from damaged tissue sites into surrounding areas, thereby walling off the inflamed tissue from surrounding tissue. This isolation of damaged tissue is especially important if the causative agent is infectious (for example, bacteria or a virus), since it limits the agent's spread.

The swelling and pain can result from cellular edema caused by the trauma-inducing agent. Pain can be due to the edematous tissue cells exerting pressure against and/or stretching nerve endings. Changes in the pH and the osmotic pressure of tissue can also contribute to the stimulation of nerve fibers.

When inflammation is localized, the clinical manifestations consist of an irritating "rash." When the response is systemic, the reasons for the symptoms, such as edema and increased blood flow to tissue banks, can inhibit life-support organs such as the heart and the lungs, thereby causing a life-threatening situation.

The exact progression of the biochemical reactions leading to the triggering of an inflammatory response as a result of immunological trauma are not yet fully understood. The general understanding is that *in vivo reactions between the causative agent (biological or chemical) and histological and cytological body defensive mechanisms (such as antibodies) result in cellular destruction*. The major reason for the actual damage is the formation and release of *histamine* from insulted tissue. Disruption of cellular, proteinaceous tissue (tissue that contains nitrogen) activates the enzyme histidine decarboxylase, which transforms the normally present amino acid histidine into histamine. Histamine in turn is released into surrounding tissue.

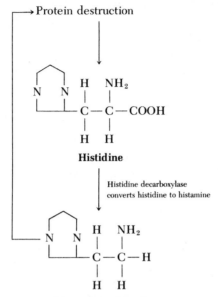

Histamine released

Histamine then acts to destroy more tissue which, in turn, activates more histidine decarboxylase, and so on. The effect of in vivo released or in vitro applied histamine on tissue cells is devastating, but varies according to species.

When histamine is injected or otherwise allowed to penetrate through the skin, the reaction in dogs and monkeys mimics a localized inflammatory response. Within seconds a red spot develops at the entrance site. This is believed to be due to an arteriolar dilating effect that histamine exhibits in some animals. With time a diffused red "flare" develops, followed by localized edema. This secondary redness and edema are the inflammatory response of the animal to the presence of histamine. Interestingly, the arteriolar response to histamine changes as one descends the zoological scale—from marked dilation in dogs and monkeys to strong constriction in rodents.[2]

Histamine's effect on the cardiovascular system also varies according to species. In rabbits histamine's generalized vasoconstricting effect leads to elevated blood pressure, while in dogs and cats it causes a sharp fall in blood pressure. High systemic concentrations of histamine in dogs and cats promote cardiac fibrillation, which results in more heart beats and a decrease in the volume of blood pumped per minute.

Histamine stimulates smooth muscle in a variety of tissue. The bronchioles in certain species are very sensitive to histamine; they respond with marked constriction, thus endangering lung function.

The sudden release of histamine by damaged cells throughout the body produces symptoms of anaphylactic shock (drop in blood pressure, pain, impaired breathing) in more highly developed animals. Other endogenous biochemicals, just beginning to be understood, have also been associated with triggering the inflammatory response. Kininogens, which can cause severe smooth muscle spasms, are released concurrently with histamine during times of cellular destruction. Prostaglandins, naturally occurring fatty acids found in the tissue of many animals, are believed to play a significant role in reducing capillary integrity, acting like necrosin to allow excessive blood flow to damaged tissue. In addition, prostaglandins mediate reactions that result in painful stimuli. The concurrent release of histamine, kinnigens, and prostaglandins can elicit the symptoms of the inflammatory response. When these endogenous substances are released by small, clustered groups of damaged cells, the inflammatory response is localized and usually not life threatening. Systemic release of these biochemicals, as can occur in an immunological crisis, or release of them by blood cells, results in a systemic, pronounced reaction, which endangers the animal's life.

EPINEPHRINE AND THE INFLAMMATORY RESPONSE

In order to moderate the effects of histamine, higher animals are able to produce and secrete large amounts of epinephrine. Epinephrine antagonizes many of the symptoms of the inflammatory response. Epinephrine causes generalized arteriolar constriction, as opposed to the vasodilation indicative of histamine. Thus cutaneous redness in localized inflammatory reactions is minimized. Epinephrine also elevates blood pressure after it has dropped as a result of the presence of histamine. In addition, epinephrine is a powerful direct cardiac stimulant. It causes the cardiac musculature to beat more rapidly (increased chronotropic activity) as well as more forcibly (increased inotropic activity). This combination of increased chronotropic and inotropic activity reverses precipitous drops in blood pressure, which are indicative of trauma-induced shock. Epinephrine is also a potent bronchiolar muscle relaxant and therefore can combat the bronchiole-constricting action of histamine. In addition, epinephrine causes an elevation in blood glucose level. This effect is related to epinephrine's ability to decrease liver glycogen levels by converting glycogen to glucose, which is transported via the bloodstream. The need for glucose is increased during trauma, since glucose is ultimately converted to energy, which is needed in greater amounts to bring about not only the biological reactions associated with the inflammatory process but also the production of more epinephrine, which is used to offset the effects of the inflammatory reaction.

Epinephrine is rapidly degraded and must be constantly produced by the adrenal glands if effective blood levels are to be maintained. The adrenal glands themselves require energy, which is received from the conversion of glycogen to glucose. Since glycogen supplies are limited, glycogen cannot serve as a prolonged source of energy for any of the processes associated with the inflammatory response or epinephrine release.

It is not beneficial for high levels of epinephrine to persist in the bloodstream for long periods of time. The dramatically increased chronotropic and inotropic activity cannot be tolerated by the myocardium for sustained periods. Eventually, irreversible damage and/or cardiac arrest will occur.

ADRENOCORTICAL HORMONES

Like epinephrine, adrenocortical hormones are produced by the adrenal glands. Epinephrine is secreted by the medulla of the adrenal gland, while the outer portions (cortex) produce adrenocortical hormones.

The adrenocortical hormones (adrenocorticosteroids) are chemically and structurally similar to each other (see Table 6-2), but they can be academically divided into three categories on the basis of their most pronounced biological functions. The adrenocortical hormones that primarily regulate the electrolyte balances of potassium, chloride, and especially sodium are called mineralocorticoids (since electrolytes are collectively referred to as minerals) or, more commonly, mineralocorticosteroids. Glucocorticosteroids affect the metabolism and catabolism of carbohydrates, fat, and protein. Sex hormones, such as androgens, which will not be considered here, are almost exclusively concerned with the development of sexual functions and characteristics. It must be emphasized that no adrenocorticosteroid has absolute glucocorticosteroidal or mineralocorticosteroidal activity. Adrenocortical hormones that affect tissue metabolism more than electrolyte levels have been termed glucocorticosteroids, while those having primarily electrolyte-regulating properties are called mineralocorticosteroids. A single adrenal hormone can exhibit both properties; however it is classified according to its predominant ability—either to influence electrolyte balance or to influence tissue metabolism. For example, although hydrocortisone influences the reabsorption of sodium, its primary role is to regulate cellular metabolism, and thus it is classified as a glucocorticosteroid. Table 6-1 shows the relative mineralocorticosteroidal and glucocorticosteroidal activity of some natural and synthetic corticosteroids.

Release of endogenous adrenocorticoids

The rate of secretion of minor mineralocorticosteroids by the adrenal cortex is controlled by the sodium concentration in extracellular fluid. The secretion of aldosterone, the major mineralocorticosteroid, is influenced by serum sodium and potassium levels.[3] The overall mechanism for electrolyte, especially sodium, uptake involves the secretion of aldosterone and at least two other, "minor" adrenal hormones having primarily mineralocorticosteroidal activity. Low systemic electrolyte (especially sodium) concentrations stimulate the release of adrenocorticosteroids having primarily mineralocorticosteroidal activity. These corticosteroids stimulate renal tu-

TABLE 6-1

Comparison of corticosteroids in terms of activity

	Relative anti-inflammatory (glucocorticoid) potency*	Relative sodium-retaining (mineralocorticoid) potency†
Cortisone	0.8	4+
Hydrocortisone	1	3+
Prednisone	3.5	3+
Prednisolone	4	2+
Methylprednisolone	5	2+
Triamcinolone	5	1+
Betamethasone	30	1+
Dexamethasone	30	1+

Modified from Murphy, J.P., editor: Where corticosteroids stand today, Patient Care, vol. 15, no. 8, April 30, 1981, p. 13.

*Hydrocortisone is the most commonly occurring adrenocorticosteroid that exhibits glucosteroidal activity and thus is usually considered the standard of comparison for anti-inflammatory drugs; hence it is given the arbitrary value of 1. As would be expected, glucosteroids that contain a fluorine atom, such as betamethasone, dexamethasone, and triamcinolone, exhibit the highest degree of anti-inflammatory activity.

†On a scale where 4+ is most potent and 1+ least potent.

bular enzymes to reabsorb sodium and probably other electrolytes, such as magnesium, chloride, phosphate, and potassium.

Fig. 6-2 summarizes the biological scheme for the release of adrenal hormones. Glucocorticosteroids are released in response to inflammation resulting from non-immunological or immunological trauma of any substantial degree—from acute anaphylactic reactions to long-term joint deterioration caused by arthritis. The first-line, short-term response to such conditions is the release of epinephrine. The effects of epinephrine are mimicked and expanded upon by the second-line defense substances, the glucocorticosteroids.

Damaged tissue releases intracellular substances, such as histamine, that stimulate chemoreceptors. Pressoreceptors are also stimulated, because edematous conditions lead to hydraulic pressure buildup in the inflamed area. Energy receptors are stimulated by the excessive heat that exists in the traumatized area as a result of increased blood flow. The overall conscious interpretation of these different modalities is pain and/or discomfort. It has been theorized that these impulses are initially directed to an ill-defined area in the hypothalmus, known as the "stress interpretation center." This site secretes the substance "corticotropin-releasing factor" (CRF), which is transported by micro vessels of the hypothalamic-hypophysial portal system into the pituitary gland. CRF, in turn, causes pituitary cells to secrete adrenocorticotropin (also known as corticotropin and adrenocorticotropic hormone [ACTH]), which is transported via the bloodstream (as all hormones are) to the

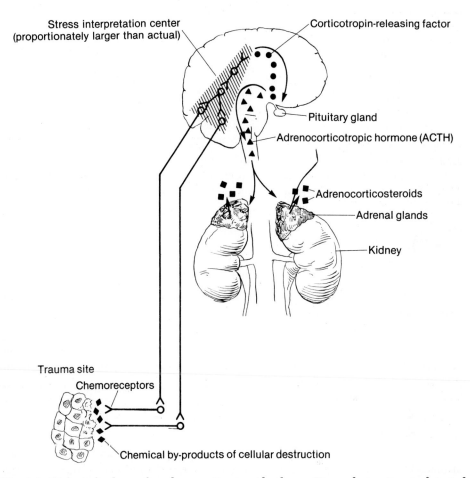

Stress interpretation center
(proportionately larger than actual)

Corticotropin-releasing factor

Pituitary gland

Adrenocorticotropic hormone (ACTH)

Adrenocorticosteroids

Adrenal glands

Kidney

Trauma site

Chemoreceptors

Chemical by-products of cellular destruction

Fig. 6-2. Biological scheme for adrenocorticosteroid release. Tissue destruction is detected by pressoreceptors and energy receptors as well as chemoreceptors. Sensory impulses are transmitted to the stress interpretation center, which, through the release of corticotropin-releasing factor, activates the pituitary gland to secrete adrenocorticotropic hormone (ACTH). ACTH stimulates the secretion of adrenocorticosteroids by the adrenal glands. The degree of tissue damage is apparently determined by the stress interpretation center, since the amount of adrenocorticosteroids released is proportional to the amount of tissue damage.

adrenal glands. Here it causes the secretion of hydrocortisone, the most important endogenous glucocorticosteroid, and other, less important glucocosteroids. *Generally, the secretion of both mineralocorticosteroids and glucocorticosteroids occurs in response to neuronal interpretation of need by the body.*

Mineralocorticosteroids

As has already been stated, the concentrations of electrolytes, particularly sodium, in the body are a function of the secretion of mineralocorticosteroids, and, similarly, the secretion of mineralocorticosteroids is influenced by the electrolyte concentrations. It will be recalled from Chapter 3 that the enzymes responsible for active reabsorption of electrolytes, especially sodium, are activated by mineralocorticosteroids (especially aldosterone). If electrolyte retention is desirable (as in malnutrition), mineralocorticosteroids are secreted and electrolyte reabsorption is promoted. If the excretion of electrolytes is desirable, mineralocorticosteroids are not released, or they are released in smaller amounts. It should be understood that *the release of mineralosteroids occurs continually and cyclically, in response to dietary habits and needs, rather than only in response to traumatic conditions, when their concentrations increase sharply.*

Glucocorticosteroids

Like the secretion of mineralosteroids, the secretion of glucocorticosteroids (glucosteroids) is a continual event that is necessary for combatting inflammation as well as for day-to-day regulation of cellular metabolism and maintainence of general homeostasis. The earliest recorded effect of glucocorticosteroids was their ability to elevate the blood glucose level. Further investigation indicated that this phenomenon is caused by the catabolism of carbohydrate, fat, and protein, which are converted to glucose. Normally, carbohydrates are readily converted to glucose and ultimately to energy. Degradation of fat and especially protein into glucose, a process called "gluconeogenesis" or "glyconeogenesis," is not a normal occurrence when the diet is satisfactory. It is indicative of normal carbohydrate stores being exhausted, secondary supplies of tissue (fat) being converted into an energy source, and, finally, tertiary sources (protein) being sacrificed to produce energy. Catabolism of protein to produce energy represents a very unhealthy situation, known as "negative nitrogen balance," and indicates that proteinaceous tissue is being destroyed, to make glucose, faster than it is being replaced.

As outlined previously (and summarized in Fig. 6-3), immunological trauma is the condition that initiates all the biological responses leading up to and including the release of glucocorticosteroids. Before glucocorticosteroids reach therapeutic blood levels, much of the carbohydrate stores are catabolized as a result of epinephrine production. Glucocorticosteroids then degrade protein and fat from body stores (and any remaining carbohydrate) to form glucose, which is converted to a usable form of energy. This energy powers biological reactions that (1) synthesize new tissue to replace damaged tissue and (2) produce more glucosteroids, which in turn degrade more tissue to ultimately form more energy.

As long as trauma and the resulting inflammation persist, glucosteroids will exert their gluconeogenic action in proportion to the degree of inflammation. If the inflammation is significant and remains for a long period, a great deal of body weight can be lost as a result of fat and protein catabolism. *Since inflammation of any degree inhibits normal biological processes, nature places top priority on minimizing and/or reversing the inflammatory reaction.* Localized inflammation (such as that caused by an insect bite) is more irritating than life threatening. However, widespread inflammation compromises the functioning of vital organs.

Glucosteroid production in response to inflammation is paramount. If inflammation is long term and extensive, the synthesis of glucosteroids will often occur

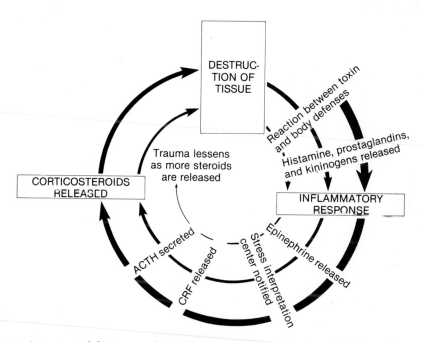

Fig. 6-3. Overview of the immunological trauma cycle. Destruction of tissue, inflammatory response, and corticosteroid release are the three major events in the immunological trauma cycle. The biological responses associated with each event are listed in chronological order. It should be noted that as more glucosteroids are released, the degee of trauma (indicated by the width of the arrows) lessens, as does the amount of tissue damage.

at the expense of other body tissues and functions. In extreme situations gluco-steroids can even catabolize necessary proteinaceous tissue such as bone marrow in order to form glucose, if other tissue banks have been exhausted. Undoubt-edly this has an adverse effect on the integrity of bone tissue as well as on his-tological processes. The existence of a number of more specific actions of glucocor-ticosteroids has been postulated to help explain these substances' anti-inflammatory effect as well as their ability to endow an animal with the capacity to resist noxious stimuli:

1. *Enhancing the formation of adenosine monophosphate (AMP),* an interme-diate substance that contains chemical bonds capable of releasing energy when broken

2. *Producing a membrane "stabilizing" effect,* which aids in the protection and repair of damaged tissue, thereby inhibiting the spread of inflammation. It has been theorized that steroids may decrease the permeability of cell walls (membranes) thereby diminishing and/or preventing the effects of histamine, kininogens, and prostaglandins.

3. *Rendering cells more sensitive to the effects of epinephrine.* It will be re-called that epinephrine represents the first-line defense against inflammation but that it cannot be produced in therapeutic concentrations indefinitely. Moreover, its continued high concentration is a threat to the cardiovascular system. By sensitizing cells to epinephrine, steroids enable cells to take full advantage of diminished epinephrine supplies in order to offset conse-quences of the inflammatory response. Interestingly, while corticosteroids potentiate a cell's response to epinephrine and epinephrine-like substances (catecholamines), they also protect the cardiovascular system against the long-term effects of high epinephrine levels.[1]

4. *Inhibiting smooth muscle contraction,* thus lessening the potential for bron-chiospasms

5. *Inhibiting the formation of antibodies and blood elements.* By inhibiting the production of antibodies and blood cells, through the suppression of DNA, and consequently the suppression of protein synthesis, glucocorticosteroids reduce the magnitude of the interaction between in vivo defense mecha-nisms (antibodies and blood cells) and noxious agents.[2] The amount of hista-mine released seems to be proportional to the magnitude of this interaction; thus, a reduction in the amount of one of the factors (body defense agents) brings about a reduction in the amount of histamine released. As a result the potential for tissue damage is likewise diminished.

6. *Inhibiting prostaglandin synthesis* by preventing the destruction of lyso-somes, which are cytoplasmic particles containing enzymes that degrade fatty acids into prostaglandin precursors

Corticosteroids, especially those exhibiting primarily glucocorticosteroidal activity, have significant effects on the central nervous system. Generally the amounts of endogenous glucosteroids are not enough to elicit CNS-related clinical symptoms. Doses of exogenous glucosteroids can be given in large enough quantities so that steroid-mediated CNS affects are clinically apparent. The mechanism by which brain function is modified are poorly understood but seem related to changes in cerebral concentrations of electrolytes, catecholamines, and other amino acids. It seems reasonable to assume that concentrations of specific catecholamines and amino acids vary from genus to genus and possibly from species to species. The clinical result of corticosteroid therapy with respect to CNS activity is that an animal's mood changes. Cats generally become depressed and/or prefer seclusion. Dogs may become irritable and sometimes vicious. They can also exhibit CNS depressant symptoms, such as lethargy and drowsiness. In addition, some dogs may pant excessively or become "hair pullers" or "flank suckers."[2]

Consequently practitioners and technicians must always keep in mind that any unusual behavior by an animal that is receiving steroids cannot always be attributed totally to the pathological condition but may be, to some degree, a side effect of drug therapy. Only by slowly tapering the dose of the steroid and observing the resultant behavior can the condition of the animal be accurately assessed.

Natural corticosteroids and synthetic corticosteroids

The mechanism by which corticosteroids influence most biological functions, especially those associated with the anti-inflammatory process and the regulation of electrolyte and water balances, have already been described. Naturally occurring corticosteroids have glucocorticosteroidal activity as low as one-thirtieth of that of the newer synthetic ones, while their mineralocorticosteroidal activity is on the order of three to four times greater than that of the newer steroids. Only seven out of approximately 44 known endogenous steroids seem capable of providing the complete spectrum of routine needs, among which are regulation of tissue metabolism and electrolyte balances. Endogenous steroids are also called upon to combat anti-inflammatory reactions of significant magnitude. Synthetic corticosteroids that have almost exclusively glucocorticosteroidal activity are used to augment the anti-inflammatory activity of the naturally occurring steroids. When the results of a traumatic incident are too overwhelming for endogenous corticosteroids, therapy with synthetic steroids becomes necessary. Consequently the goal of pharmaceutical research has been to develop corticosteroids that are (1) many times more potent in glucocorticosteroidal activity than endogenous steroids, and (2) devoid of mineralocorticosteroidal side effects. As will be discussed in more detail later, the major effect of mineralocorticoid activity is sodium reabsorption and consequently water retention. This effect is undesirable in most clinical situations.

Structure-activity relationships

The basic molecular structure common to all corticosteroids is shown in Table 6-2. Chemically it is referred to as the "17,21-dihydroxy-4-pregnene-3,20 dione" structure, but most people prefer to call it the "three rooms and a bath" molecule. All corticosteroids require this core structure for their general pharmacological activity. Substitutions are usually limited to the bond between carbons 1 and 2 and the bonds on carbons 6, 9, 11, and 16. Manipulation of other parts of the molecule either severely reduces activity or enhances it only marginally.

Certain structural changes in the basic corticosteroid molecule result in predictable biological responses:

1. Introduction of a double bond between carbons 1 and 2 increases glucosteroidal activity without additional mineralosteroidal effect.
2. Generally, the addition of a methyl group ($-CH_3$) to carbon 6 will enhance glucosteroidal activity; however, the effect on sodium reabsorption is variable, depending on the species.

TABLE 6-2

Comparative steroid structures

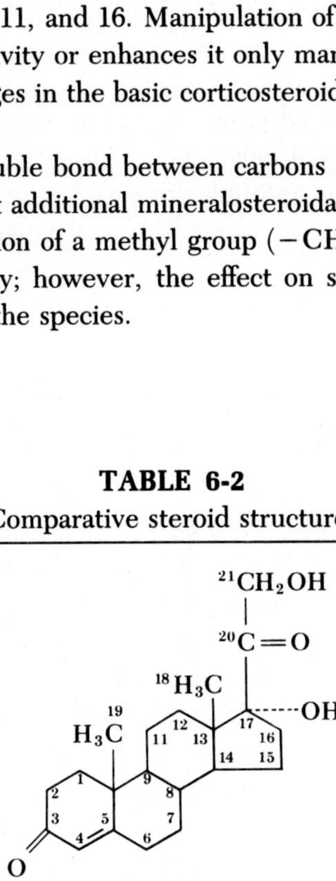

Basic structure

Drug	Carbons 1 and 2	Carbon 6	Carbon 9	Carbon 11	Carbon 16
Betamethasone	Double bond	—	F	$-OH$	$-CH_3$
Cortisone	—	—	—	$=O$	—
Dexamethasone	Double bond	—	F	$-OH$	$-CH_3$
Hydrocortisone	—	—	—	$-OH$	—
Methylprednisolone	Double bond	$-CH_3$	—	$-OH$	—
Prednisolone	Double bond	—	—	$-OH$	—
Prednisone	Double bond	—	—	$=O$	—
Triamcinolone	Double bond	—	F	$-OH$	$-OH$

3. The addition of a halogen atom (usually fluorine) to carbon 9 prolongs the steroidal effect because the halogen atom inhibits biodegradation in the liver. The consequently increased half-life of fluorinated steroids is at least in part responsible for their high degree of activity.
4. The presence of an oxygen atom on carbon 11 is indispensable for significant anti-inflammatory activity. This activity can be enhanced by bonding a hydrogen atom to the oxygen atom, thus forming a hydroxyl group (−OH). Neither the oxygen atom nor the hydrogen atom is required for mineralocorticosteroidal activity.
5. The addition of a methyl group to carbon 16 signicantly diminishes sodium retaining properties, but only slightly diminishes anti-inflammatory activity.
6. All presently available anti-inflammatory steroids have a hydroxyl group on carbon 17. Although some glucosteroidal effects occur without this hydroxyl group, they are clinically negligible. Other, nonadrenal, steroidal hormones, such as the sex hormones, also lack the carbon 17 hydroxyl group and thus, as would be expected, have little or no glucocorticosteroidal effects.
7. All natural corticosteroids and their synthetic analogues have a hydroxyl group on carbon 21, which is necessary for significant sodium retention but produces only marginally effective anti-inflammatory activity.

Pharmacokinetics

Natural and synthetic corticosteroids are all acid stable and thus can be administered orally. They are completely absorbed from the gastrointestinal tract. The natural ones, and some synthetics, however, are so rapidly degraded in the liver and in other, extrahepatic sites that they are only marginally effective when given by the oral route; hence they should be administered parenterally.

Attaching large, lipid-soluble organic molecules to the basic or modified steroidal structure decreases solubility and allows for slower absorption from the injection site. Conversely, the addition of water-soluble molecules to the steroidal molecule increases the absorption rate and, in some instances, even allows the drug to be given by the intravenous route.

All glucocorticoids are readily absorbed through either decompensated or intact skin. The amount of drug degradation is proportional to the time required for absorption. Consequently, if a corticosteroid ointment or cream is applied to paws or other areas of dense epidermal tissue, its effect will be localized, since most of the drug will be degraded as it penetrates the many tissue layers. Application to areas where the dermis is thin or to abraded skin, however, promotes systemic absorption and thus increases the possibility of side effects. Occlusive dressings also increase the rate and amount of absorption.

Undoubtedly the dramatic biological effect of corticosteroids is related to their ability to penetrate all tissues. Their accessibility to kidney, cardiac, fat, and proteinaceous tissue as well as to carbohydrate stores has already been suggested, since they affect the metabolism of these tissues. The corticosteroids' inhibition of the production of blood elements is related to their capacity to penetrate and affect the functions of lymphoid tissue. The ability of adrenocorticoids to catabolize lymphoid tissue to glucose and finally to energy is illustrated dramatically in mice. This species may lose up to 30% of its lymphoid tissue during starvation-induced trauma. Corticosteroids readily pass placental barriers and gain access to the fetus. This fact is of great concern if corticosteroids are administered to pregnant animals, since they can induce a condition known as "iatrogenic secondary adrenocortical insufficiency," which results in the offspring requiring steroidal therapy for the rest of its life, both before and after birth. (This condition will be discussed further in the section dealing with side effects of corticosteroid therapy.)

Biotransformation (degradation, detoxification) by hepatic microsomal enzymes as well as by nonhepatic tissue breaks double bonds and reduces molecules attached to carbons 3, 11, 17, and 20 to hydroxyl groups (if they are not already hydroxyl groups), which are more water soluble. These reduced compounds can then be conjugated with glucuronic acid to further increase their water solubility and enhance renal excretion. The rate of biotransformation is decreased if lipid-soluble molecules are attached to the steroidal structure and increased if water-soluble molecules are attached to the structure. Most species convert 99% of an administered steroid to some biodegraded form.[1]

Therapeutic uses

The dramatic and extensive effects of glucocorticosteroidal therapy have prompted at least one practioner to conclude: "There is probably no organ system in the body that does not suffer from one or many diseases that require glucocorticoids for their proper management. On the other hand, abuse of these drugs is attributable to ignorance and neglect."[2] Rational and prudent use of these drugs, along with constant surveillance of animals receiving steroids, can minimize such abuse. Avoiding the temptation for a quick reversal of symptoms that do not indicate a need for exogenous corticosteroidal therapy is fundamental to judicious use of this class of drugs. Like other potent medications, however, a practioner should not hesitate to use them in accepted or even heroic doses when conditions demonstrate an obvious need for them.

Adrenocorticosteroidal therapy is generally reserved for two indications—*replacement therapy* and *anti-inflammatory activity*. The need for replacement therapy is unqualified when an animal is unable to produce sufficient quantities of adrenocorticosteroids to sustain a healthy condition. The general term for such a situation is "hypoadrenocorticism" (or "hypoadrenalism"), commonly called "Addison's disease." Treatment with corticosteroids should be immediate and complete;

otherwise death is almost certain. Proper coverage of the animal's steroidal needs requires administration of corticosteroids that have glucosteroidal and mineralosteroidal activity. Postacute therapy generally centers on a mix of natural and synthetic steroids, since no single steroid can cover the daily needs of the animal. A canine usually requires oral sodium chloride tablets (to meet its sodium requirement) in addition to a mineralocorticosteroid such as fludrocortisone acetate. If the dog becomes sluggish or exhibits poor appetite, then life-long glucocorticosteroidal therapy, with cortisone and/or methylprednisolone, is mandatory. During times of trauma (for example, surgical insult, infection, anaphylactic shock), the need for additional amounts of parenteral glucocorticoids (which should be given parenterally) should be anticipated in order to the avoid life-threatening episodes that occur as the result of inadequate glucocorticosteroid levels.[2]

The decision to administer exogenous glucosteroids to a traumatized animal that has normal adrenal function is much more subjective than the practice of replacement for frank adrenal insufficiency. Clearly the degree of trauma must be assessed; the dosage must be adequate but not excessive. Nonreplacement therapy is done for two related reasons. One is to reduce inflammation and/or stabilize threatened cells. Another, much less frequently employed, practice in veterinary medicine is to intentionally suppress an animal's normal immune response mechanism (immunosuppressive therapy). Various aspects of the immune system are affected by the inhibiting action of steroids on the production of blood elements and antibodies. If an animal is to receive an organ transplant, aggressive therapy with glucocortiocsteroids severely interferes with the animal's ability to mobilize antibodies used to attack and cause rejection of the organ. In the true sense, this can be considered anti-inflammatory therapy, since the organ represents the agent that elicits the inflammatory response. Admittedly most of such work with animals is done to collect data that may be applicable to human problems rather than for clinical veterinary requirements.

A fundamental fact to remember is that corticosteroids do not cure the conditions for which their use is indicated. Their purpose is either (1) to inhibit the natural inflammatory response that occurs as the result of a traumatic experience or (2) to serve in place of endogenous adrenocorticosteroids to maintain body homeostasis.

Incorrect use of steroids can result in serious, life-long adverse side effects and even death. If an animal is to receive long-term corticosteroid therapy, close observation of its overall behavior as well as frequent blood tests are needed to avoid the problems that will be described in the section on side effects.

Thus far our discussion has centered on systemic uses of corticosteroids; however, there is a wide range of indications for topical corticosteroid administration. Corticosteroids are used topically for various skin conditions, which may be due to localized inflammation or to systemic problems such as arthritis.

Glucosteroids have proved effective in reducing ocular inflammation and preventing scarring of the cornea. Application of corticosteroids to the eye must be closely monitored, since their use can promote increased ocular pressure (drug-induced glaucoma) and has been associated with cataract formation.

There are many legitimate indications for intra-articular and joint injections of corticosteroids. Rheumatoid arthritis can result in intermittently swollen, "red hot," painful joints, which may prevent or hinder ambulation. Aspiration of excess fluid from the joint and injection of an appropriate glucocorticoid can relieve (but not cure) the problem. Site injection avoids the need to give oral doses, which predispose an animal to serious adverse side effects. While site injection does not avoid all side effects, it does allow high concentrations of the drug at the pathological site after only one administration. This avoids long-term administration, which may never achieve the same concentration at the localized area. Tendonitis likewise can be treated with direct site injections of a corticosteroid.

Localized injections of steroids are not without complications. Although glucosteroids can decrease inflammation within a joint, they also decrease the regenerative ability of proteinaceous cartilage. This side effect is related to glucosteroids' depressant effect on protein synthesis. Furthermore, since corticosteroids are crystalline products, often in suspension, injection of these particulates can physically irritate joint membranes, producing a type of arthritis known as "crystalline arthropathy."

After symptoms have subsided, movement of a joint that had been inflamed before corticosteroid therapy should be done carefully. Normal use of a joint that requires continuous symptomatic relief of inflammation through repeated steroidal injections can cause irreversible degeneration of the joint as a result of a combination of excessive exercise and drug therapy.

As is always true of steroidal therapy, localized application or injection of these drugs will not generally cure the condition. The disappearance of a rash or the reduction of a swollen, painful joint does not mean that the cause has been eliminated but only that the symptoms of the problem have been relieved, sometimes only temporarily.

Side effects

Unlike the situation with regard to the other classes of drugs thus far considered, serious side effects from steroidal therapy can develop even when doses are not excessive. Prolonged therapy with recommended doses can result in irreversible side effects, such as iatrogenic secondary hypoadrenalism. (The term "iatrogenic" refers to an abnormal state produced as a result of therapy. Indeed, in some cases the "cure" can be worse than the original pathological condition.)

This is perhaps the most insidious, devastating side effect of glucocorticoid therapy. Although not common, iatrogenic secondary hypoadrenalism is worth discussing, since it can be life threatening and at the very least requires an animal to receive steroid replacement therapy for years and sometimes for the rest of its life.

It will be recalled that the release of adrenocortical steroids is preceded first by the release of CRF from the "stress interpretation center," located in the hypothalamic area of the brain, and second by ACTH secretion from the pituitary gland. This triad of areas—hypothalamus, pituitary, and adrenals—as well as the substances they produce—CRF, ACTH, and adrenocorticosteroids, respectively—is referred to as the "HPA (hypothalamus, pituitary, adrenal) axis" or the "HPA function." Administration of exogenous steroids, most of which are many times more potent than the naturally occurring ones, suppresses the HPA axis, since the stress situation is dealt with by the medication. Consequently the HPA-related functions have no reason to occur, since synthetic steroids are replacing endogenous ones. The degree of HPA suppression is related to (1) the particular glucosteroid being administered (the more potent the steroid, the greater the suppression), (2) the dose (the higher the dose, the greater the suppression), (3) duration of therapy (the longer the therapy continues, the greater the suppression), and (4) the route of administration (the parenteral route causes the greatest suppression, followed by the oral and topical routes, in that order).

Unlike classical hypocorticism (Addison's disease), which is marked by electrolyte and metabolic disturbances, drug-induced hypocorticism does not affect endogenous mineralocorticosteroidal secretion or activity but only activity associated with glucocorticosteroidal release.

If exogenous steroids are given in sufficient quantity to induce symptoms of hypercorticism (actually iatrogenic hypercorticism), also known as "Cushing's syndrome," then it should be assumed that significant adrenal atrophy has occurred as a result of adrenal disuse. The fact that the hyperadrenalism is drug-induced means that more than the therapeutic steroidal need has been met and that the adrenals have had no reason to be functioning during the therapy period. It can further be anticipated that since the HPA axis is significantly suppressed, rapid withdrawal of medication will cause an acute hypoadrenocortical crisis. In such a case, ironically, an animal is simultaneously suffering from both hyperadrenocorticism and hypoadrenocorticism. The amount of steroid required to induce hypercorticism, and automatically secondary hypocorticism, varies among animals and breeds. In one instance, involving a pug, hypercorticism was documented after only three monthly doses of betamethasone.[2]

Although cats are apparently quite resistant to the development of iatrogenic hyperadrenocorticism during glucocorticosteroidal therapy, they are very susceptible to iatrogenic secondary hypocorticism. Thus they do not exhibit symptoms of hyperadrenocorticism while they are receiving steroidal therapy, but they can be expected to exhibit marked adrenal atrophy once the drugs are discontinued. Cats therefore should be considered especially susceptible to adrenal atrophy induced by exogenous steroids.

Rarely is suppression of the HPA axis in dogs and cats irreversible. Usually it is corrected by tapering off the dose of glucosteroid over a 3-month period; however, suppression may persist for more than a year, thus necessitating supportive steroidal therapy during this time.[1] During HPA suppression it is vital to increase the dose of glucosteroids in proportion to the severity of any stressful episode the animal may encounter (for example, infectious or noninfectious injury), since its ability to mobilize increased amounts of endogenous adrenocorticoids is compromised.

Side effects that are more commonly encountered will be discussed next. Unlike secondary hypoadrenalism, these side effects can occur to some degree (even subclinically) during most courses of steroid therapy. Only when one or more of these symptoms become apparent should the therapy with a particular steroid be reevaluated.

Side effects involving water and electrolyte balances—that is, sodium and water retention and potassium depletion—are more pronounced in humans than in dogs or cats. Some glucocorticoids (triamcinolone, betamethasone, and methyprednisolone) actually enhance sodium excretion in animals, thereby promoting water loss. Likewise some practioners have not seen hypokalemia (excessive potassium loss) in dogs with diagnosed steroidal drug-induced hyperadrenalism, even after long-term glucocorticoid therapy.[2] Nevertheless it is important to remember that these side effects can occur even if the degree is minimal.

Corticosteroid therapy can produce various side effects involving carbohydrate, protein, and lipid metabolism. Among these side effects are skeletal muscle wasting and weakness; hyperglycemia; decreased immune response and resultant increased susceptibility to infections; lameness and bone pain, with increased propensity for fractures; poor wound healing; and thin, alopecic skin that bruises easily. The ability of glucosteroids to form glucose (glucogenesis) from all types of tissue and foodstores is the common thread linking these seemingly unrelated side effects to each other. Proteinaceous, muscle tissue can be degraded to form glucose after more accessible body stores of carbohydrates and fat (lipids) have been exhausted. As was mentioned earlier, the breakdown of vital tissue stores into glucose (gluconeogenesis) represents a pathological condition; it must be corrected by reducing the dosage, changing the particular drug(s) being used, and/or enriching the diet with protein. Muscle wasting is manifested by weakness, fatigue, and inability to walk properly.

Hyperglycemia is to be expected, as a result of excessive glucose in the bloodstream because of steroid-induced (1) tissue breakdown and/or (2) inhibition of tissue synthesis. In the latter situation, foodstuffs are shunted from forming tissue to being converted to glucose. For most animals the hyperglycemia is usually not extreme or dangerous, but it can become so if an animal is a latent diabetic. If steroid-induced diabetes requires treatment, the use of oral antidiabetic drugs (oral hypoglycemics), such as acetohexamide, chlorpropamide, tolazamide, or tolbutamide, and/or insulin, should be considered. Oral hypoglycemics promote cellular uptake of glucose, thereby reducing its concentration in the blood. Their ease of administration, as opposed to the situation with insulin, is clearly an advantage, especially if an animal is not hospitalized. Insulin also accelerates glucose uptake by cells, but it has other physiological actions that inhibit the catabolic effects of steroids. Glucosteroids promote lipid degradation (lipolysis) by breaking lipids down, to produce, first, free fatty acids and, finally, glucose. Insulin enhances fat formation (lipogenesis), thereby inhibiting steroid-mediated lipolysis. In addition, insulin promotes protein synthesis, while steroids act to degrade protein or to prevent its formation by converting amino acids to glucose rather than to protein.

A vast amount of protein is associated with the blood and immune systems. Either by catabolization or by inhibition of their synthesis, blood cells and antibodies are adversely affected by glucocorticoid administration. Glucosteroids classically produce neutrophilia, eosinophilia, lymphopenia, and, to lesser degrees, erythrocytosis and thrombocytosis. The following elements of the immune system are adversely affected most often:

1. Macrophages and monocytes. Inhibition of their synthesis results in decreased phagocytosis and decreased ability to process antigens.
2. Lymphocytes. Because glucosteroids are lymphocytolytic, host defenses for fighting infectious agents are compromised. Also, formation of red blood cells is impeded, since lymphocytes may enter bone marrow and become red blood cells. Lymphocytes can also be converted into precursors for connective and supportive tissue. Thus their destruction diminishes the ability of the skeletal frame to function properly.
3. Humoral antibodies. Glucosteroids depress their formation, partly as a result of these drugs' lymphocytolytic activity.

The overall consequences of these hematological and immunological side effects are that an animal becomes more susceptible to infections because it is less able to combat an infectious agent; nor can the animal as effectively form antibodies to prevent subsequent infections. In addition, wound healing is retarded, probably because of the combination of compromised hematological factors and inability to neutralize infectious agents in the wound. The ability of glucocorticoids to compromise an animal's natural anti-infective defense mechanisms, which was discussed earlier when "immunosuppression" was mentioned, is a practical, clinical consideration rather than an academic curiosity. During steroidal therapy the increased susceptibility to disease should be anticipated, and various anti-infectives should be available for administration if needed. Oftentimes an infection of nuisance value to an animal not receiving steroids becomes a serious, possibly life-threatening, condition to an animal receiving significant amounts of a glucocorticosteroid. Although the occurrence of these side effects varies according to dose, duration of treatment, and species, the hematological and immunological systems of any animal receiving steroids on a regular basis are compromised. In addition, frank symptoms of drug-induced hyperadrenalism should signal a technician that an animal's humoral defenses could be decompensated.

Glucocorticosteroid-induced alteration of protein metabolism and decreased calcium absorption account for the side effects associated with bones. Bone marrow (a rich protein source) and calcium support bone formation and function; the marrow lends a certain degree of flexibility to bones, while calcium provides rigidity. Together these two qualities help bones endure impact-type injuries without fracturing. Concurrent loss of marrow (through conversion to glucose or inhibition of synthesis) and calcium (as a consequence of steroidal therapy) weakens bone, making it brittle and more prone to fracture.

Drug-induced alterations in protein metabolism can affect the amount of protein and fat deposited in the skin and hair. Protein and fat lend elasticity to skin. In addition, fat serves a protective function by limiting the penetration of many agents through the skin. Protein is also instrumental in the seating of hair follicles in skin. Diversion of protein and fat from skin and hair cells, or preventing its deposition in these areas by inhibiting its formation, results in skin that bruises and bleeds easily and alopecia (hair loss).

Glucocorticosteroids, except for triamcinolone, increase the appetite in most animals, thereby promoting weight gain. The appetite stimulation complements the steroids' ability to increase the production of glucose. Since an animal eats more, food intake is increased and tissue is thereby spared from being catabolized. In order to promote digestion, glucosteroids also increase the production of pepsin and gastric acid. Unfortunately, steroids decrease the rate of gastric mucosal cell replenishment.[2] The increased acidity accelerates the destruction of stomach mucosal lining, and since its replacement is retarded, the animal is predisposed to gastric ulceration (see Chapter 1). Irritation of the gastrointestinal tract is a common side effect of oral glucocorticoid therapy. To minimize the irritation, oral steroids should always be administered with food or milk. Any indication of gastrointestinal disturbance, such as diarrhea (bloody or nonbloody) or bloody stools, should be reason enough to discontinue steroidal therapy until the animal has been examined.

Dosage concepts

Many attempts have been made to minimize the side effects associated with glucosteroid therapy. While modifications of the basic steroidal molecule have altered the type and degree of activity, none have had a significant effect in lowering the magnitude and incidence of side effects. Consequently practioners have turned to experimenting with different dosage regimens. After 33 years of clinical experience with adrenocorticosteroids, certain fundamental concepts regarding dosage have developed:

1. *Doses are rarely definitive; they should be based on clinical response rather than on a fixed number of milligrams per kilogram.*
2. *(Long-term) administration should bring about only the clinical response desired, without inducing signs of iatrogenic secondary hyperadrenalism.*
3. *For life-threatening situations, massive doses (sometimes up to 25 times the otherwise recommended doses) may be required.* Experience has indicated that a few massive, parenteral doses do not elicit any long-term side effects.
4. *Intermittent ACTH therapy should be used when glucosteroidal therapy is prolonged.* ACTH is most beneficial when used to *avoid* secondary drug-induced depression of the adrenals rather than as a means to cure it. If functional capacity of the adrenal glands is suppressed, ACTH may actually hinder their revitalization. Recent data suggest that the most enduring block to adrenal stimulation is not reactivation of the adrenals themselves, but the ability to release CRF. Apparently the sensory and/or motor cortical mechanism(s) associated with receiving or reacting to a stress signal are most lastingly depressed when exogenous steroids are administered. Administration of ACTH would stimulate the adrenals but would do nothing to stimulate the mechanism(s) needed for CRF release.[2]
5. *Intermittent ACTH administration is beneficial to test the functional capacity of the adrenals.*
6. *Administration should never be stopped abruptly, but always tapered off over a number of days.* If the adrenal glands or other elements of the HPA axis have been suppressed, clinical signs of hypoadrenalism will be manifested as the dosage of the exogenous steroid is reduced. Gradual reduction in dosage over a number of days provides the animal with some steroidal protection if symptoms of hypoadrenalism occur.

A newer, more sophisticated approach to the administration of glucosteroids is "alternate day steroidal dosing" (ADSD). By making use of an animal's own 24-hour cyclic pattern (circadian cycle) of release of endogenous steroids, most notably cortisone, a practitioner can give a lower-than-usual amount of a steroid without apparently sacrificing beneficial clinical effect. For most nonnocturnal animals, cortisone levels are highest in the morning (7 AM to 10 AM) and lowest at night (10 PM to midnight). By administering small doses of a glucosteroid in the morning, a practitioner does not overly depress HPA functions. In addition, it seems that with some steroids (the longer-acting ones), supplementation of already high endogenous cortisone levels affords adequate coverage even on the days when medication is not given. Thus far the only oral glucocorticosteroids that can be given with this dosage pattern are prednisolone, prednisone, and methylprednisolone. As would be expected, endogenous steroidal circadian cycles in cats are the opposite of what has just been discussed; concentrations are highest at night and lowest in the morning.

Contraindications, drug interactions, and drug incompatibilities

Except in life-threatening disorders, glucocorticosteroids should not be used in animals with any of the following conditions:

1. Peptic ulcers, because of steroids' ability to increase gastric acid secretion and inhibit stomach mucosal cell regeneration
2. Erratic or abnormal behavior. Because steroids may alter the concentrations of electrolytes and amino acids in the brain, they can induce unanticipated behavioral changes in animals, possibly intensifying an already abnormal pattern.
3. Infections not controlled by anti-infectives. In such situations host defense mechanisms cannot afford to be compromised, which is the effect steroids will have.
4. Osteoporosis, which can increase in intensity because of excessive excretion of calcium and phosphate as a result of steroidal therapy
5. Diabetes mellitus, which will be aggravated by the hyperglycemic activity of glucocorticosteroids
6. Blood dyscrasias, which can be intensified because steroids depress blood cell formation and have a direct lymphocytolytic activity

Because of their propensity to exhibit some mineralocorticosteroidal side effects, glucosteroids should be used with caution in animals with hypertension or congestive heart failure.

Although data for all animals are not available, it has been demonstrated that high doses of steroids in pregnant rabbits cause fetal abnormalities and abortion. Thus the use of steroids should be avoided whenever possible in pregnant animals.

Some drugs that may be indicated in conjunction with steroids, such as antibiotics or other anti-infectives, neither minimize nor potentiate steroidal activity. Insulin and oral hypoglycemic drugs, however, exhibit a direct antagonistic effect, which can minimize the magnitude and spectrum of glucocorticosteroidal activity. Diuretics compensate for any mineralosteroidal activity without diminishing the anti-inflammatory effect of a steroid. Antihistamines promote the biodegradation of steroids, probably through a mutual enzyme induction type of reaction (see Chapter 2), thereby reducing the steroidal effect. Adding a CNS drug that is intended to alter behavior to a drug regimen that already includes glucosteroids can lead to unpredictable results. If the animal is depressed as a result of steroidal therapy, the addition of a CNS depressant can be expected to increase the depression. The addition of a CNS stimulant may evoke overly aggressive behavior and therefore cannot be considered acceptable therapy. Phenytoin, an anticonvulsant, inhibits steroidal activity, probably as a result of altering cerebral electrolyte movement and concentrations. Because the exact pharmacological action of many CNS drugs has yet to be determined, the best policy would seem to exclude concurrent administration of these drugs with steroids unless therapeutic benefit outweighs potential or actual behavioral effects.

As was mentioned previously, organic or inorganic molecules can be bonded to the steroid nucleus at certain reactive centers. These reactive centers can also chemically react in vitro with other medications, as could occur in intravenous solutions when steroids are mixed with other drugs. Generally, high-molecular-weight substances like steroids can react with other high-molecular-medications, such as antibiotics, when they are present in the same intravenous fluid. Other in vitro chemical interactions result from steroids being mixed with drugs that have significantly different pH values. For a detailed review of medications considered incompatible with steroids, refer to Appendix A, at the back of this book. It should be noted that the interactions listed there pertain only to the in vitro mixture of the drugs. Thus, drugs considered chemically or physically incompatible could possibly be given if they are administered in separate intravenous solutions. (Also note that Appendix A does not take therapeutic incompatibilities into consideration.)

Individual glucocorticoids

From the glucosteroids thus far mentiond it can be seen that they, like many hormones, share the ending, "-one." One is tempted to assume that since steroids are horm*ones*, the ending "-one" is used to emphasize this fact. It should be realized, however, that the "-one" ending is not used exclusively for corticosteroids but is also used for most of the sex hormones (tetosterone, progesterone, and so on) and for a related class of drugs termed the anabolic steroids (for example, oxymetholone and norethandrolone), which are used to promote weight gain by means of increased tissue synthesis rather than water retention.

See Table 6-2 for a summary of the similarities and differences between the steroids that will be discussed individually here.

Betamethasone

Betamethasone, a fluorinated glucosteroid, is typical of the newer synthetic steroids, which display little or no mineralocorticoid side effects. When animals are converted from another glucosteroid to betamethasone, diuresis usually follows. Since betamethasone is approximately 30 to 33 times more potent than hydrocortisone, animals receiving this drug should be observed closely for development of side effects indicating hypercorticism. Like other steroids, betamethasone is not recommended in presence of acute infection. In addition, its use has been associated with weight gain, presumably because of increased appetite and anabolic activity, much like the effects of the anabolic steroids. Like other steroids, betamethasone is a very stable molecule, being capable of withstanding temperatures as high as 150° F (65° C). Because of this stability, the drug has been produced in many dosage forms, including tablets, ointments, creams, syrups, and injectables. One injectable form is a mixture of two betamethasone salts—betamethasone sodium phosphate and betamethasone acetate. The phosphate salt provides rapid attainment of therapeutic blood levels, while the insoluble acetate form is more slowly dissolved, thereby providing prolonged duration of effect. Some injectable forms are suspensions; when they are used for intrasynovial or intra-articular administration, pain can be initially expected, because of the presence of drug particulates.

The parenteral dose for dogs ranges from 0.013 to 0.023 mg/kg (13 to 23 µg/kg), with no subsequent doses recommended. Because of the high propensity for cats to develop hypocorticism, betamethasone is not recommended for this species.

Cortisone acetate

Cortisone acetate is a naturally occurring adrenocorticosteroidal hormone; in most animals it is probably second in abundance to hydrocortisone. Cortisone acetate is prepared commercially by synthetic modification of naturally occurring plant steroids rather than by extraction from animals.

Absorption is poor following subcutaneous or intramuscular injection, and in small animals the oral route is usually used to attain a rapid clinical effect. Topical application to skin or eyes results only in localized, largely superficial effects. Intra-articular injection provides a rapid local effect and accompanying "particulate pain." After absorption cortisone acetate is metabolized to hydrocortisone, which is responsible for the drug's predominantly glucosteroidal effect; however, this drug also has notable mineralocorticoid effects.

Cortisone acetate affects carbohydrate, fat, and protein metabolism. In addition, the functional capacity of the HPA axis should be closely monitored, as should hematological parameters. One of the most important side effects of cortisone acetate is depression of HPA axis, even when the drug is used topically for skin diseases. If steroids are required for dermal conditions, it is recommended that the newer steroids, which exhibit little adrenal depression, be used.

As is true of any steroid causing HPA axis depression, withdrawal of the drug should be done gradually, to avoid symptoms of hypocorticism.

Water retention may occur during the first few days of therapy with cortisone acetate, but if therapy is continued, diuresis may follow. Cortisone acetate influences the water shift more than it causes frank water retention, oftentimes increasing the volume of extracellular fluid at the expense of intracellular fluid.

Desoxycorticosterone acetate

Desoxycorticosterone acetate, a naturally occurring steroid, has very limited glucocorticosteroidal activity but significant mineralocorticoid activity. It is mentioned here only to point out that it is not generally accepted to be effective as an anti-inflammatory drug if the pathological condition is significant. Since it is, for all clinical purposes, a mineralosteroid, its side effects are largely the result of sodium reabsorption—namely edema, pulmonary and cardiac congestion, and hypertension. This drug's mineralocorticoid activity is estimated to be 15 to 30 times greater than that of cortisone. Neither the blood glucose level nor the metabolism of fat, carbohydrate, or protein is significantly affected by this drug.

Dexamethasone

Dexamethasone is structurally and clinically very similar to betamethasone, both being fluorinated steroids. The difference, if any, in their anti-inflammatory activity is academic; for all clinical purposes both can be considered 30 to 33 times more potent than hydrocortisone. In therapeutic doses, dexamethasone rarely causes sodium or water retention; however, animals should be observed for development of less obvious side effects indicating hypercorticism, especially behavioral changes and tissue wasting.

Dexamethasone is available in oral dosage forms (tablets and syrup), as injections, and as sprays for instillation into either the nasal passages or the throat. Application in these last two instances is done with a hand-held, pressurized atomizer that has adapters suited for nasal or throat instillation. The depth of penetration of the medication depends upon droplet size. (Review Chapter 1 for a detailed discussion of droplet size and penetration.) Topical application of dexamethasone with such a device is contraindicated in the presence of an acute infection that is not controlled by antibiotics or other anti-infectives. The parenteral form of dexamethasone—the sodium phosphate salt—is a solution that lends itself to intraarticular injection. Because dexamethasone sodium phosphate is freely soluble in water, particulates are not present upon injection and thus administration of the drug by this route is not associated with as much pain as results from the injection of suspensions of steroids. Unfortunately, because the drug is in solution, its anti-inflammatory effects following intrasynovial or intra-articular injection persist for only about 24 hours. Doses can be repeated from once every 3 days to once every 3 weeks, depending on the degree of inflammation.

Hydrocortisone

First known as "compound F," hydrocortisone is usually considered the standard by which other glucosteroids are compared. On a milligram-to-milligram basis, hydrocortisone is approximately one and one-half times stronger than cortisone in glucocorticosteroidal activity, and it has a quicker onset of activity than cortisone when injected. Parenteral forms include a suspension (hydrocortisone acetate) and a solution (hydrocortisone sodium succinate). The suspension is preferred for intraarticular use. Particulate pain is less than with cortisone acetate. Local relief from pain and stiffness in the area of the injected joint usually occurs within 24 hours and may persist for 96 hours or longer. Articulating joint temperature is decreased, as is the total cell count of the synovial fluid. The main contraindication to the intra-articular use of hydrocortisone is the presence of infection in or near the joint. If rapid and intense systemic blood levels are required, the sodium succinate salt is preferred. Hydrocortisone acetate suspension should never be administered by the intravenous route, since it is highly insoluble and the prolonged presence of partic-ulates will predispose the animal to emboli formation.

The mineralocorticoid activity of hydrocortisone is approximately 3 times greater than that of betamethasone or dexamethasone but somewhat less than that of cor-tisone. Hydrocortisone is acid stable and well absorbed from the gastrointestinal tract. It is also effective when applied topically to the skin or the eye.

Doses for dogs range from 5 mg/kg given intravenously in cases of shock to 5 mg given intramuscularly once monthly. Usual long-term oral doses range from 0.25 to 1.25 mg daily. It should be remembered that, as with all steroids, these ranges should serve only as guidelines and that doses should consist of the minimal amount necessary to achieve the effect desired. The dosage for shock in cats is the same as that for dogs. Oral, intravenous, and intramuscular doses in cats range from 0.125 to 0.5 mg daily.

Methylprednisolone

The glucocorticosteroid methylprednisolone is available in oral and injectable forms. The oral form is the free base, while the parenteral forms consist of a sus-pension (methylprednisolone acetate) and a solution (methylprednisolone sodium succinate). The longer-acting acetate salt is used primarily for intracutaneous, intra-articular, or intralesional administration. After intra-articular injection, effects of methylprednisolone acetate persist for at least 1 week. The sodium succinate salt is generally intended for short-term, emergency therapy, with an intravenous bolus or intravenous infusion usually being preferred for initial treatment. Methylpred-nisolone sodium succinate can also be injected by the intramuscular route.

Side effects such as increased appetite, gastrointestinal ulceration, and psychic changes are somewhat less common with methylprednisolone than with most of the other synthetic glucosteroids. Like betamethasone, methylprednisolone is a potent glucocorticosteroid and thus has little tendency to cause sodium and water reten-tion; however, an animal should be observed for less obvious side effects, such as protein wasting (negative nitrogen balance).

Doses of methylprednisolone in dogs generally range from 1 mg/kg, given intra-muscularly every 2 weeks, to 0.5 mg/kg, given orally or intramuscularly twice a day for allergic conditions. If suppression of the immune system is the goal of therapy, then doses on the order of 2 mg/kg given orally or intramuscularly twice a day, are used. When doses of this magnitude are employed for prolonged periods (3 to 5 days), significant hypocorticism is very possible. Noncritical conditions in cats gen-erally response to one dose of 20 mg.

Prednisolone and prednisone

Prednisolone and prednisone were the first synthetic glucocorticosteroids to be commercially available. They rapidly became popular because of their low sodium-retaining potency in comparison to their anti-inflammatory activity; both are four times more potent in the latter regard than hydrocortisone. With time, newer synthetic steroids, such as betamethasone and methylprednisolone, became available; these drugs have even less mineralosteroidal activity than prednisone or prednisolone. Clinical experience indicates that the newer corticosteroids exhibit approximately the same side effects, with the exception of sodium retention, as these older drugs.

For clinical purposes, prednisolone and prednisone are considered identical in anti-inflammatory capability. Prednisolone is more soluble than prednisone and hence is used for liquid dosage forms such as injections and ophthalmic preparations, although it is also used in topical ointments and creams. Prednisone is somewhat less prone to cause gastric ulceration and thus is used exclusively for oral administration.

Parenteral doses in larger animals (horses and cattle) range from 100 to 400 mg, given intramuscularly; in these animals the drugs are usually intended for treatment of ketosis and inflammatory conditions. Although the causes of ketosis vary, a common symptom is hypoglycemia. Glucocorticosteroids are therefore used to stimulate gluconeogenesis (providing glucose from noncarbohydrate sources), thereby correcting the low blood glucose level.

Doses for dogs and cats usually are 20-25 mg, given intramuscularly for 3 to 5 days, followed by 2.5-1 mg given orally each day.

Prednisolone and prednisone are prepared commercially by microbiological conversion of hydrocortisone and cortisone, respectively.

Triamcinolone

Triamcinolone is structurally very similar to betamethasone, the only difference being that triamcinolone has a hydroxyl (—OH) group on carbon 16 rather than a methyl (—CH$_3$) group. This subtle difference, however, accounts for triamcinolone having only about one-sixth the anti-inflammatory activity of betamethasone while exhibiting the same degree of mineralocorticoid activity. Perhaps more than any other glucosteroid, triamcinolone has been incorporated into many different dosage forms (primarily as its acetonide salt), both alone and in combination with other drugs. A popular topical ointment and cream includes triamcinolone and antifungal and antibacterial drugs (triamcinolone, neomycin, nystatin, and gramicidin) for identified as well as nonspecific dermatitis. (Glucocorticoids in topical dosage forms should not be applied to infected areas of skin unless antibiotics are applied concurrently, either in the same product or separately. Triamcinolone is also effective for intra-articular, intrasynovial, and intralesional injection, the effects appearing within a few hours and lasting from 1 week to several weeks. Like other injectable synthetic glucocorticoids, triamcinolone (as the hexacetonide salt) may be diluted prior to intra-articular administration with 1% or 2% lidocaine or a similar *preservative-free* local anesthetic, to reduce pain resulting from the injection method.

Oral doses for dogs range from 0.25-2 mg, once daily for 7 days. Intramuscular or subcutaneous doses in dogs and cats can be as high as 0.22 mg/kg. Oral doses for cats should not exceed 0.5 mg daily for 7 days.

Once again it should be remembered that doses depend more on clinical evaluation of an animal than on general guidelines. The evaluation and resultant doses should reflect not only the extent of pathogenicity but also the degree of HPA functioning.

NONSTEROIDAL ANTI-INFLAMMATORY DRUGS (NSAID)

The number and severity of side effects associated with glucosteroidal therapy have prompted clinicians to use certain nonsteroidal drugs that mimic the anti-inflammatory effects of the glucosteroids. Reduction of inflammation without the worry of depressed HPA function, protein wasting, or the the other major debilitating side effects attributed to steroids is obviously advantageous. Many NSAID are relatively new, while others have been used almost from the time glucosteroids became available.

Pharmacology and therapeutic indications

While the NSAID are not devoid of serious side effects, which primarily involve the central nervous system and the gastrointestinal tract, they do reduce inflammation without accompanying alterations in cellular metabolism or HPA function.

The oldest group of NSAID is the pyrazolone derivatives, which include the drugs oxyphenbutazone and phenylbutazone. It will be recalled that this group was discussed in Chapter 4, in the section dealing with analgesics. Both the older NSAID and the newer ones have the dimension of analgesia as well as anti-inflammatory action. Glucocorticosteroids are not capable of producing analgesia. It has been theorized that the analgesic properties of the NSAID are due to their ability to depress neuronal transmission of impulses both peripherally and centrally, the latter effect occurring after the drugs have penetrated the blood-brain barrier. The exact mechanism of their anti-inflammatory activity is not known; unlike the situation with regard to the steroids, the mechanism probably varies somewhat from drug to drug. *It seems probable that their anti-inflammatory action is exclusively limited to localized inflamed tissue (whether inside or outside the CNS) and does not involve either direct or indirect stimulation of organs to release endogenous substances that act against the inflammatory process.* The anti-inflammatory effect is mediated by the drugs' ability to antagonize the biological reactions that promote the inflammatory process. Indomethacin, one of the NSAID whose structures are shown in the boxed material on p. 193, exemplifies this direct antagonistic action.

Besides having antipyretic activity, it appears to inhibit the development of cellular exudates in injured tissue and to reduce increased vascular permeability.[1] These last two effects result in the inhibition of the intercellular spread of endogenous irritants such as the prostaglandins.

Likewise ibuprofen, another NSAID, is believed to inhibit peripheral synthesis and/or release of prostaglandins. Naproxen, a relatively new NSAID and analgesic, has also demonstrated that it acts directly at inflamed tissue sites to inhibit the synthesis of prostaglandins by inhibiting the enzyme(s) responsible for their release and/or function. Like all other NSAID, ibuprofen does not possess glucocorticoid or adrenal cortex–stimulating abilities.

Structures of nonsteroidal anti-inflammatory drugs*

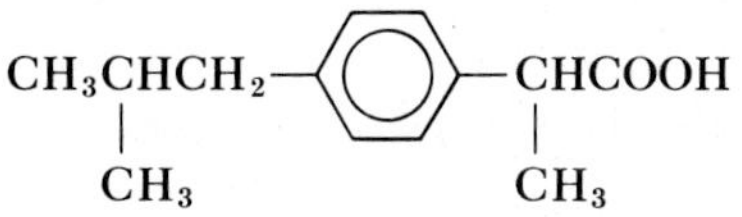

Ibuprofen

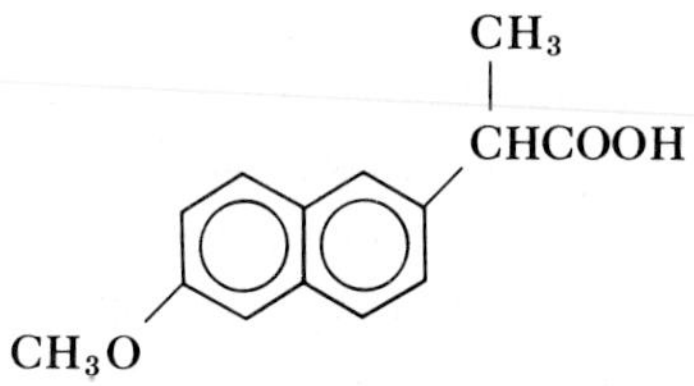

Naproxen

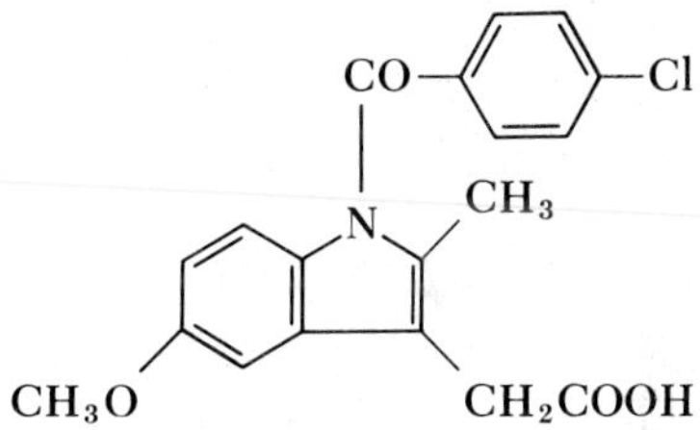

Indomethacin

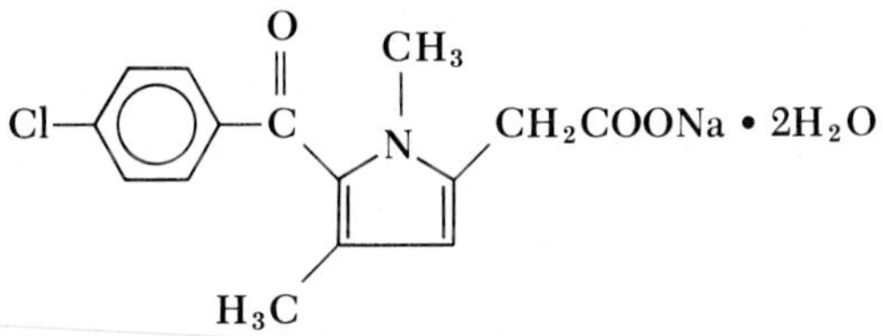

Zomepirac sodium

*Since these drugs are also moderately potent nonnarcotic analgesics, they are also listed in Fig. 4-2.

Interestingly, recent investigation into the pharmacological activity of the oldest group of NSAID, the pyrazolones, indicates that these drugs also have a direct anti-inflammatory action and that their activity is limited to inflamed tissue.

Likewise, the newest NSAID, zomepirac, exhibits antiprostaglandin activity by inhibiting synthesis at inflamed tissue sites, whether they be located outside or inside the CNS. And therapeutic doses of zomepirac in humans have significant analgesic activity, usually equivalent to 8 to 16 mg of morphine given intramuscularly.

As the box on p. 193 shows, no core structure is shared by the most common NSAID; yet they all apparently have the ability to diminish the activity of prostaglandins, either by inhibiting their formation or by preventing their release. Since prostaglandin synthesis is carried on by an enzyme or enzymes that apparently can be inhibited by these drugs, it would seem that receptor sites on these enzymes are relatively nonspecific and can accommodate a variety of chemical structures. This opens the possibility that in the future, NSAID that do not exhibit the serious side effects of the present ones can be developed.

It is well recognized that aspirin also exerts a significant anti-inflammatory action and that it is probably used more often for this indication than any one of the other NSAID mentioned thus far. Aspirin justifiably serves as the standard of comparison for the anti-inflammatory action of the other NSAID. Preliminary trials designed to compare the clinical anti-inflammatory effectiveness of NSAID with that of the glucocorticosteroids or the salicylates (such as aspirin) have not yielded conclusive results and only indicate that response to the NSAID varies not only among species, but from animal to animal and from time to time (the latter finding probably being linked to the circadian cycle of steroid levels). Claims that dosages of corticosteroids can be reduced and their use gradually terminated during NSAID therapy have not been substantiated in all situations. Since the NSAID have no effect on corticosteroid levels, they cannot be used to supplement mineralocorticoid activity.[1]

Although it was hoped initially that NSAID could replace glucosteroids for long-term administration, it is doubtful that this will be realized. In addition to the fact that NSAID have some significant side effects that restrict the duration of their use, they cannot elicit all the biological reactions attributed to steroids. As a result they are not indicated for acute shock situations, regardless of the cause. To date their use has been largely suggested for the treatment of inflammation accompanying musculoskeletal disorders such as capsulitis, bursitis, arthritis, and uncomplicated lameness. Clinically all NSAID are given by the oral route, and therefore data concerning their intra-articular or intrasynovial administration are not available.[1]

If a veterinarian is faced with the need to administer glucosteroids to an animal for an extended time, it would seem appropriate that the possibility of at least intermittent therapy with NSAID be considered.

Side effects and drug interactions

While the NSAID do not have the range of side effects that the glucosteroids have, their use nevertheless must be closely monitored. Their ability to cross the blood-brain barrier results in their tending to cause side effects associated with CNS dysfunction—specifically, behavioral patterns associated with CNS depression, such as fatigue and malaise. The effects are not common but can occur. Paradoxically, insomnia has also been reported occasionally in humans. In addition, animals may also become anxious and appear confused and disoriented, to the point of staggering or falling. Coordination can also become compromised as a result of visual disturbances such as amblyopia (dimming of vision and/or blurred vision). Rarely, cases of deafness have been reported; in some the deafness was irreversible, while in others the deafness ended after doses were reduced or discontinued.

The most serious side effects limiting dosage and duration of therapy are associated with the gastrointestinal tract. Gastrointestinal irritation demonstrated by nausea, vomiting, anorexia, diarrhea, constipation, stomatitis, flatulence (bloating), and epigastric and abdominal pain should be anticipated. In some cases gastrointestinal irritation has progressed to ulcerations, which eventually have perforated, causing internal bleeding. Concurrent administration of milk, food, or antacids may be of some help but rarely will prevent irritation over extended dosage periods.

As would be expected, the ulcerogenic (ulcer forming) potential is increased if more than one NSAID is administered concurrently, and increased even more if salicylates are added to the regimen. Unlike the situation in regard to the sulfa drugs, no evidence exists that equivalent clinical effects can be reached by administering more than one NSAID in doses lower than recommended, as opposed to administering the recommended dose of a single NSAID. Consequently, concurrent administration of multiple NSAID only increases the possibility of gastrointestinal irritation without improving the therapy. An empirical rule of thumb for determining the suitability of administering NSAID to an animal is that they should not be administered if the animal has shown gastrointestinal or any other, related problems as a result of aspirin. It is also prudent to intermittently do routine blood workups, since NSAID use is also associated with hemolytic anemia and bone marrow depression, which can result in various blood dyscrasias.

A unique side effect of the pyrazolone-type anti-inflammatory drugs is fluid and electrolyte disturbances, including sodium retention, which can result in edema. The cause of this electrolyte imbalance is not fully understood, but it does not seem to be associated with the release of endogenous steroids. Rather it is suspected to be related to renal enzyme activity. Strangely enough, the pyrazolone-type analgesic/anti-inflammatory drugs have been shown to cause conditions they are supposed to alleviate. Specifically they have been linked to inflammatory conditions such as pericarditis, optic neuritis, and diffuse interstitial myocarditis. In addition, since NSAID inhibit the synthesis and release of prostaglandins, these drugs can affect labor and parturition. Thus the administration of NSAID to pregnant animals is not recommended. NSAID have also been found in the milk of nursing animals.

All of the aforementioned side effects of NSAID seem to be dose related; they usually diminish or disappear as dosages are reduced.

Like the anticonvulsant drugs, NSAID are notorious for interacting with concurrently administered drugs. NSAID have the potential to decrease blood levels of anticoagulant drugs such as warfarin; although this tendency has not been demonstrated clinically, it should be remembered if an animal is receiving an oral anticoagulant drug. Such an interaction is probable because detoxification of NSAID occurs largely in the liver, which utilizes the microsomal enzyme systems common to the degradation of the oral anticoagulants.

In animals, blood levels of some NSAID have decreased when aspirin has been concurrently administered.

Undoubtedly the NSAID offer an alternative to glucocorticosteroidal therapy for some conditions, but it should always be kept in mind that their use, like that of the steroids, can be marked by serious side effects.

ANCILLARY DRUGS USED FOR INFLAMMATORY CONDITIONS
Antihistamines

It is often the case that drugs having no direct anti-inflammatory action are beneficial when given along with the true anti-inflammatory drugs, such as corticosteroids or NSAID. Antihistamines exemplify such a class of drugs; they do not have direct anti-inflammatory action but nevertheless may be useful in curbing the effect and spread of an inflammatory condition.

Pharmacological activity and structure-activity relationships

Both the steroids and the NSAID act to minimize damage done by the release of histamine and prostaglandins—by directly or indirectly preventing their production or by reversing the damage done to tissue. Neither type of drug acts to directly protect tissue. Antihistamines, however, are specific competitive inhibitors of histamine; they function (1) by preventing histamine from attaching to tissue receptors not yet exposed to histamine and (2) by displacing histamine from receptor sites of tissue already affected by it. To date no evidence suggests that antihistamines are effective against the prostaglandins.

Like other substances that influence cellular function, histamine must first become attached to a cell by the "lock and key" method, which was described in Chapter 1. Histamine must find specific receptor sites on the cellular surface and become attached to them. Once contact is made, histamine can begin to alter the functioning of the cell.

Thus far two different types of histamine receptors have been identified. The H_1 receptors, found on blood vessels and nonvascular smooth muscle, are responsible for the classical inflammatory symptoms attributed to histamine. Namely, stimulation of H_1 receptors by histamine causes (1) vasodilation and vascular permeability in higher animals, (2) smooth muscle spasm, and (3) increased chronotropic activity.

Another class of histamine receptors, called H_2 receptors, are responsible for mediating the secretion of gastric acid and pepsin into the stomach. Traditional H_1 antihistamines do not block H_2 receptors. Only one drug to date, namely cimetidine, acts to reduce the secretion of gastric acid into the stomach by blocking H_2 receptors. As would be expected, cimetidine is used to alleviate gastrointestinal irritation and ulceration. By decreasing the amount of acid in the stomach, cimetidine increases the pH, thereby providing a more suitable environment for healing to occur. A higher pH also prevents further irritation of stomach lining.

Fig. 6-4 summarizes the cycle of tissue destruction and the other side effects caused by histamine and also shows the sites of antihistamine blocking. Trauma to tissue cells causes the conversion of histidine to histamine by the enzyme histidine decarboxylase. The action of histamine is then competitively inhibited by antihistamines, which occupy H_1 receptor sites; hence inflammatory effects caused by histamine are prevented or at least diminished. As the activity of histamine is lessened because of its degradation by histaminase and as its effects are decreased by antihistamines, the extent of further trauma is reduced. Consequently fewer cells are damaged, less histidine is converted to histamine, and side effects diminish in number and intensity.

In order to successfully compete with histamine for H_1 receptor sites, antihistamines require the core structure shown in the box on p. 199. R_1 can be a ring structure, as is found in the antihistamine chlorpheniramine, or it can be other heterocyclic groups, as illustrated by the structure of promethazine. If a halogen atom (either chlorine or bromine) is attached to the ring structure, the antihistaminic action of the drug is increased. X is a nitrogen, oxygen, or carbon atom. This replacement atom has an effect on the degree of CNS depression, while the ethylamine portion ($-CH_2-CH_2-N=$) is largely responsible for antihistaminic activity. Antihistamines are structurally classified on the basis of what atom is in the X position. If it is nitrogen, the antihistamine is called an "ethylenediamine." The phenothiazine-type H_1 antihistamines (illustrated by promethazine) also have a nitrogen atom in this position, but since it is part of a heterocyclic structure, these drugs are not considered ethylenediamine-type antihistamines. When oxygen is in the X location, the antihistamine is referred to as an "ethanolamine," and when a carbon is present, the drug is called an "alkylamine," or a "propylamine" (since three noncyclic carbon atoms are attached to each other).

Ethylenediamines are moderately effective in competing for H_1 receptor sites and consequently are good antipruritics (medications that relieve itching). Ethanolamines and phenothiazines are potent antihistamines but unfortunately exhibit significant CNS depressant side effects. Oftentimes side effects are so intense that

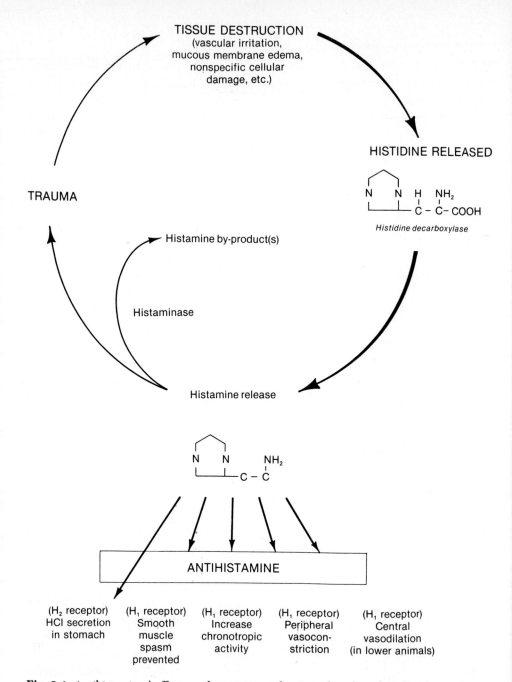

Fig. 6-4. Antihistamines' effect on the trauma cycle. Once histidine decarboxylase converts histidine to histamine, the enzyme histaminase degrades histamine into various by-products. Even though histamine is short lived, it still causes the trauma cycle to continue by its contact with tissues via H_1 receptor sites. Antihistamines occupy H_1 tissue receptors, inhibiting histamine from affecting tissue. Antihistamines are not effective in blocking histamine from occupying H_2 receptors. Stimulation of H_2 receptors causes the secretion of hydrochloric acid into the stomach. To date only one commercially available drug, cimetidine, has been effective in blocking H_2 receptors from the effects of histamine. As would be expected, cimetidine is used for the treatment of gastric ulceration.

Comparison of antihistamine types

Core antihistamine structure for H_1 blockers

x = nitrogen
Ethylenediamine type

x = nitrogen in a ring
Phenothiazine type

EXAMPLE: tripelennamine
OTHERS: methapyrilene, pyrilamine

EXAMPLE: promethazine
OTHERS: temaril

x = oxygen
Ethanolamine type

x = carbon
Alkylamine (propylamine) type

EXAMPLE: diphenhydramine
OTHERS: doxylamine

EXAMPLE: chlorpheniramine
OTHERS: brompheniramine

therapy with these particular antihistamines must be discontinued. This is not surprising for the phenothiazines, since (as was mentioned in Chapter 4) these drugs are also potent tranquilizers. Although the alkylamines (or propylamines) are generally considered the mildest of the major antihistamines, they do exhibit good antipruritic activity.

Although it is customary to classify antihistamines according to relative potencies, the ratings vary from clinician to clinician. Clinicial end points are difficult to determine, and reactions to the different histamines varies considerably from species to species. Usually the determining factor as to which antihistamine is selected is the intensity of the side effect(s) rather than the amount of histamine-blocking activity, which can only be judged by the relative lack of symptoms.

The pharmacological action of antihistamines, within normal dosage ranges, can be summarized as follows:

1. Antihistamines competitively antagonize most actions of histamine by occupying histamine H_1 receptor sites, thereby preventing action of histamine on the cell.
2. Antihistamines do not stimulate the cell per se but rather perform a blocking action.
3. Antihistamines do not chemically react with histamine to neutralize or degrade it.

In practice the antihistamines have largely been confined to treating dermatological responses to inflammatory reactions (for example, pruritis and uticaria); they have been administered by parenteral, oral, and topical routes. Antihistamines should never be the only drugs used to treat serious inflammatory reactions, since other, more potent medications (such as the glucosteroids and epinephrine) are initially required to control the myriad side effects associated with an acute inflammatory reaction. Although antihistamines can be injected, but only by the intramuscular route, as well as given orally, it still requires time for a therapeutic concentration to accumulate on receptor sites. Intravenous administration of antihistamines results in excessive CNS stimulation, such as convulsions. If an inflammatory reaction occurs before the administration of antihistamines, higher doses are needed to effectively displace histamines from H_1 receptor sites. With higher oral or intramuscular doses comes CNS depression, which is not advantageous in situations of acute inflammation such as anaphylactic shock.

With the exception of the phenothiazine antihistamines, all H_1 antihistamines contain the suffix "-amine" in their names. Like the phenothiazine-type tranquilizers, phenothiazine antihistamines end in "-azine."

Side effects and drug interactions

Central nervous system depression is commonplace within normal dosage ranges, especially with the phenothiazine and ethanolamine types of antihistamines. As would be expected this depression is manifested by lassitude, drowsiness, and dizziness, and sometimes by muscle weakness. In addition, anticholinergic effects such as dryness of mucous membranes and smooth muscle relaxation can be expected. The anticholinergic actions are useful in controlling the bronchospastic effects of histamine.

Acute antihistamine overdoses are rare; they require massive amounts of the drug. However, when such an overdose does occur, it is marked by CNS *stimulation* rather than excessive depression.[2] Presumably this is due to the ability of excessive antihistamine drug concentrations to either directly or indirectly cause cellular stimulation rather than act passively as a blocking agent, as antihistamines do in therapeutic doses. This reaction is just the opposite of morphine's effect on cells. It will be recalled from Chapter 4 that morphine causes initial CNS stimulation followed by deep depression.

Paradoxically, idiosyncratic side effects of antihistamines have included dermal hypersensitivity, resulting in skin rashes. It is also well documented that some antihistamines cross the placental barrier, resulting in teratogenesis; thus systemic therapy with antihistamines should be avoided in the early stages of pregnancy.[2] Concurrent administration of CNS depressants such as sedatives and/or tranquilizers (to manage an animal) will have an additive effect on the CNS-depressant capabilities of antihistamines, and vice versa. While these drugs are not contraindicated for simultaneous use with antihistamines, once must be aware of the increased CNS depression that will occur and take appropriate measures, such as reducing the dose of the tranquilizer or sedative. A reduction in the antihistamine's dose is counterproductive, since its competitive inhibition capability is directly proportional to the dose (the higher the dose, the greater the blocking effect).

Animals receiving oral anticoagulants, such as warfarin, may have to be retitered to ensure that blood levels of the anticoagulant are not excessive. Since hepatic microsomal enzymes necessary for the biotransformation of antihistamines and oral anticoagulants are the same, the addition of an antihistamine may temporarily overload the enzyme system(s), resulting in slower degradation rates and therefore higher-than-normal anticoagulant blood levels. The higher antihistamine levels that may also occur initially are not as critical as the levels of the anticoagulant. More important, if the dose of the anticoagulant is decreased to offset the reduced detoxification rate, it must be increased when the antihistamine is discontinued.

Miscellaneous drugs

Other medications, such as topical astringents or protective ointments and creams, may be helpful in managing dermal complications of inflammatory reactions. In acute situations medications intended to support life systems, such as cardiac stimulants (discussed in the following chapter) and pulmonary medications (designed to allow air exchange) may also be required. Tranquilizers or sedatives may prove beneficial, to prevent an animal from causing self-inflicted damage to affected skin areas.

* * *

The treatment of inflammatory conditions requires an in-depth knowledge of their cause as well as an acute awareness of the side effects that can occur because of drug therapy. A proper balance of medication to fit the degree of inflammation is the key to successful therapeutic results without serious side effects.

REFERENCES

1. American Society of Hospital Pharmacists: Hospital formulary, vol. 2, 68:00, Washington, D.C., 1980, The Society.
2. Kirk, R.W.: Current veterinary therapy, Philadelphia, 1980, W.B. Saunders Co.
3. Murphy, J.P., editor: Where corticosteroids stand today, Patient Care, vol. 15, no. 8, April 30, 1981, p. 13.

7

Cardiovascular drugs

PERFORMANCE OBJECTIVES

After completion of this chapter the student will:

- Explain the difference between contractile and conductile tissue
- Explain the process of myofibril contraction as it relates to electrical stimuli, catecholamines, and calcium
- Define and describe the three major types of pathological conditions of the heart
- Describe the differences in pharmacological activity between catecholamines and beta blockers in regard to receptor sites
- Compare the pharmacological actions of the cardiac regulators and depressants with respect to the following:
  1. Overall clinical effect
  2. Impulse conduction velocity
  3. Stimulation threshold
  4. Refractory period
  5. Calcium
  6. Electrolyte shifts across cellular membranes
- Describe the effect calcium has on electrical excitation and mechanical contraction

This consideration of cardiovascular drugs assumes that the reader is already familiar with the mechanics of blood flow through the heart. This discussion will concentrate on the transmission of electrical impulses through the myocardium and how they are enhanced or inhibited by various drugs.

The two major stages of cardiac function—contraction (systole) and subsequent relaxation (diastole)—are directly and indirectly dependent upon the transmission of impulses throughout the myocardium. If the flow of impulses is interrupted by nonconductive tissue (for example, scar tissue resulting from myocardial infarcts), the efficiency of the pumping action will be compromised. Likewise, in higher animals, if the two areas of impulse origination—the sinoatrial (SA) node and the atrioventricular (AV) node—are not coordinated with each other, the efficiency of the pumping action will be compromised.

Most cardiac drugs discussed in this chapter either directly or indirectly influence the movement of electrolytes across myocardial tissue. In this way they help to correct problems affecting the chronotropic (rate of contraction) and/or inotropic (force of contraction) activity of the heart. Because the heart is intimately responsible for the well-being of the whole animal, cardiac dysfunction results in fluid imbalance disorders such as cardiac and pulmonary edema. Cardiac problems therefore rarely can be treated only with the medications discussed in this chapter but also require concurrent use of drugs already mentioned elsewhere in this book. Diuretics (see Chapter 2), usually are required to relieve edematous conditions resulting from cardiac dysfunction. (It may be a good idea at this point to review the chapter on diuretics in order to see how they complement the action of cardiac drugs.) Some of the drugs discussed exert noticeable and beneficial effects on blood vessels; therefore discussion of only their cardiac actions would not provide a true picture of their entire biological effect. As a result, discussions of the pharmacological action of drugs used in cardiac treatment will also include, when appropriate, their effect on blood pressure.

CARDIAC RHYTHM

In order to pump efficiently, the heart must maintain a recurring alternate rhythm of relaxation and contraction. Blood enters the heart's chambers (atria and ventricles) during relaxation and is forced out when the heart contracts. The timing of contractions is the result of complex electrical interrelationships between specialized muscle fibers called "nodes" or "sinuses" and myofibrils, which are fibrous strands of cardiac tissue that contract when stimulated. The pattern of alternating contraction and relaxation is inherent in cardiac muscle itself and not dependent upon outside factors such as hormonal influence. It should be noted, however, that changes in the pattern of contraction and relaxation are influenced by endogenous biochemicals or impulses, such as the impulses reaching the heart by way of the vagal nerve. The innate rhythm of the heart can be demonstrated simply by observing an exposed heart isolated from an animal. It can be seen that contractions continue even though the heart is removed from its biological environment. In vivo cardiac contractions are timed to coincide with the filling of chambers, thereby allowing the maximum amount of blood to be pumped per contraction.

In higher animals electrical impulses originate in areas of the heart known as the SA node and the AV node. In such animals the electrically functional areas of the heart are the SA node, the AV node, the AV bundle, the Purkinje fibers, and the myofibrils. Fig. 7-1 shows the general locations of these structures and their relationships to the other, more familiar anatomical features of the heart. In lower animals such as turtles, a distinct sinus exists—that is, a specialized grouping of fibers that automatically emits electrial impulses that radiate out from the sinus, causing contraction of the atria and ventricles. In higher animals no distinct sinus exists. However, located in the posterior wall of the right atrium of most animals is a small area known as the SA node, which is the embryonic remnant of the "sinus" in lower animals. Cardiac muscle fibers (myofibrils) excised from the SA node contract faster than those taken from atrial tissue, and atrial myofibrils beat faster than venticular myofibrils. Because the SA node has a faster rate of contraction than other sections of the heart, impulses originating from the SA node spread to the atria and ventricles (via the Purkinje fibers); hence the SA node is often referred to as the "pacemaker" of the heart.

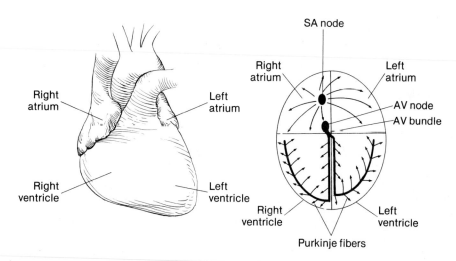

Fig. 7-1. Electrically functional areas of the heart. The location of the SA node, which initiates the electrical impulse leading to a heart beat, facilitates emptying of the atria. Myofibril contraction (the path of which is indicated by arrows) in the atria is responsible for effectively pushing blood from the atria into the ventricles. Likewise, contraction of ventricular myofibrils (see arrows) effectively pumps blood from the ventricles into the lungs and the systemic circulation. Effective movement of blood minimizes complications of sluggish blood flow, such as pulmonary or cardiac edema.

IMPULSE CONDUCTION THROUGH THE HEART

Myofibrils are interconnected (as shown in Fig. 7-2) so firmly that cellular walls are often not distinguishable; under a microscope myofibrils appear to constitute a single, multinucleated cell. Such a maze of interrelated fibers is called a "syncytium," or muscle mass. In the heart the atrial myofibrils form a separate syncytium from the ventricular myofibrils; thus two distinct syncytia make up the heart. An electrical stimulus (action potential) initiated in any fiber (for example, a fiber in the SA nodal area) will be transmitted over the membranes of all fibers in that particular muscle mass. The electrical potential or impulse spreads in a manner similar to that described in Chapter 4 in regard to muscle contraction. As in neuronal conduction of impulses, a shift in sodium and potassium ions is involved, but unlike the situation with regard to neuronal transmission, the myofibrils are muscle tissue and therefore contract as a result of ionic shifts across their membranes.

The heart's two distinct syncytia (the atria and ventricles) are joined together by the Purkinje system, which conducts impulses from the atrial muscle mass to the ventricular muscle mass. Conduction of the impulse along the Purkinje system resembles typical neuronal impulse transmission, since Purkinje fibers do not contract as a result of ionic shifts. One of the functions of the Purkinje system is to rapidly conduct impulses throughout the ventricles so that all ventricular areas con-

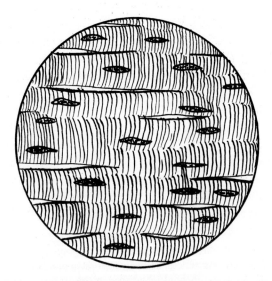

Fig. 7-2. Interconnection of myofibrils. The lack of distinct boundaries between individual myofibrils promotes smooth transmission of an impulse from one myofibril to the next and helps to provide a uniform intensity of inotropic response over the myocardiaum.

tract as nearly simultaneously as possible. Without the Purkinje system an impulse would travel much more slowly through the ventricular myofibrils, allowing some of them to contract (depolarize) and relax before others. This would cause an uncoordinated compression of blood in the chambers, resulting in decreased, inefficient pumping action. Because of the Purkinje system, once an impulse is initiated in the SA node it can travel throughout the heart in a pattern that provides efficient pumping of blood from all chambers. The recurrent action of the heart, in fact, represents that of any muscle tissue—contraction (depolarization), refractoriness, and repolarization.

PATHOLOGICAL CONDITIONS OF THE HEART

Cardiac dysfunction is not absolute. Even though conditions may exist that reduce the efficiency of the heart, there are also biological compensating mechanisms that try to offset the problem(s). For example, the inhibition of the arteriolar blood supply to the heart, as a result of coronary artery blockage, causes new coronary arterioles to form. Heart enlargement (to a certain extent) can compensate for inadequate circulation, as can increased chronotropic activity. Only when natural compensating factors are not sufficient to maintain proper blood pressure and adequate blood oxygenation is there a need for drug support.

For our purposes pathological conditions of the heart can be divided into three major categories:

1. Diseases of the myocardium, which result in large portions of the myocardium being nonfunctional or less than optimally effective
2. Anatomical defects, which include valvular malfunction, causing blood to be pumped at the wrong time, and faults in cardiac walls or associated vessels, causing restricted or misdirected blood flow[4]
3. Abnormal initiation and/or conduction of impulses, resulting in arrthymias (loss of normal cardiac rhythm), which are manifested as changes in chronotropic and/or inotropic activity

Problems in the conduction of impulses may be related to disease and/or anatomical problems; thus the three categories can be interrelated to some extent.

With the exception of the use of indomethacin, in humans, for the treatment of patent ductus arteriosus (failure of a vessel connecting the aorta and a pulmonary vessel to constrict after birth), conditions in the first two categories generally do not respond to drug therapy and usually necessitate surgery.[4] The primary use for cardiac drug therapy is the management of arrhythmias. It is not the purpose of this book to describe the multitude of arrhythmias and their origins and then match them to the drugs that are most beneficial in their treatment. Instead, the pharmacological categories of cardiac drugs will be reviewed. It is hoped that this general information will provide an understanding of the rationale behind the prescribing of certain drugs for specific arrhythmias.

CARDIAC STIMULANTS (SYMPATHOMIMETIC AMINES)
Pharmacological actions and individual drugs

In acute cardiac failure medications that enhance stimulation and hence contraction of myofibrils are needed so that blood pressure can be restored and/or maintained. The immediate need in cardiac arrest is to regain some pattern of contractions, with the hope of subsequent stabilization to a normal or near normal rhythm. At one time, irritant chemicals called "reflux stimulants" were injected, the logic being that chemical irritation of myofibrils would mimic the normal electrical potential in their effect on the myofibrils, thereby causing them to contract. These reflex stimulants included ammonia-like compounds, camphor, and ether. As time passed, these compounds were dropped in favor of injectables that caused systemic stimulation, such as caffeine, theophylline, and picrotoxin.[1] With the advent of the sympathomimetic amines, the first class of sophisticated compounds that are analogues of epinephrine became available; these drugs stimulate receptors on cardiovascular tissue rather than causing generalized, nonspecific stimulation. The more commonly used sympathomimetic amines, which are compared in Table 7-1, have a structural similarity to epinephrine, which is a natural amine (nitrogen-containing compound) released by the sympathetic nervous system; hence the name "sympathomimetic amines" ("mimetic" meaning to mimic the action of).

Explanation of the pharmacological activity of the sympathomimetic amines (also known as catecholamines) as well as some of the other cardiac drugs, centers on the theoretical presence of "alpha" and "beta" receptors located on cardiovascular tissue. Stimulation of alpha and beta receptors on different tissues by epinephrine or other sympathomimetics elicits certain types of biological responses. Stimulation of these same receptors by parasympathomimetics (sympatholytics), such as acetylcholine, usually evokes an opposite response or at least a different response from adrenergic (sympathomimetic) stimulation. Blocking of alpha and beta receptors by certain drugs lessens the adrenergic effect. The sympathomimetic amines are fairly consistent in the cardiovascular responses they evoke in higher animals. This is to be expected, since epinephrine is a natural sympathetic mediator and both isoproterenol and levarterenol are analogues of epinephrine.

The biological response to the sympathomimetics may involve every organ or tissue mass; however, this discussion will be restricted to consideration of the cardiovascular system. It has been theorized that the sympathomimetic amines listed in Table 7-1 act in generally the same fashion but with varying potencies. Specifically, they stimulate beta and/or alpha receptors, which in turn lower the threshold resistance needed to be overcome before a cell can be stimulated to contract or transmit impulses. (This aspect of their function is similar to the action of the CNS stimulants, mentioned in Chapter 4.) In addition, sympathomimetic amines may also enhance the activity of the sodium pump and/or facilitate ionic shifts across

TABLE 7-1

Comparison of sympathomimetic amines*

Drug	Route and dosage (dogs and cats)	Inotropic activity	Chronotropic activity	Blood pressure
Epinephrine (1:1000 solution)	SC, IM, IV, IC†: 0.1-0.5 ml (dogs) 0.1-0.2 ml (cats)	+++‡	++	+
Isoproterenol (1:5000 solution)	SC, IM: 0.5-1 ml every 6 hours; IV: 5 ml in 200 ml D_5W, to effect	++++	++++	+
Levarterenol (1:1000 solution)	IV: 1 ml in 250 ml D_5W, to effect	+	+	+++

*Isoproterenol and levarterenol, two synthetic sympathomimetic amines, are structurally similar to naturally occurring epinephrine. Substitution on the nitrogen atom affects the intensity of inotropic and chronotropic activity as well as the degree of vasoconstriction. The degree of vasoconstriction is one determinant of how much the blood pressure will be elevated by administration of any one of these drugs.

†Intracardiac.

‡The plus signs provide a relative indication of how much activity occurs or how much the blood pressure is increased. One plus sign indicates the least response, and four signs indicate the greatest response.

membranes; the latter effect may be related, at least in part, to increased sodium pump activity.

The ultimate effect is that direct intracardial injection or intravenous infusion of sympathomimetic amines encourages nonfunctioning myofibrils and pacemaker fibers to resume activity.

Epinephrine

Epinephrine, a powerful cardiac stimulant, acts directly on myofibril and pacemaker beta receptors as well as on conducting tissue such as the Purkinje fibers. Chronotropic and inotropic activity are both increased, as is oxygen consumption by the heart in response to the increased workload. The acceleration of cardiac activity results in shorter but more forceful contractions. Conduction speed by noncontractile fibers, such as the Purkinje fibers, is increased as a result of the same pharmacological effects that promote the contraction of myofibrils. Epinephrine also causes the dilation of coronary vessels. This effect enhances cardiac activity by allowing more oxygenated blood to reach the myocardium. In addition, blood vessels supplying other parts of the body, such as skin, abdominal viscera, and skeletal muscle, are constricted, thereby causing more blood to be shunted into dilated coronary vessels.

This constriction of arterioles also serves to increase blood pressure. Indeed, when epinephrine is given by rapid intravenous injection, it causes a dramatic rise in blood pressure, in proportion to the dose. In acute cardiac failure rapid intravenous administration or direct intracardial administration is recommended. Intramuscular or subcutaneous injection, in some animals, will cause vasoconstriction at the injection site, thereby increasing the time required for the drug to reach the heart.

The first commercially available epinephrine was called "Adrenalin," and over the years this term has become synonomous with the term epinephrine.

Isoproterenol

Isoproterenol is the only synthetic sympathomimetic amine that is used extensively. It is the most active of the three listed in Table 7-1 and functions almost exclusively to stimulate beta receptors. This reduces the severity of side effects, such as abdominal cramping, that are associated with alpha receptor stimulation. Intravenous infusion causes increased cardiac output as a result of (1) increased inotropic and chronotropic action and (2) increased return of venous blood to the heart. Therapeutic doses usually result in an increase in systolic pressure if some cardiac activity is present. Large doses (such as 1 μg/kg), however, cause a dramatic drop in blood pressure. As is true of epinephrine, intravenous administration results in rapid response times while the oral route is unreliable (because of erratic gastric acid degradation) and thus not recommended in cases of heart block.

Isoproterenol is less toxic than epinephrine when given to animals having normal cardiac activity. As will be discussed at the end of this section, administration of sympathomimetic amines to animals with adequate or normal cardiac function can lead to serious arrhythmias and heart failure.

Levarterenol (norepinephrine)

Like epinephrine, levarterenol is a natural chemical mediator secreted by postganglionic adrenergic neurons. In dogs and cats it is a less potent cardiac stimulant (actually depressing cardiac activity in some animals) than either epinephrine or isoproterenol. However, levarterenol is one to four times more active than these drugs as a vasopressor (drug that elevates blood pressure), presumably because its stimulation of alpha receptors results in marked vasoconstriction. Levarterenol has weak cardiac stimulatory action, and thus its use should be restricted to elevating blood pressure in hypotensive states resulting from trauma (immunological or nonimmunological), hemorrhage, CNS depression, or acute cardiac failure. Like epinephrine, levarterenol is largely ineffective by the oral route and thus should be administered intravenously. Careful monitoring of blood pressure is essential to avoid acute, dangerous hypertensive episodes.

• • •

Table 7-1 lists dosage ranges for isoproterenol, epinephrine, and levarterenol.

Administration precautions and drug interactions

Intravenous infusion of any sympathomimetic requires close supervision. Long-term infusion, especially of levarterenol, can cause irreversible damage to extremities as a result of prolonged, intense, peripheral vasoconstriction produced by alpha receptor stimulation. Such constriction deprives tissues of adequate oxygen and can ultimately cause necrosis.

Only one sympathomimetic should be administered parenterally at a time. Simultaneous infusion or injection of more than one can cause excessive cardiac stimulation, leading to tachycardia (rapid heartbeat), fibrillation (excessive twitching of heart muscle rather than definitive beating), and finally cardiac arrest. The overstimulation caused by the additive effect of more than one sympathomimetic being administered at a time results in the heart literally burning itself out.

The administration of epinephrine or isoproterenol to an animal with adequate cardiac function (for noncritical conditions, such as minor inflammatory reactions) likewise carries with it the possibility of "cardiac burnout." The use of any sympathomimetic should be clinically warranted, and the animal should be closely monitored for signs of cardiac hyperstimulation. In addition, large doses of epinephrine or isoproterenol may lead to cardiac enlargement and/or myocarditis (inflammation of the heart wall).

Normal, anticipated reactions to parenteral administration of sympathomimetics should be limited to cardiac palpitations and tachycardia. If these signs do occur, the animal should be treated so as to avoid further increases in chronotropic activity. (Table 7-1 compares the potencies of the three sympathomimetics in terms of inotropic and chronotropic activity as well as ability to increase blood pressure.)

Sympathomimetics are sensitive to pH changes and will degrade rapidly outside their normal range of 4 to 5 (especially in an excessively alkaline environment). During times of cardiac arrest there is the temptation to medications in the same intravenous-administration bottle. Other acute-need cardiopulmonary drugs, such as bronchodilators (for example, aminophylline), have pH ranges in the vicinity of 11. Thus their mixture with sympathomimetics immediately destroys the sympathomimetics.

Since the sympathomimetics are usually the most important drugs given during cardiac failure, their full potency should be safeguarded by not mixing any other drugs with them in the same bottle.

CARDIAC REGULATORS (DIGITALIS GLYCOSIDES)

Digitalis glycosides are neither stimulators nor depressants of cardiac activity. They act to control arrhythmias by increasing inotropic activity while decreasing chronotropic activity; the net result is increased cardiac output, or, as it is often called, "increased functional capacity." Older textbooks refer to this as a "tonic" or "cardiotonic" effect, and as a result digitalis drugs are sometimes called "cardiotonic glycosides." Digitalis glycosides are obtained from plant sources, the most common being *digitalis purpurea* (named for its small purple flowers), commonly called "foxglove."

All the glycosides have the same core structure:

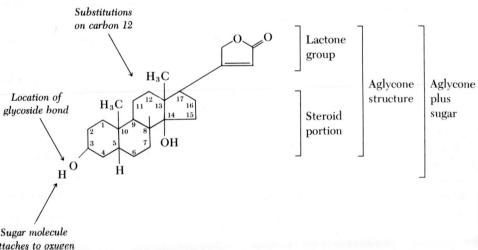

This structure is curiously similar in part to that of the steroidal hormones. The major difference is the addition of a lactone ring on carbon 17. The combination of the steroid portion and the lactone ring is called an "aglycone" or "genin" structure. In addition, all the digitalis-derived cardiac glycosides have a sugar molecule attached to the steroidal portion, usually at carbon 3. The attachment is by means of a glycoside bonding type of reaction, in which the particular sugar and the genin join, release a water molecule, and are consequently bonded by an oxygen atom; hence the name cardiac glycosides: "cardiac" for their pronounced action on the heart and "glycoside" for the chemical bond that forms the active drug. All glycosides obtained from the genus *digitalis* have the same basic aglycone and differ only in the substitutions at the carbon 12 position and the type of sugar substitution. Digitoxin, for example, has two hydrogen atoms attached to carbon 12, while digoxin has a hydroxyl group ($-OH$) and a hydrogen atom attached to carbon 12. Both drugs have the same sugar molecule, digitoxose. The sugar portion affects the potency of a glycoside by influencing its solubility and pharmacokinetic properties. It must be emphasized that *Digitalis* plants are considered *poisonous* (as is the medication derived from them) if consumed in large enough amounts, since they affect normal cardiac rhythm.

Like all other medications, digitalis glycosides are not benign in excessive doses, which can lead to "digitalis intoxication" and death.

Pharmacological action

As was mentioned in the opening remarks to this section, it is more correct to call the cardiac glycosides "cardiac regulators" rather than stimulators or depressants. Their clinical effect is to correct various arrhythmias in a way that strengthens the inotropic activity (myocardial contraction) while decreasing the chronotropic activity (rate of contraction). As the *force* of systole is *increased*, the *rate* of myofibril contraction is *decreased*, and thus the heart has more time to rest between beats; consequently it has more time to adequately fill its chambers with venous blood. Contractions thus will pump more blood into the systemic circulation to sustain blood pressure, avoid edema, and attain adequate oxygen perfusion of all tissue.

The exact mechanism that produces this result is not fully understood; however, certain definable effects of the glycosides on myofibril activity give us insight into the etiological basis for this clinical response. The contractile force of myofibrils is dependent on calcium ion concentration in the myocardium. Once calcium enters a contractile cell, such as a skeletal muscle fiber or myofibril, it initiates a series of reactions that end with activation of the enzyme adenosine triphosphatase (ATPase). ATPase releases the energy needed for contraction (shortening) of the fibril. Up to a certain concentration, the more calcium available the more energy released and therefore the stronger the inotropic effect. Digitalis glycosides increase the concentration of calcium ions within the fibril, presumably by facilitating their entrance at the time of depolarization. The increase in the number of calcium ions promotes a more forceful contraction.

The early view that digitalis's ability to increase oxygen uptake by myocardial tissue was responsible for the increased inotropic activity has not been substantiated by newer testing techniques.

Digitalis glycosides also (1) depress chronotropic activity, by decreasing the conduction velocity of impulses arising primarily from the AV node, and (2) reduce the number of impulses emitted from the SA node per unit of time. The decrease in the velocity of impulse conduction is believed to be due to the glycosides' effect on the movement of potassium ions in the myocardium. Digitalis glycosides promote potassium migration out of the fibril (potassium efflux) while also promoting sodium ion entrance (sodium influx) into the fibril. The greater the potassium efflux, the longer it will take the sodium pump to reestablish the ratio of sodium and potassium across the membrane that existed before stimulation. In other words, a longer refractory period will be required before the fibril becomes polarized and thus able to contract again. As with neuronal and skeletal muscle tissue, myofibrils cannot be stimulated during most of the refractory period. Hence, the longer the refractory period, the smaller the number of contractions that can occur during a period of time; the result is decreased chronotropic activity. Another in vivo action of digitialis glycosides that is believed to somewhat affect chronotropic activity is their ability to increase vagus stimulation of the myocardium. Increased vagus nerve stimulation results in a slowing of the nodal impulse emission rate.[2] However, this does not seem to be as important a factor as the role digitalis glycosides play with respect to electrolytes—specifically calcium, sodium, and potassium. In summary, *changes caused by the digitalis glycosides in calcium ion concentration are responsible for the effect on inotropic activity, while changes in potassium ion movement affect the rate of electrical conduction of impulses and thus the chronotropic activity.*

Pharmacokinetics

The clinical effects of cardiac glycosides are due to their accumulation in the body. No effect is demonstrable until adequate amounts have accumulated in myocardial tissue. Unlike the situation with regard to most drugs, the therapeutic effects of the glycosides are not related to blood levels. Administration is usually by the oral route; however, absorption varies among the individual cardiac glycosides. Intravenous administration likewise produces variable results; even this route of administration does not produce consistent results in terms of onset of activity and myocardial tissue concentrations of the drugs. This is due to differences in protein binding and penetration among the various glycosides. These differences result largely from the different sugar molecules attached to the aglycone portion of the drug.

The glycosides are distributed to most tissue, with highest concentrations found in myocardium, intestine, liver, and kidneys. They cross placental barriers. Studies in dogs demonstrate that concentrations of digitoxin (one of the cardiac glycosides) in the heart of a fetus can be up to twice those found in the heart of the mother, while concentrations of digoxin (another glycoside) in fetal blood have been found to be equivalent to the concentrations in the blood of the bitch. This situation is indicative of the difference in elimination rates between digitoxin and digoxin. In addition, arrthymias resulting from cardiac glycoside intoxication have been observed to appear simultaneously in the mother and fetus.[2] Cardiac glycosides also appear in the milk of nursing animals. Since they have a dramatic impact on cardiac function, a practitioner who contemplates their administration to nursing animals should consider the inevitable effects on the developing heart of the offspring. The sugar molecule also affects the cardiac glycosides' rate of detoxification in the liver and at other sites. Considerable variation in the degree of hepatic detoxification is exhibited among the cardiac glycosides. As would be expected, those requiring longer times to be eliminated are the ones that generally accumulate faster in the system and thereby exhibit a clinical effect sooner. Detoxification by the liver includes hydroxylation and/or conjugation, as evidenced by the cardiac glycosides' glucuronide derivatives being found in urine. The cardiac glycosides' elimination rates closely correlate with the degree of accumulation; the longer it takes to attain therapeutic blood levels, the quicker the drugs are eliminated.

Currently the two most commonly used digitalis glycosides are digoxin and digitoxin. Equal concentrations of digitoxin and digoxin within the myocardium elicit equivalent responses. Both are preferably administered by the oral route. The oral dose of digitoxin is the same as its intravenous dose, indicating good absorption from the gastrointestinal tract. The oral dose of digoxin exceeds its intravenous dose because of erratic absorption from the gastrointestinal tract. However, oral water-and-alcohol solutions (elixirs) of digoxin require a lower dose than do tablets, presumably because alcohol enhances the movement of the glycoside across the intestinal walls. For both drugs, absorption from intramuscular and intravenous routes is erratic and intramuscular injection is painful.[2] Digitoxin is detoxified much slower than digoxin and thus accumulates quicker. Clinically this results in a quicker onset of measurable activity and a longer duration of action. This also makes digitoxin a potentially more toxic drug than digoxin, and for this reason digitoxin is used less often than digoxin.

As is true of other medications, factors such as an animal's age and general health (especially hepatic and kidney function) are considerations that affect the dose and the administration schedule.

Indications

Digitalis glycosides are used chiefly in the prophylactic management and treatment of clinical congestive heart failure and in controlling the rate of ventricular contractions in animals with atrial fibrillation. The rationale for the use of these drugs in congestive (edematous) conditions is that an increase in functional capacity will cause increased movement of blood in the cardiovascular system. This relieves sluggish circulation, which causes excessive pooling of blood. The pooling of blood is responsible for edematous conditions of the lungs as well as the heart. By suppressing the initiation of atrial impulses as well as their conduction velocity, digitalis glycosides depress the rate of ventricular contractions, since the SA nodal tissue acts as pacemaker for the heart's chronotropic activity. Generally, cardiac glycosides exhibit their best clinical responses in cases of diminished cardiac output and hyperstimulation of atrial fibrils resulting from a variety of reasons.

Side effects and drug interactions

Since digitalis glycosides have a low therapeutic index (see Chapter 2 for an explanation of therapeutic index), side effects are to be expected. As was indicated previously, the general health of an animal determines the dose; poor health predisposes an animal to digitalis glycoside intoxication (poisoning) by reducing the margin between toxic and effective doses. Conditions such as hypercalemia (high calcium level) and hypokalemia (low potassium level) tend to mimic the effects of the glycosides, thereby potentiating these drugs' effects. The longer the duration of heart disease prior to treatment, the smaller the margin between toxic and effective doses; hence the lower the therapeutic index. Davis reports that in such cases it is "not uncommon to encounter a patient in which the effective dose of a glycoside may be 90% of the toxic dose."[2] This produces a therapeutic index of 1.1!

Initial signs of excessive digitalis glycoside accumulation in dogs and cats are usually anorexia, vomiting, and diarrhea; these symptoms are more severe with digoxin than with the other glycosides. Other signs that usually follow include depression, muscle weakness, stupor, and visual disturbances. Almost any cardiac arrhythmia can occur with or after these latter symptoms.[2] A slowing of cardiac activity, to the point of heart block, can occur, or paradoxical hyperstimulation (for example, ventricular tachycardia) may be observed. At this point, therapy is usually discontinued and the dose is reevaluated on the basis of serum electrolyte levels. How long the administration of the drug is discontinued, if it is not stopped entirely, depends upon the drug's rate of elimination.

As would be expected, drugs that act to increase the rate of detoxification of cardiac glycosides are the ones that stimulate the microsomal enzymes responsible for degradation of the glycosides; these drugs include barbiturates, primidone, and phenylbutazone. This increased rate of detoxification causes quicker-than-anticipated elimination of the glycosides—and of the other, enzyme-inducing drugs—thereby resulting in subtherapeutic concentrations of all the drugs.

Certain non-enzyme-inducing drugs, when administered concurrently with the glycosides, act to *decrease* the glycosides' absorption rate. This effect is separate from liver-related activity, it is concerned with activity in the gastrointestinal tract.

Generally, non-enzyme-inducing drugs either destroy bacteria responsible for absorption or bind (by adsorption) the cardiac glycosides so that they are not absorbed. Examples of these drugs are the anti-infectives neomycin and salicylazosulfapyridine (a sulfa drug). Adsorbent drugs include preparations containing kaolin and/or pectin, which are used as antidiarrheals, and most antacids.

Inhibition of microsomal enzymes causes the opposite effect, thus predisposing an animal to digitalis intoxication. Specifically, drugs that depress microsomal activity are considered incompatible with cardiac glycosides; these drugs include quinine, chloramphenicol, and all the tetracylcines.[2]

Cardiac glycosides generally are used with other medications, such as diuretics, and with diet regimens, such as low-sodium diets, to reduce the propensity for edema. As a result, it is difficult to assess the actual impact of a glycoside on the heart. Undoubtedly the use of glycosides as cardiac regulators will continue for many years, as will the controversy about their benefits as compared to their risks— namely digitalis glycoside intoxication. It seems doubtful, however, that the glycosides will be dropped from use. Instead their use may become more restricted, being limited to cases of heart failure resulting from unquestionable atrial hyperstimulation.[4]

CARDIAC DEPRESSANTS

Like the cardiac regulators, the drugs belonging to the cardiac depressant group— namely lidocaine, procainamide, propranolol, quinidine, phenytoin, and verapamil—all depress one or several aspects of cardiac activity. The fundamental difference between the cardiac depressants and the cardiac regulators is that the *depressants do not exhibit significant positive inotropic activity*. The inclusion of quinidine and phenytoin in this group can be controversial. Quinidine, as will be discussed shortly, can increase chronotropic activity. Phenytoin likewise tends to increase chronotropic activity, but by a different mechanism than quinidine. However, both quinidine and phenytoin have significant depressant actions on abnormal, hyperactive hearts. Therefore, for our purposes, they will be considered as antiarrhythmic drugs that function, at least in part, by depressing myocardial activity.

Quinidine

Pharmacological action

Although a majority of quinidine's pharmacological effects are concerned with depressing the myocardium, in therapeutic doses the drug can increase chronotropic activity. This increase results from (1) inhibition of vagal stimulation to the heart and (2) the response of the heart to decreased arterial blood pressure as a result of quinidine administration.[4] By pumping faster, the heart attempts to maintain blood pressure through increased blood flow rate.

Unquestionably quinidine's primary action on the myocardium is to depress its activity. This action is accomplished in the following ways:

1. By decreasing the rate of impulses emitted from pacemaker tissue
2. By slowing the velocity of impulse conduction through the contractile and conductive heart tissue (myofibrils and Purkinje fibers respectively)
3. By increasing refractory time of contractile and noncontractile heart tissue

These functions seem equivalent to those produced by the cardiac glycosides. The mechanism by which they are accomplished, however, seems to be related more to increasing the threshold for stimulation of cells (contractile and noncontractile) than to directly affecting electrolyte movement as is done by the glycosides. This is not to imply that electrolytes such as calcium are not affected in some way by quinidine. It may be that increasing the excitability threshold (action potential) of cells is partially related to inhibiting calcium influx into the cells. It also appears that quinidine may indeed share some of the actions of the glycosides, especially those related to prolongation of the refractory period.

Like the digitalis glycosides, quinidine is obtained from a botanical source the bark of trees of the genus *Cinchona*. As is evident from the boxed material on p. 219, quinidine's chemical structure is unlike that of the digitalis glycosides.

Pharmacokinetics

Quinidine is predictably and well absorbed from the gastrointestinal tract, with peak plasma levels in dogs occurring within 60 to 90 minutes. Its half-life in dogs and cats is 5.6 and 1.9 hours, respectively. Like the glycosides, quinidine depends upon accumulation in the myocardium to exert its action. Since it is eliminated much quicker than the glycosides, in order to obtain a cumulative effect it is usually administered ever 4 to 6 hours, in dogs.[2] Like digitalis glycosides, quinidine depends upon accumulation for an optimal response. Like the steroids and the digitalis glycosides, doses of quinidine are largely empirical, depending upon beneficial as well as adverse reactions by the animal. Quinidine is detoxified in the liver in both dogs and cats.[2] It is effective when administered intramuscularly or intravenously. Injectable and oral solutions of quinidine slowly acquire a brownish tint on exposure to light, which may also result in precipitation of the drug. Thus only colorless, clear solutions of quinidine (usually the gluconate salt) should be administered. Unlike the glycosides, quinidine must be used with caution in cases of heart congestion. *If inotropic activity is already compromised, quinidine will decrease it even more.* Although some forms of arrhythmias require concurrent administration of both glycosides and quinidine, the latter cannot always be considered as a substitute for the glycosides in cases of digitalis glycoside intoxication.

Structures of commonly used cardiac depressants*

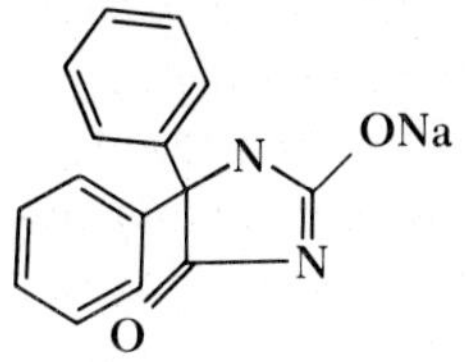

Phenytoin

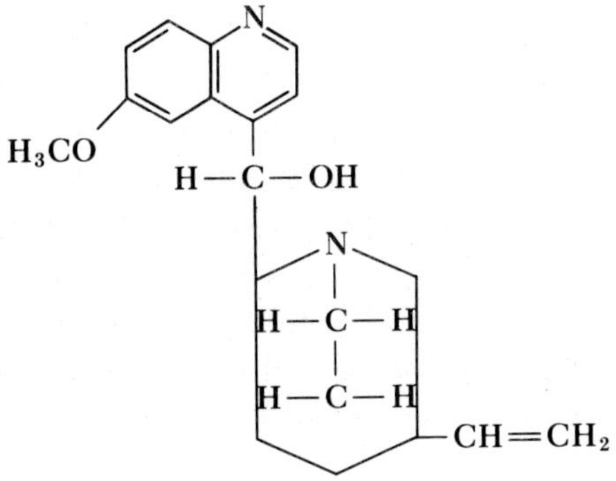

Quinidine

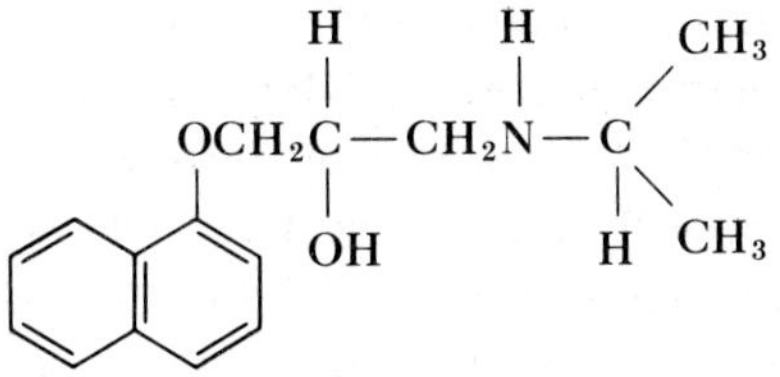

Propranolol

PROCAINE AND ITS DERIVATIVES

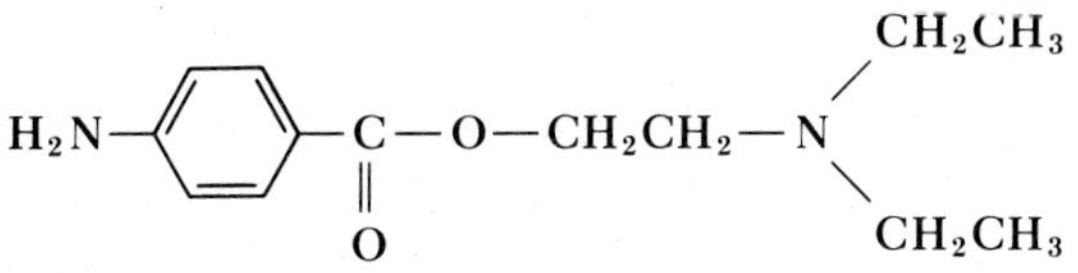

$$H_2N-\langle\ \rangle-C-O-CH_2CH_2-N\begin{matrix}CH_2CH_3\\\\CH_2CH_3\end{matrix}$$

Procaine

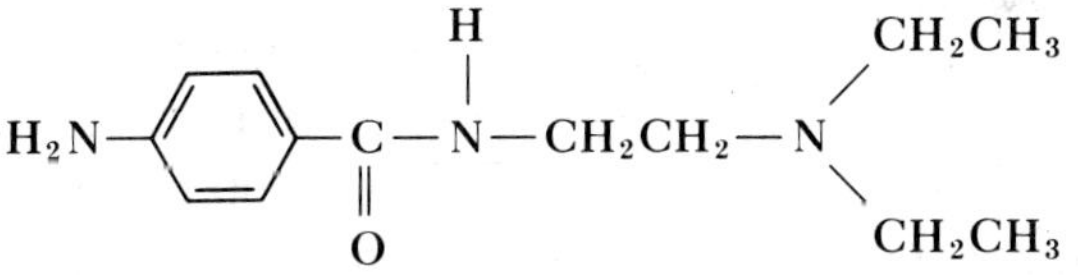

Procainamide

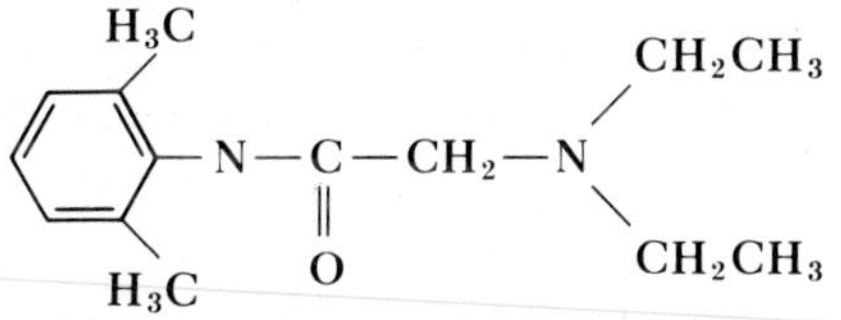

Lidocaine

*Procainamide and lidocaine are derived from procaine; their relationship is more apparent if one looks at the structure of procainamide and compares it to that of procaine. Propranolol, unlike any of the other cardiac depressants, acts by competitive inhibition to block beta receptors from becoming stimulated by cardiac stimulants such as epinephrine.

Indications

Quinidine is used in the prophylactic management and treatment of certain atrial and ventricular arrhythmias. Initially the intravenous route is preferred, especially for emergency treatment. Quinidine can be combined with another cardiac depressant and/or a digitalis glycoside in patients in whom increases in the dosage of either drug would result in toxic reactions.

Side effects and drug interactions

Signs of quinidine intoxication mimic those of the glycosides, both in the nature of the symptoms and in the time of onset. Specifically, they include vomiting (as a result of CNS vomit center stimulation rather than any direct action on the stomach mucosa), diarrhea, depression, uncoordination, and occasionally convulsions.[4] Other serious side effects directly related to cardiac function include AV block (impairment of impulse conduction between atria and ventricles) and bradycardia (significant decrease in chronotropic activity).

Quinidine is a potent inhibitor of hepatic microsomal enzymes; thus it can dramatically intensify and prolong the pharmacological effects of drugs that are degraded by these enzymes, most notably the CNS depressants.

Procainamide

Procainamide is a derivative of the local anesthetic procaine (see the box on p. 219). Although the exact mechanism of its antiarrhythmic action is not fully understood, it appears to be very closely related to that of quinidine. Like quinidine, procainamide appears to depress the susceptibility of cardiac muscle to electrical stimulation, probably by raising the threshold resistance capacity. Also like quinidine, procainamide decreases the velocity of impulse conduction and prolongs the refractory period.

Procainamide is effective by the oral route, with clinical results usually being apparent within 30 minutes in dogs. It is also effective when administered by the intramuscular and intravenous routes. Since the drug can produce significant peripheral vasodilation, its administration by the intravenous route should be closely monitored. Too rapid infusion can result in marked hypotension as a result of the drug's vasodilating properties. Thus the intravenous administration of procainamide to dogs with preexisting low blood pressure should be done with constant monitoring.

Procainamide is widely distributed in the body, with highest concentrations appearing in the heart and the kidneys. It undergoes degradation in plasma and the liver.

This drug is primarily used to abolish premature ventricular beats and to manage ventricular tachycardia. The usual intravenous dose for life threatening tachycardia is 100 mg/minute[9]; administration is continued until a more normal heart rate develops. Symptoms of procainamide toxicity are similar to those of quinidine toxicity. If a dog receiving procainamide becomes anorexic, vomits, or develops electrocardiographic abnormalities that specifically indicate depressed cardiac function, the drug should be discontinued.[4]

Lidocaine

Lidocaine is also a derivative of procaine. Lidocaine's mechanism of action was discussed in Chapter 4, in the section dealing with local anesthetics. It was postulated that the drug may prevent depolarization by interfering with enzymatic activity responsible for shifts of sodium and potassium across cell membranes. This same mechanism could account for its ability to depress the excitability of myofibrils. As a result of this depression, the fibrils are less prone to contract in response to premature impulses (which are not always as strong as scheduled ones). Lidocaine differs from procainamide and quinidine in that it does not reduce the velocity of impulse conduction or increase the refractory period.[2] Like the other cardiac depressants, lidocaine does not significantly affect the inotropic action of the heart. Unlike procainamide, lidocaine is not indicated for long-term treatment, since its half-life (in dogs) is only about 11 minutes, with clinical effects lasting for only 10 to 20 minutes after administration is stopped. Lidocaine is intended for short-term control of ventricular arrhythmias. Clinically this drug is given by the intravenous route; usually a loading dose of 2 mg/kg is followed by a constant infusion of 120 μg/kg/minute,[2,4] which is continued until a more normal heart rate is achieved. Intravenous administration is not usually associated with hypotensive episodes. Toxic concentrations of lidocaine initially cause vomiting; if such concentrations are not reduced, convulsions will follow. Generally these symptoms are reversible if administration is stopped or the dosage reduced. The development of seizures is especially dangerous in animals that are predisposed to arrhythmias. Seizures place an added burden on the heart, which results in increased chronotropic activity. This hyperactivity of the myocardium promotes the development of arrhythmias.

Phenytoin

Phenytoin was also mentioned in Chapter 4. It has long been used as an anticonvulsant in humans and animals and more recently as an antiarrhythmic. As an anticonvulsant phenytoin suppresses renegade impulses, which are spontaneously emitted from clusters of pathogenic cerebral cells. Its use as an antiarrhythmic drug parallels its use as an anticonvulsant. Phenytoin is indicated for arrhythmias that result from impulses emitted from areas other than the SA node. Like cerebral tissue, the myocardium can give rise to areas capable of sending out electrical impulses. The resultant heart beat has its origin therefore in an abnormal area or "focus." The extra beat compromises cardiac output, since it occurs at a time when the chambers are not yet filled with blood; extra contractions thus result in less than a normal volume of blood being pumped. These abnormal locations are called "ectopic foci" (ectopic = out of place).

Phenytoin's action in the myocardium is similar to its cerebral activity. Its CNS action prevents unwanted impulses from spreading over the brain by depleting cerebral sodium concentrations. An imbalance in the sodium-to-potassium ratio compromises the ability of a cell to depolarize. As is true of its action in the brain, phenytoin seems to be somewhat selective for abnormal myocardial tissue foci. In the heart it reduces the ability of ectopic pacemakers to emit impulses. Part of this action is related to sodium depletion, which "stabilizes" fibrils and thus prevents depolarization. Fibrils of ectopic foci have threshold (membrane potential) values lower than normal fibrils and as such are more prone to become "self-stimulating." Stabilization of these fibrils as a result of sodium depletion may depress self-stimulation by decreasing the electrical potential across the membrane. The effect produced mimics that of raising the threshold resistance value so that it approaches normalcy. Phenytoin apparently does not significantly affect the membrane potential of normal cells, since it does not slow down impulse conduction in normal cardiac musculature. In this respect it differs from procainamide and quinidine, since they do decrease the velocity of impulse conduction.[2]

As a result of its somewhat characteristic affinity for pathological cardiac tissue, phenytoin can be used for management of ventricular arrhythmias resulting from premature electrical impulses emitted from ectopic pacemakers. It has not been of value in treating atrial fibrillation. Phenytoin is also useful in treatment of arrhythmias resulting from digitalis glycosides or procainamide therapy.[2]

As was noted in the discussion of this drug as an anticonvulsant, phenytoin's use in dogs and cats is limited because of the way it is detoxified. In dogs it has a relatively short half-life (3 hours). Since the half-life is dose dependent, increasing the dose increases the duration of effect. Clinically, approximately 30 mg/kg is needed every 6 to 8 hours to control arrhythmias for which phenytoin is indicated. The resultant doses are on the high side of accepted values, thereby promoting side effects of ataxia (loss of muscle coordination), nystagmus (repeating oscillation of the eyeball), and gingival hyperplasia. In addition, excessively rapid intravenous infusion can cause hypotension.

The pH of an intravenous solution of phenytoin is approximately 11, and therefore the solution is extremely irritating to tissue. As a result pain, tissue necrosis, and inflammation at the injection site can be expected. Injections of the drug should be followed by administration of sodium chloride injection through the same needle or catheter (if it is to remain in the vein) to flush out residual phenytoin solution so that local irritation can be avoided. Because of phenytoin's high pH, other drugs should not be mixed with it in the same intravenous-administration bottle, since they would, in most cases, be degraded in the alkaline environment. Because the solution is so irritating, it should not be given by the intramuscular route.

Propranolol

The discussion of cardiac stimulants (catecholamines) pointed out the theoretical presence of beta receptors on myocardial tissue. Their stimulation by catecholamines is thought to be responsible for contraction of the fibril. A class of drugs known as beta receptor blockers has been developed, and as their name implies, they function to block stimulation of the fibrils by endogenous substances such as epinephrine released by the sympathetic (adrenergic) system. Like other drugs that function by competitive inhibition, the beta blockers have an affinity for certain tissue receptor sites, migrate to them, and inhibit receptor stimulation by occupying the receptor sites. Lack of stimulation causes depression of cellular function, in this case resulting in depressed cardiac activity. Specifically, competitive inhibition of the beta receptors that are normally stimulated by catecholamines results in decreased chronotropic and inotropic activity. The conduction rate through the SA and AV nodes is decreased, and systolic pumping time is increased. Prolonging the systolic time enables a maximum volume of blood to be pumped, thereby maximizing cardiac output. As a result, even though inotropic action is decreased, cardiac efficiency is still improved, because of the extension of contraction time.

Initially the blockade of beta receptors in the vascular system causes constriction of blood vessels, leading to some resistance to blood flow; however this tends to decrease after long-term administration of the beta blockers. Like the catecholamines, the beta blockers also exhibit a multitude of other effects on the body, but their most significant effects known to date are concerned with the cardiovascular system.

The first commercially available beta blocker was propranolol (its structure is shown on p. 219), which has become the standard of comparison for the newer agents. As newer drugs become available, it is expected that one of their advantages will be that they are more selective to cardiac tissue than propranolol. Increasing cardiac selectivity decreases the scope of side effects resulting from the blockade of beta receptors on other organs.

Propranolol is useful as an anti-arrhythmic drug for various types of cardiac hyperstimulation (tachyarrhythmias). It can also be used with digitalis glycosides in reducing the ventricular rate and atrial fibrillation. Propranolol should not be given if quinidine levels are detectable in the bloodstream, since the effects of the two drugs are additive; overt cardiac depression leading to heart failure is likely.

Propranolol is effective by the oral and intravenous routes. In dogs, up to 5 mg/kg can be given intravenously (at a rate of 1 mg every 1 to 2 minutes); oral doses in dogs range from 5-40 mg. Subsequent oral doses may have to be reduced after the initial dose to avoid accumulation to concentrations that may lead to excessive depression of the myocardium. Although the bioavailability of orally administered propranolol is low, longer periods of time are required to eliminate equal amounts of the drug as administration continues.[2]

As would be expected, propranolol will interfere with the actions of the cate-cholamines, and vice versa. In fact, if the effects of propranolol must be reversed, surprisingly large doses of isoproterenol will be required. Phenothiazine-type drugs (tranquilizers, antihistamines, and anthelmintics) may have an additive hypotensive action if they are administered concurrently with propranolol.

Since propranolol has a negative inotropic action, its use in animals with inad-equate myocardial function should be monitored closely. Congestive heart failure could rapidly occur in such circumstances.

Verapamil

Verapamil is one of a group of drugs known as calcium channel blockers, which represent the newest approach to management of arrthymias resulting from hyper-stimulation of myocardial tissue.

Depolarization, sodium influx, and potassium efflux are accompanied by the influx of calcium ions into contractile and noncontractile (conductile) cells such as those of the myocardium. As was explained more fully in the section on digitalis glycosides, the degree of inotropic activity is proportional to the amount of calcium in the fibril. Likewise, electrical activity through the SA and AV nodes depends on calcium ion influx. Inhibition of this influx (1) slows AV conduction, (2) prolongs the refractory period, and (3) diminishes the ionotropic activity of contractile myo-cardial cells. As has been discussed before, two major processes occur in the heart: (1) electrical excitation, induced by pacemaker cells and conducted by noncontrac-tile tissue, and (2) mechanical contraction of fibrils, produced by electrical excita-tion. The calcium ion is needed for both processes. If the availability of calcium within the contractile or conductile cell is reduced, the magnitude of contraction and impulse initiation is reduced.

By inhibiting the influx of calcium ions through "channels" in the cell mem-brane, verapamil reduces the calcium concentration in contractile and conductile cells.[3] To date verapamil has proved beneficial in treating ventricular tachyarrhyth-mias. Intravenous administration must be accompanied by constant monitoring for signs of excessive cardiac depression. Verapamil has been used in humans, along with concurrent, oral administration of a digitalis glycoside, quinidine, procainam-ide, and/or propranolol, without serious side effects, although strict monitoring for cardiac depression is required because of the additive effects of the drugs. Whether verapamil will become a standard drug for the treatment of arrhythmias, in both humans and animals, has yet to be determined.

• • •

In the drug treatment of any pathological conditions, the effects of the drug(s) chosen must be proportional to the severity of the condition. Some cardiac condi-tions are best not treated with drugs, while others require aggressive drug therapy.

The risk associated with treatment must always be weighed against the risk posed by the pathological condition. Proper management of pathological conditions of the heart is especially crucial, since even a momentary delay in the functioning of the heart can result in permanent alteration of its functioning or in death. Proper therapy thus should be based on the ancient adage "First do no more harm."

REFERENCES

1. Brander, G.C., and Pugh, D.M.: Veterinary-applied pharmacology and therapeutics, ed. 2, London, 1971, Baillière Tindall.
2. Kirk, R.W.: Current veterinary therapy, Philadelphia, 1980, W.B. Saunders Co., vol. 7, Small animal practice.
3. Knoll Pharmaceutical Company: Calcium in cardiac metabolism, publication 1011, Whippany, N.J., 1980.
4. Spinelli, J.S., and Enos, L.R.: Drugs in veterinary practice, St. Louis, 1978, The C.V. Mosby Co.

A

Guide for intravenous administration of drugs

The following chart lists medications discussed in this book that can be administered by the intravenous route. A symbol is used for medications that should not be mixed together in the same container or that are therapeutically antagonistic when given at the same time. *It is important to note that the absence of a symbol does not mean that the two drugs are compatible, but only that no data have been found to document their incompatibility.*

The mixing of intravenous medications in the same container should always be done with strict aseptic technique. Before the drugs are added to the solution, glass bottles should be checked for cracks, especially around and under where the hanging ring is attached. Intravenous-administration bags should be lightly squeezed to determine if pinhole-size punctures are present.

Rarely will intravenous drug incompatibilities result in a visible change in a solution. The overwhelming number of interactions between medications result in the creation of a new substance(s) that is water soluble and thus invisible. It is not wise, therefore, to determine the compatibility of mixed drugs solely on the basis of visual inspection. Intravenous-administration procedures must be based on complete, up-to-date information about the compatibilities of drugs in solution.

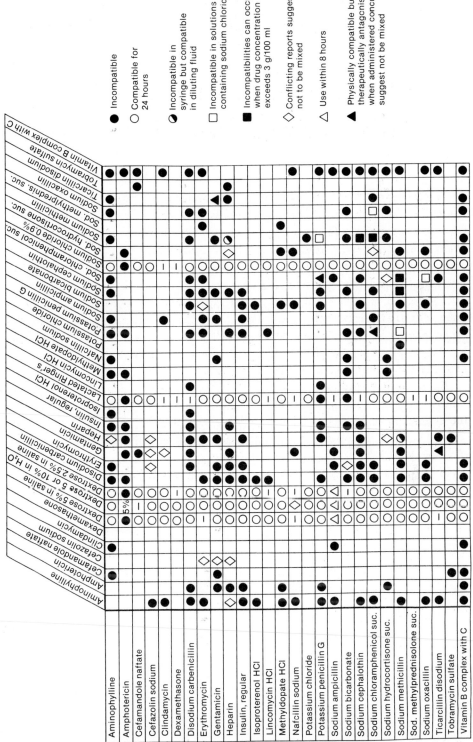

Legend:

● Incompatible

○ Compatible for 24 hours

◑ Incompatible in syringe but compatible in diluting fluid

□ Incompatible in solutions containing sodium chloride

■ Incompatibilities can occur when drug concentration exceeds 3 g/100 ml

◇ Conflicting reports suggest not to be mixed

△ Use within 8 hours

▲ Physically compatible but therapeutically antagonistic when administered concurrently; suggest not be mixed

B

Federal classification of and regulations for addictive drugs

Since some drugs that affect the central nervous system are considered to be addictive to humans, persons who prescribe and/or handle them must conform to regulations set forth by the federal and state governments.

The Drug Enforcement Agency (DEA), a division of the Treasury Department, regulates drug prescribing, handling, and storage. Drugs that are considered addicting are categorized by the DEA into five "schedules." Any drug that is considered a "schedule drug" must have a "C" on the label of its container. In addition, the roman numeral I, II, III, IV, or V must be present. For example, a drug listed in Schedule II would have the designation "CII" on its label. *The lower the roman numeral, the more potentially addicting the drug*.

The following table lists some of the more commonly used drugs in each schedule. When possible, drugs have been listed under headings used in this book. For example, morphine is listed under opiate analgesics, as it is in Chapter 4.

It should be noted that the information listed in this appendix is based on federal regulations. State regulations are allowed to be stricter, but not less strict, than federal regulations. Thus a state may decide to place a particular drug in Schedule II while federal regulations place it in Schedule III.

	Drugs	Comments regarding regulations
Schedule I C_I	Heroin Lysergic acid diethylamide (LSD) Marijuana Mescaline Peyote	Drugs in Schedule I are considered to have the highest potential for abuse and to have no recognized medical use in the treatment of disease. Although marijuana is currently under investigation for its anti-glaucoma and anti-nausea properties, to date evidence indicating that it is safe and efficacious for these indications is inconclusive. Drugs in Schedule I are not generally available to medical practitioners.

Schedule II C_{II}	Opiate analgesics
	  Codeine
	  Morphine
	  Opium tincture
	Semi-synthetic opiate analgesics
	  Dihydrocodeine
	  Oxycodone
	  Oxymorphone
	Nonopiate analgesics
	  Fentanyl
	  Fentanyl with droperidol
	  Meperidine
	Short-acting barbiturate hypnotics (oral and injectable)
	  Pentobarbital
	  Amobarbital
	  Secobarbital
	Stimulants
	  Dextroamphetamine
	  Methylphenidate
	Cocoa leaves and derivatives
	  Cocaine
		Drugs in this schedule are considered potentially less addicting than those in Schedule I but more addicting than those in Schedule III.
		They are available for use by medical practioners.
		No more than a 30-day supply may be prescribed in most situations.
		Prescriptions for drugs in this schedule must be filled within 5 days of the time they are written or they automatically are considered void.
		Prescriptions for these drugs should always be written.
		These drugs must be stored in a locked container or a vault.
		Records as to what has been received and what has been used must be maintained.
		Written documentation of inventory must be done annually.

Continued.

	Drugs	*Comments regarding regulations*

Schedule III
 	
C_{III}
	Opiate and nonopiate analgesics
	  In amounts smaller than those required for Schedule II classification (alone or combined with nonscheduled drug[s])
	Short-acting barbiturate hypnotics
	  In amounts smaller than those required for Schedule II classification (alone or combined with nonscheduled drug[s])
	  In any amount, but in suppository form
	Intravenous anesthetics
	  Thiamylal
	  Thiopental
		Prescriptions may be telephoned to a pharmacy.
		Schedule III drugs are not required to be locked in a container or a vault, but it is good practice to do so.
		Schedule III drugs do not have to be inventoried annually, and records of receipts and issues do not have to be kept; however, it is good practice to do so.

Schedule IV
 	
C_{IV}
	Tranquilizers
	  Chlordiazepoxide
	  Diazepam
	Nonbarbiturate hypnotics
	  Chloral hydrate
	  Ethchlorvynol
	  Ethinamate
	  Flurazepam
	  Paraldehyde
	Long-acting barbiturate hypnotics
	  Phenobarbital
		Prescriptions for Schedule IV drugs may be refilled.
		Prescriptions for these drugs may be telephoned to a pharmacy.

Schedule V **C**_V	Opiate derivatives In amounts smaller than those required for Schedule III classification	The drugs and/or their amounts in this schedule are considered to have the lowest potential for addiction or abuse. Although not required by federal law, it is good practice to keep a list of patients receiving these drugs and the frequency with which they obtain them.

Index

A

Acetaminophen, 65-66
  action of, 66
  as analgesic, 62
  detoxification of, 65-66
  dosage of, 66
Acetanilid, 65
Acetazolamide, 50
Acetylcholinesterase, 69-70
Acetylpromazine, 94
Acetylsalicylic acid, 65
Acetylsulfisoxazole, 148
ACTH; *see* Adrenocorticotropic hormone
Actinobacillus, 133
Actinomyces, 138
Addison's disease, 178, 181
Adenosine monophosphate, 174
Adipose tissue
  barbiturate distribution in, 80-82
  drug distribution in, 32
  excessive, effect of, on drug, 34
Adrenalin, 210
Adrenocortical hormones, 169-192
  glucocorticosteroids, 172-175
  mineralocorticosteroids, 172
Adrenocortical insufficiency, 178
Adrenocorticoids, 169
  endogenous, release of, 169-172
Adrenocorticotropic hormone, 170, 185
Adrenocorticotropin, 170
Aerobacter, 117, 121, 137
Aldosterone, 54, 169
Alkaloids, 69
Allergens, 155
  in immunological trauma, 165
Alpha-endorphin, 75
Amikacin, 131, 133
  indications for use, 134
7-Aminocephalosporonic acid, 116
Aminoglycosides, 131-136
  absorption of, 132
  administration of, routes of, 136
  antibacterial spectrum and resistance to, 132-133

Aminoglycosides—cont'd
  distribution of, 132
  dosage patterns for, 134
  indications for use, 134-136
  ototoxicity of, 132
  pharmacokinetics of, 133-134
  pharmacological activity of, 132
6-Aminopenicillanic acid, 111
Aminophylline
  as gastrointestinal tract irritant, 8
  with penicillin, 40
  pH of, 9
Amobarbital, 87
Amoxicillin
  as acid-stable drug, 5
  antibacterial spectrum of, 113
  resistance to, 108
Amphotericin B, 139
Ampicillin, 108
  as acid-stable drug, 5
  antibacterial spectrum of, 113
  half-life of, 116
  structure of, 110
Analgesics
  acetaminophen, 65-66
  classification and comparison of, 63
  endogenously secreted, 75
  fentanyl, 74-75
  function of, 62
  ibuprofen, 68
  indomethacin, 68
  meclofenamic acid, 68
  meperidine hydrochloride, 74
  naproxen, 68
  narcotic, 68-75
    purpose of, 59
  nonnarcotic, 62-68
    purpose of, 59
  nonopiate, 73-75
  opiate, 69-73
  pentazocine, 68
  potencies of, relative, 76
  pyrazolone derivatives, 66-67

Anaphylactic reaction, 165
  histamine in, 168
Anesthetic equilibrium, 85
Anesthetics, 76-85
  administration of, routes of, 76
  categories of, 76
  dibucaine, 77
  ethylaminobenzoate, 77
  ethyl chloride, 77
  general, 76, 78-84
    vs narcotics, 78
    purpose of, 59
  intravenous, 78-84
  lidocaine, 77
  local
    with hyaluronidase, 78
    purpose of, 59
    with vasoconstrictors, 77-78
  procaine, 77
  volatile, 84-85
Anhydrotetracycline, 120
Aniline, 62, 63
Antacids, 6
  magnesium ions in, 42
  with tetracyclines, 23
Anthelmintics, 23, 93, 153-154
Antibiotics, 105-147
  acid-stable, 5
  vs antibodies, 157
  discovery, detection, and isolation of, 106
  dose determination for, 39
  as endotoxins, 105
  guidelines for therapy, 146
  inhalation of, 21
  narrow vs wide spectrum, 106
  organisms producing, 106-107
  resistance to, 107-111
  for ruminants, 14
  side effects of, 145-147
  with steroidal therapy, 18, 186
  with vitamin administration, 18
Antibodies, 154
  antibacterial, 161
  vs antibiotics, 157
  antitoxic, 161
  classification of, 161
  exotoxin stimulation of, 155
  glucocorticosteroid effect on, 183
  inhibition of formation of, 174
  in serum, 161
  synthesis of, 156
Anticancer agents, 41
Anticoagulants, 67

Anticonvulsants, 97-102
  chemical classification of, 99
  imidazole-derived, 100-101
  purpose of, 59
  pyrimidine-derived, 101-102
Antifungal antibiotics, 18, 138-141
Antigens, 154
  antibody formation from exposure to, 156, 157
  bacterial, 159
  as exotoxins, 155
  in immunological trauma, 165
  as vaccines, 159
Antihistamines
  pharmacological activity of, 196-200
  and pyrazolone derivatives, 67
  side effects and drug interactions, 200-201
  in steroidal biodegradation, 186
  structure-activity relationships of, 196-200
  in trauma, 198
Anti-infective drugs, 105-154
  antibiotics, 106-147
  classification of, 109
  sulfonamides, 147-154
Anti-inflammatory drugs, 164-202
  antihistamines, 196-202
  betamethasone, 187-188
  corticosteroids, 175-187
  cortisone acetate, 188
  desoxycorticosterone acetate, 188-189
  dexamethasone, 189
  hydrocortisone, 189-190
  methylprednisolone, 190
  nonsteroidal, 192-196
    pharmacology and therapeutic indications, 192-194
    side effects and drug interactions of, 195-196
  prednisolone and prednisone, 191
  triamcinolone, 191-192
Antineoplastics, 41
Antiserum, 161
Antispasmodics, 69
Antitoxins, 161
Arrhythmias, 207
  digitalis glycosides for, 212
  lidocaine for, 221
  phenytoin for, 221, 222
  quinidine for, 220
Arthritis, 170
  corticosteroids for, 180
Arthropathy, crystalline, 180
Aspirin
  absorption of, in stomach vs small intestine, 10
  anti-inflammatory action of, 101

Aspirin—cont'd
  in delayed-release dosage form, 7
  as gastric irritant, 8
  toxicity from, 65
Ataractics, 90-102
  acetylpromazine, 94
  anticonvulsants, 97-102
  benzodiazepines, 95-97
  biochemical activity changes with, 91-92
  butyrophenones, 95
  chlorpromazine, 94
  CNS electrical function changes with, 92
  CNS neurotransmitter concentration changes
      with, 91
  meprobamate, 96
  perphenazine, 94
  pharmacology of, 91-92
  phenaglycodal, 96
  phenothiazines, 93-95
  promazine, 94
  trimeprazine, 94, 95
Ativan, 96
Atria, 206
Atrioventricular node, 204, 205
Atropine, 72
Attenuation of organisms, 158
Azaperone, 95

B

Bacillus, 121
Bacillus anthracis, 113
Bacillus cereus, 117
Bacillus subtilismesentericus, 113
Bacitracin, 136, 138
  absorption of, 21
Bacterin, 159
Bacteroides, 121
Barbital, 87
Barbiturates, 32, 34
  in adipose tissue, 80-82
  detoxification of, 83
  duration of activity, 87
  for epileptic seizures, 98
  as hypnotics, 86-89
  long-acting, 80
  oxybarbiturates, 80, 83
  partition coefficients of, 87
  pharmacology, distribution, and excretion of, 80,
      88-89
  with phenylbutazone, 42
  and pyrazolone derivatives, 67
  structure of, 78, 79, 80
  thiobarbiturates, 80, 83

Barbiturates—cont'd
  ultra-short-acting, 80, 82, 83
Benzhydroflumethiazide, 52
Benzocaine, 77-78
Benzodiazepines, 95-97
Benzothiadiazides, 52
Benzthiazide, 52
Benzyl alcohol, 83
Benzylpenicillin, 111
  as acid-labile drug, 3
Beta-endorphin, 75
Beta lactamase, 117
Betamethasone, 187-188
  relative activity of, 170
Bile, 36-37
Bioassay, 162
Biologicals, 154
Brain, drug distribution in, 33
Bromides, 98
Bronchodilators, 21
Brucellosis, 121
Butabarbital, 88
Butyrophenones, 95

C

Caffeine, 208
Calcium and tetracycline, 42
Candida albicans, 141
Capsules, 2
Carbenicillin, 108
  antibacterial spectrum of, 113
  half-life of, 116
  structure of, 110
Carbohydrates, 172
Carbonic anhydrase inhibitors, 48-50
  acidosis from, 50
  average dosage of, 50
  mechanism of action, 49
  side effects of, 50
Cardiac arrest, 208, 211
Cardiovascular drugs, 203-225
  depressants, 217-225
    lidocaine, 221
    phenytoin, 221-222
    procainamide, 220-221
    propranolol, 223-224
    quinidine, 217-220
    verapamil, 224-225
  regulators, 212-217
    indications for, 215-216
    pharmacokinetics of, 214-215
    pharmacological action of, 213-214
    side effects and drug interactions of, 216-217

Cardiovascular drugs—cont'd
  stimulants, 208-212
    administration precautions, 211-212
    drug interactions with, 211-212
    pharmacological action of, 208-210
Catecholamines
  phenothiazine effect on, 93
  as sympathomimetic amines, 208
  tranquilizer effects on, 91-92
Cefazolin, 117
Central nervous system
  corticosteroid effects on, 175
  drugs affecting, 58-103
    analgesics, 62-76
      narcotic, 68-75
      nonnarcotic, 62-68
      secreted endogenously, 75-76
    anesthetics, 76-85
      general, 77-85
      local, 77-78
    hypnotics, 85-90
      barbiturates, 86-89
      nonbarbiturates, 89-90
    tranquilizers, 90-102
      anticonvulsants, 97-102
      benzodiazepines, 95
      butyrophenones, 95-97
      pharmacology of, 91-92
      phenothiazines, 93-95
  modalities in, 60
  motor activity of, 59
  physiology of, 59-62
  receptor neurons of
    chemical, 59
    energy, 59
    exteroceptors, 60
    postganglionic, 59
    preganglionic, 59
    pressure, 59
    proprioceptor, 60
    visceral, 60
  sensory activity of, 59
  stimulants of, 102
Cephalexin, 5
Cephaloglycin, 119
  as acid-stable drug, 5
Cephaloridine, 117, 118-119
Cephalosporin, 116-119
  administration of, routes of, 117
  antibacterial spectrum and resistance to, 117
  classification of, 118
  discovery of, 106
  dosage ranges for, 117
  hematologic side effects of, 145

Cephalosporin—cont'd
  indications for use of, 118
  pharmacokinetics of, 117-118
  pharmacological activity of, 116-117
  renal tubular secretion of, 36
Cephalosporinases, 117
Cephalosporium cremonium, 116
Cephalothin, 117, 118-119
Cephapirin, 119
Cerebral cortex, 60
Chemoreceptors, 59
  activation of, 60
Cheyne-Stokes breathing, 84
Chlamydia, 121
Chloral hydrate, 89
Chloramphenicol, 141-143
  administration of, 142
  antibacterial spectrum and resistance, 142-143
  distribution of, 142
  dosages of, 143
  indications for use, 143
  pharmacological activity and pharmacokinetics of,
    141-142
Chlordiazepoxide, 90
  tranquilizing effect of, 95
Chloride
  hormonal regulation of, 169
  thiazide effect on, 51
  vs urine output, 47
Chlorothiazide, 52
Chlorpheniramine, 197
Chlorpromazine, 94
Chlortetracycline, 119
  bacterial spectrum of, 123, 124
  indications for use, 124
  pharmacokinetics of, 122
Cimetidine, 197
Citrobacter, 133
Clindamycin, 143-144
Clostridium, 113, 121, 138
Cloxacillin, 113
  as acid-stable drug, 5
Codeine, 73
  in opium, 69
Colitis, ulcerative, 14
Colon, drug absorption in, 15
Convulsions
  etiology of, 97-98
  pharmacology of, 98-100
Corticosteroids
  contraindications to, 186
  dosage concepts of, 184-185
  drug incompatibility with, 186-187
  drug interactions with, 186

Corticosteroids—cont'd
  natural and synthetic, 175-187
  ocular pressure increased with, 180
  pharmacokinetics of, 177-178
  side effects of, 180-184
  structure-activity relationships of, 176-177
  therapeutic uses of, 178-180
Corticotropin, 170
Corticotropin-releasing factor, 170
Cortisone, 188
  circadian cycle of, 185
  relative activity of, 170
Corynebacterium, 113, 121, 138
Crystalluria, 33, 151
Cushing's syndrome, 181

D

Dehydrobenzperidol, 95
Desoxycholate, 139
Desoxycorticosterone acetate, 188-189
Dexamethasone, 189
  as gastrointestinal tract irritant, 8
  relative activity of, 170
Dextroamphetamine, 102
Diabetes, 182-183
  and glucocorticosteroids, 186
Diastole, 204
Diazepam, 90
  administration of, 95
  intramuscular administration of, 15
  tranquilizing effect of, 95
Dibucaine, 77-78
Dichlorphenamide, 50
Dichlorvos, 153
Dicloxacillin
  acid resistance of, 113
  as acid-stable drug, 5
Diet in drug distribution, 33-34
Digestive systems, differences in, 13-14
Digitalis, 212-217
  efficacy of, in ruminants, 14
  indications for, 215-216
  pharmocokinetics of, 214-215
  pharmacological action of, 213-214
  side effects and drug interactions of, 216-217
Digitoxin, 213, 215
  biliary excretion of, 37
Digoxin, 215
Dihydrostreptomycin, 134-135
  dosage of, 136
  indications for use, 134
Dioctyl sodium sulfosuccinate, 23
Diphenoxylate, 70
Diphenylhydantoin, 98

Diphtheria, calf, 123, 143
Dipyrone, 67
Diuretics, 46-57
  for cardiac dysfunction, 204
  crossing placenta, 49-50
  ethyl alcohol, 54
  factors affecting strength of, 48
  mannitol, 56
  organomercurials, 53-54
  osmotic, 54-57
  spironolactone, 54
  tubular resorption inhibitors, 48-53
  urea, 56-57
Dopamine, 91
Dosages, drug, 23
Doxycycline, 124
Droperidol, 74-75
  as tranquilizer, 95
Drugs
  absorption of, 2-21
  acid-labile, 3
    biodegradation of, 3-4
    chemical alteration of, 4
  acid-stable, 4
  addictive, 228-230
  administration of, with food, 6
  affected by gastric secretions, 3-4
  affecting CNS, 58-102
    analgesics, 62-76
    anesthetics, 76-85
    hypnotics, 85-90
    purpose of, 59
    tranquilizers, 90-102
  affecting environmental pH, 42
  antagonism in actions of many, 40
  bacteriostatic vs bacteriocidal, 40
  bioavailability of, 23-24
  bioequivalence of, 24
  bound, 25
  carrier concept in movement of, 12, 13
  coating of, with acid-resistant agents, 6
  crossing placental barrier, 28, 29-31
  cumulation of, 39
  definition of, 2
  detoxification of, 26
    age as factor in, 27
    health status as factor in, 27-28
    limits of, 42-43
    sex as factor in, 28
  dissociation of, 9
  distribution of, 22-34
    in adipose tissue, 32
    blood-brain barrier in, 33
    concentration gradient in, 25

Drugs—cont'd
  distribution of—cont'd
    in fetal circulation, 28-31
    metabolic mechanisms in, 26-28
    nutritional status in, 33-34
    plasma-binding ability in, 25-26
  dosage of, 23
    determination of, 38-45
  efficacy of, vs bioavailability, 23
  elimination of, 35-45
    via biliary excretion, 36-37
    via intestinal excretion, 37
    via kidney excretion, 35-36
  enteric delayed-release forms of, 6
  enteric sustained-release forms of, 6-7
  free, 26
    in crossing placental barrier, 28
  frequency of administration, 38-45
  half-life of, biological, 26
  vs immunologicals, 154
  incompatibility of, 17-18
  inhalation of, 21
  interactions between, 41-43
  intravenous administration of, guide for, 226-227
  ionization of, 9
  kinetics of, 44
  lipid solubility of, 11
  loading dose of, 39
  metabolites of, 35
  multiple, in therapy, 39-40
  oral administration of, 2-14
    acid stability and lability with, 3-5
    differences in digestive systems and, 13-14
    enzymatic activity and membrane transport
      and, 11-13
    irritability with, 5-8
    partition coefficient in, 10-11
    pH in, 8-10
  parenteral administration of, 15-19
    via intradermal injection, 15
    via intramuscular injection, 16-17
    via intravenous injection, 17-19
    via subcutaneous injection, 16
  pH of, 8-10
  plasma-binding ability of, 25, 33
  protein-binding ability of, 25
  receptors for, 23
  rectal administration of, 14-15
    vehicle considerations, 15
  solubility of, 11
  summation in administration of many, 39
  topical administration of, 19-20
  toxic levels of, 39
  unbound, 20

E
Edema
  cardiac and pulmonary, 204
  in drug distribution, 34
Electrolytes
  furosemide effect on, 52
  hormonal regulation of, 169
  imbalance of, with pyrazolone-type anti-inflam-
    matory drugs, 195
  inhalation of, 21
  in membrane potentials, 61
  osmotic diuretic effect on, 55
  reabsorption of, in kidneys, 36
  vs urine output, 47-48
Emboli, 15, 17
Enema, 14
  steroidal, 15
Energy receptors, 59
Endorphins, 75
Endotoxins, 105
Enkephalin, 75
Enteritis, regional, 15
Enterobacter, 117, 133
Enzymes, 11-13
  conjugation, 27
  degrading drugs, 108
  in drug metabolism, 26
  hydrolysis, 27
  induction of, 28
    for drug detoxification, 42-43
  intestinal, 11
  mucolytic, 21
  oxidation, 27
  reduction, 27
  in renal drug transport, 35, 36
Epianhydrotetracycline, 120
Epinephrine
  as acid-labile drug, 3
  as cardiac stimulant, 210
  glucocorticosteroids in sensitizing cells to, 174
  and inflammatory response, 168-169
  with local anesthetics, 77
  phenothiazine effect on, 93
  release of, 170
  secretion of, by adrenal gland, 169
  tranquilizer effects on, 91
Erysipelothrix rhusiopathiae, 113
Erythromycin, 124
  administration of, 128-129
  as gastrointestinal tract irritant, 8
Escherichia, 117, 121, 133, 137
Ethchlorvynol, 89-90
Ethinamate, 89-90
Ethoxzolamide, 50

Ethyl alcohol, 54
Ethyl aminobenzoate, 77-78
Ethyl chloride, 77
Exotoxins, 155
  as antigens, 159-160
Exteroceptors, 60

F

Fat, 172
Fentanyl, 74-75
  vs morphine, 74
  piperidine ring of, 63
Fentanyl citrate, 74
  with droperidol, 74
Fetal circulation, 28-31
Fludrocortisone acetate, 179
Flumethasone, 8
Fluprednisone, 8
Flurazepam, 90
Folic acid, 149
Foot rot, 128, 143
Furosemide, 52, 53
  dosage of, 53
Fusobacterium, 138

G

Gamma-endorphin, 75
Gastroenteritis, 123
Gastrointestinal tract
  drug passage from, to blood, 12, 13
  irritating drugs to, 8
  secretions of, 5
Gentamicin, 133
  dosage for, 136
  indications for use of, 134
  structure of, 131
Gentian violet, 141
Glaucoma, 56
  treatment of, 48
Glial cells, 33
Glomerular filtration
  in drug excretion, 35-36
  rate of, 47
Glucocorticosteroids, 169, 172-175
  action of, 174
  CNS affected by, 175
  release of, 170
  synthesis of, 173-174
Gluconeogenesis, 172
Glycerol, 56
Glyconeogenesis, 172
Gout, 41
Gramicidin, 191

Griseofulvin, 139-140
  as acid-stable drug, 5
  detoxification of, 140

H

Haemophilus, 121, 137
Heart
  chronotropic and inotropic activity of, 204
    digitalis effect on, 212, 213
    epinephrine effect on, 210
    lidocaine effect on, 221
    quinidine effect on, 217, 218
  electrically functional areas of, 205
  impulse conduction through, 206-207
  pacemaker of, 205
  pathologic conditions of, 207
  rhythm of, 204-205
Heparin, 17
Hetacillin, 116
  as acid-stable drug, 5
  antibacterial spectrum of, 113
  resistance to, 108
Hexobarbital, 86
Histamine
  cardiovascular effect of, 167
  in immune response, 157
  in inflammatory response, 166-167
  receptors for, 196-197
  salicylate effect on, 64
Hormones
  adrenocortical, 169-192
    glucocorticosteroids, 172-175
    mineralocorticosteroids, 172
  in electrolyte reabsorption, 36
HPA axis and functions, 181
  cortisone acetate effect on, 188
Hyaluronidase, 78
Hydantoin drugs, 100
Hydrochlorothiazide, 51
Hydrocortisone, 189-190
  function of, 169
  as gastrointestinal tract irritant, 8
  relative activity of, 170
  secretion of, 172
Hydroflumethiazide, 52
Hypnotics, 85-90
  barbiturates, 86-89
  chloral hydrate, 89
  ethchlorvynol, 89-90
  ethinamate, 89-90
  flurazepam, 90
  nonbarbiturate, 89-90
  purpose of, 59, 85

Hypoadrenalism, 178
iatrogenic secondary, 180
Hypoadrenocorticism, 178
Hypocorticism, 181
Hypothalamus, 64

I

Ibuprofen, 68
action of, 193
structure of, 63
Immune response, 155-157
Immune serum, 161
Immunity, 154
active, 157
products for, 158-161
passive, 157
products for, 161-162
Immunological trauma, 165
Immunologicals, 154-162
for active immunity, 158
from bacteria, 159
classification of, 157-158
history of use, 154-155
Indomethacin
action of, 68
as nonsteroidal anti-inflammatory drug, 192-193
for patent ductus arteriosus, 207
structure of, 63
Inflammatory response
clinical manifestations of, 166
epinephrine in, 168-169
glucocorticosteroids in, 173
and trauma, 165-168
Influenza, feline, 123
Innovar-Vet, 74
Insulin
as acid-labile drug, 3
cerebral activity with administration of, 92
and steroid therapy, 186
subcutaneous administration of, 16
Intradermal injections, 15
Intramuscular injections, 15, 16-17
Intravenous injections, 17-19
aseptic technique in, 18
bolus, 18
drug incompatibilities in, 18
guide for, 226-227
infusion of fluid in, 18
intermittent therapy, 18
Isoproterenol, 21, 210-211

K

Kanamycin, 131, 132
dosage for, 136

Kanamycin—cont'd
indications for use of, 134
Kendall's compound E, 188
Kidneys in drug elimination, 26, 35-36
Kininogens
in immune response, 157
in inflammatory response, 168
Klebsiella, 121, 133, 137

L

Lactic acid, 20
Lactose
as binder in tablet, 2
as diluent in tablet, 2
Laxatives, 23
Leptospira, 113
Leptospirosis, 123
Leukotaxine, 166
Levarterenol, 211
Librium; *see* Chlordiazepoxide
Lidocaine, 77-78, 221
Limbic area of brain, 75
Lincomycin, 143-144
Lipolysis and lipogenesis, 183
Liver
in drug metabolism, 26
in drug storage, 27
Lorazepam, 96
Lymphocytes, 183

M

Maalox, 6
Macrolides, 124-130
administration of, routes of, 130
anaphylactic reactions from, 129
antibacterial spectrum and resistance to, 127
dosages of, 130
indications for use, 128
pharmacokinetics of, 128
pharmacological activity of, 125-127
protein formation inhibition by, 126-127
Macrophages, 183
Magnesium
as lubricant in tablet, 2
and tetracycline, 42
Mannitol, 56
Mastitis, 123
streptococcal, bovine, 115
Meclofenamic acid
action of, 68
as gastrointestinal tract irritant, 8
Medroxyprogesterone, 8
Membrane potential, 61

Meperidine, 69
  administration of, 74
  indications for, 74
  piperidine ring of, 63
Mephobarbital, 101
Meprobamate, 96
Meralluride, 54
  biliary excretion of, 37
Mercaptomerin, 54
Mercurophylline, 54
Metacresol, 83
Methampyrone, 67
Methazolamide, 50
Methemoglobin, 65
Methicillin, 113
Methoxyflurane, 78
Methylcothiazide, 52
Methylparaben, 83
Methylprednisolone, 190
  as gastrointestinal tract irritant, 8
  relative activity of, 170
Metritis, 123, 128
Miconazole, 140
Microsporium, 139
Milk in drug excretion, 35, 37
Mineralocorticoids, 169, 172
Minocycline, 124
Monocytes, 183
Morphine, 69, 71-73
  action of, 71
  administration of, 72
  antidotes for, 72
  with atropine, 72
  idiosyncratic responses to, 72
  metabolism of, 72
  overdosages of, 72
  in opium, 69
  in paregoric, 70
  vs pentazocine, 68
  stimulatory phase of, 71-72
  in tincture of opium, 70
  toxicity with, 72
Mucus of gastrointestinal tract, 5
Mycobacterium, 121
Mylanta, 6
Myocardium
  diseases of, 207
  electrical impulses throughout, 214
Myofibrils, 204, 205
  interconnection of, 206

N

Nafcillin, 113
Nalbuphine hydrochloride, 71

Nalorphine, 72
Naloxone, 72
Naproxen, 68
  prostaglandins affected by, 193
  structure of, 63
Necrosin, 166
Negative nitrogen balance, 172
Neisseria, 138
Neomycin, 131, 135, 191
  dosage for, 136
Neuron, central nervous system
  depolarization of, 62
  impulse transmittance in, 61
  refractory period of, 62
  repolarization of, 62
  stimulation of, 61-62
Norepinephrine, 211
  tranquilizer effects on, 91
Nystatin, 141, 191

O

Ointments, 19-20
  endodermic bases, 19
  epidermic bases, 19
  hydrophobic vs hydrophilic, 20
Oleaginous depot for drug administration, 16-17
Oleandomycin, 124
  side effects of, 129
Opiate analgesics, 69-73
  acetylcholinesterase inhibition via, 69-70
  codeine, 73
  morphine, 71-73
  oxymorphone, 73
  paregoric, 70
  semisynthetic, 73
  tincture of opium, 70
Opium
  derivatives of, as analgesics, 62, 63, 68
  source of, 69
  structure of, 69
  tincture of, 70
Organomercurials, 53-54
Oxacillin
  acid resistance of, 113
  as acid-stable drug, 5
Oxybarbiturates, 80, 83
Oxymorphone, 73
Oxyphenbutazone, 67
  as anti-inflammatory drug, 192
Oxytetracycline, 122
  as acid-stable drug, 5
  bacterial spectrum of, 123, 124
  indications for use, 124

P

Paramethadione, 100, 101
Parasites, 153
Paregoric, 70
Pasteurella, 137
Pasteurellosis, 123
Patent ductus arteriosus, 207
Pellets, 16
Penicillin
  with aminophylline, 40
  antibacterial spectrum of, 112-113
  bacteriostatic vs bacteriocidal activity of, 112
  biliary excretion of, 37
  dosages of, 112
  general formula of, 110
  hematologic side effects of, 145
  pharmacologic activity of, 112
  with probenecid, 41
  renal tubular secretion of, 36
  resistance to, 112-113
    acid, 113-114
  semisynthetic derivatives of, 111-116
    manufacture of, 4
  with sulfonamides, 150
  temperature effect on, 112
  with vitamin administration, 18
Penicillin G, 114-115
  as acid-labile drug, 3
    alterations affecting, 4
  as acid-stable drug, 5
  administration of, routes of, 115
  distribution of, 114
  dosage ranges of, 115
  resistance to, 107
  semisynthetic derivatives of, 108, 111
  structure of, 110
Penicillin V, 5
Penicillin VK, 113
Penicillinase, 108, 113
  in affecting macrolides, 127
Pentazocine, 68
  piperidine ring of, 63
Pentobarbital
  as anesthetic, 88
  as hypnotic, 88
  as short-acting barbiturate, 87
Pepsin, 13
Perphenazine, 94
Phenacetin, 65
Phenaglycodal, 96
Phenanthrene narcotics, 69
Phenethicillin, 5, 108
Phenobarbital, 87, 101
  absorption and excretion of, 88

Phenothiazines, 93-95
  as antihistamines, 200
  effects of, 93
  recommended dose for, 94
  structure of, 93
Phenylbutazone, 67
  as anti-inflammatory drug, 192
  with barbiturates, 42
  as gastrointestinal tract irritant, 8
Phenylhydroxylamine, 65
Phenytoin, 98, 99, 100
  as cardiac depressant, 221-222
  with steroid therapy, 186
Phlebitis, 17
Picrotoxin, 208
Piperazine salts, 23
Placenta
  diuretics crossing, 49-50
  drug passage through, 28
Pneumonia, cattle, 128
Polymyxin, 136, 137-138
  absorption of, 21
  neurotoxic effects of, 137
  surfactant activity of, 137
Polypeptide antibiotics, 136-138
Polythiazide, 52
Potassium chloride
  intramuscular administration of, 15
  in tablets, 6
Potassium ions
  hormonal regulation of, 169
  in membrane potentials, 61
  in neuron depolarization, 62
  opiate effect on, 69
  renal tubular secretion of, 36
  thiazide effect on, 51
Potassium phenoxymethyl penicillin, 4
Prednisolone, 191
  relative activity of, 170
Prednisone, 191
  as gastrointestinal tract irritant, 8
  relative activity of, 170
Pressoreceptors, 59
Primidone, 100
  structure of, 101
Probenecid with penicillin, 41
Procainamide, 220-221
Procaine, 77-78
  with intramuscular injections, 16
Proenzymes, 54
Promazine, 94
Promethazine, 197
Prontosil, 147
Propranolol, 223-224

Proprioceptors, 60
Propylparaben, 83
Prostaglandins
  in immune response, 157
  in inflammatory response, 168
  inhibition of synthesis of, 174
  nonsteroidal anti-inflammatory drug effects on,
     193, 194
  salicylate effect on, 64
Protein
  catabolism of, 172
  glucocorticosteroid effect on, 184
Proteus, 133
Providencia, 133
Pseudomonas, 117, 133
Purkinje fibers, 205, 206, 207
Pyrazolone derivatives, 66-67
  action of, 66
  as analgesics, 62, 63
  metabolism of, 66
  plasma-binding ability of, 67

Q

Quinidine, 217-220
  indications for use, 220
  pharmacokinetics of, 218
  pharmacological action of, 217-218
  side effects and drug interactions, 220

R

Reticular formation of brain, 92
Ringworm, 138
Ruminants, 14

S

Salicylazosulfapyridine, 148
Salicylic acid (salicylates)
  absorption of, 64-65
  as antifungal drug, 141
  anti-inflammatory effect of, 64
  antipyretic activity of, 64
  derivatives of, as analgesics, 62
  distribution and excretion of, 64-65
  with ointments, 20
  pain relief from, 64
Saliva in drug excretion, 35, 37
Salmonella, 121, 133, 137
Secobarbital
  as anesthetic, 88
  as hypnotic, 88
  pH of, 11

Secobarbital—cont'd
  as short-acting barbiturate, 87
  solubility of, 11
Sedation, 85
  via barbiturates, 90
  via tranquilizers, 90
Sedatives, 69
Seizures, 97
  triggering of, 98
Semen, 35, 37
Serratia, 133
Shigella, 121, 133, 137
Silica gel, 2
Sinoatrial node, 204, 205
Small intestine, 9-10
Sodium bicarbonate
  in salicylate excretion, 65
  in sodium reabsorption, 49
  in tablets, 2
Sodium ions
  aldosterone in uptake of, 169
  carbonic anhydrase effect on, 49
  carbonic anhydrase inhibitors and, 49
  hormonal regulation of, 169
  hydantoin drug effects on, 100
  in membrane potential, 61
  in neuron stimulation, 61-62
  opiate effect on, 69
  thiazide effect on, 51
  vs urine output, 47-48
Sodium pump, 62, 69
Sodium salicylate, 65
Spironolactone, 54
Status epilepticus, 97
Steroids
  with antibiotics, 18
  inhalation of, 21
  intramuscular injections of, 16
  and pyrazolone derivatives of, 67
Stomach, 3
Strangles, 123
Streptomycin, 131
  biliary excretion of, 37
  dosage for, 136
  indications for use, 134-135
  with sulfonamides, 150
  toxic reactions from, 135
Subcutaneous injections, 16
Succinylcholine, 132
Sulfacetamide, 100
  structure of, 148
Sulfadimethoxine, 148
Sulfamethazine, 148
Sulfapyridine, 147

Sulfisoxazole, 147
  for ophthalmic use, 150
Sulfonamides, 147-154
  action of, 149
  antibacterial spectrum of, 150
  blood dyscrasias with, 151
  detoxification of, 151
  dose determination of, 39
  indications for use, 152-153
  nutritional status as factor in distribution of, 33
  partition coefficients for, 150, 157
  pharmocokinetics of, 150-151
  pharmacological activity of, 149
  principles of therapy with, 152
  with pyrazolone derivatives, 67
  renal precipitation of, 42
  resistance to, 150
  side effects of, 150, 151-152
  structure of, 147-148
    vs PABA structure, 149
  toxicity of, 152
  with warfarin, 42
Superinfections, 146
Suppositories, 15
Sweat, 35, 37
Sympathomimetic amines, 208-212
  administration precautions and drug interactions, 211-212
  epinephrine, 209, 210
  isoproterenol, 209, 210-211
  levarterenol, 209, 211
  pharmacological actions of, 208-210
Syncytium, 206
Systole, 204

T

Tablets, 2
Talwin, 68
Tetracycline
  as acid-stable drug, 5
  administration of, routes of, 123
  adverse effect of, on teeth, 130
  antibacterial spectrum and resistance of, 121-122
  biliary excretion of, 37
  with calcium or magnesium ions, 42
  chelating ability of, 120
  dosage ranges for, 123
  inactivation of, with milk, 6
  indications for use, 123, 124
  pH of, 9
  pharmacokinetics of, 122
  pharmacological activity of, 120
  structure of, 119

Thalamus, 64
Theophylline, 208
Therapeutic index, 40-41
Thiabutazide, 52
Thiamylal sodium, 83-84
Thiazides, 51-52
  acidosis from, 51
  side effects of, 51
  toxicity of, 52
Thiobarbiturates, 80, 83
  administration of, 84
Thiopental, 83-84
  and diluents, 83
  distribution of, 81
  plasma concentration of, 81
Ticarcillin, 113
Tincture of opium, 70
Tobramycin, 131, 133
  indications for use, 134
Toxins, 165
Toxoids, 158, 160, 161
Tranquilizers, 90-102
  acetylpromazine, 94
  anticonvulsants, 97-102
  benzodiazepines, 95-97
  biochemical activity changes with, 91-92
  butyrophenones, 95
  chlorpromazine, 94
  CNS electrical function changes with, 92
  CNS neurotransmitter concentration changes with, 91
  meprobamate, 96
  minor, 96
  perphenazine, 94
  pharmacology of, 91-93
  phenaglycodal, 96
  phenothiazines, 93-95
  promazine, 94
  purpose of, 59
  and pyrazolone derivatives, 67
  trimeprazine, 94-95
Trauma
  antihistamine effect on, 198
  and inflammatory responses, 165-168
  types of, 165
Triamcinolone, 191-192
  relative activity of, 170
Trichlormethiazide, 52
Trichophyton, 138
Trimeprazine, 94, 95
Trimethadione, 100
d-Tubocurarine, 132
Tylosin, 124, 129
  structure of, 125

U

Ulcer, gastric, 5
  glucocorticosteroid effect on, 184
Ulcer, peptic, 186
Ulcerative colitis, 14
Undecylenic acid, 141
Urine
  alkalinization of, 151
  excretion of, 47
Urea, 56

V

Vaccination, 155
Vaccine, 158, 159
  autogenous, 159
  bacterial, 159

Vaccine—cont'd
  monovalent vs polyvalent, 159
Vagus nerve, 204
Valium; *see* Diazepam
Ventricles, 206
Verapamil, 224-225
Vibriosis in cattle, 123
Visceral receptors, 60
Vitamins, 18
  K, in drug interaction, 43

W

Warfarin, 42
Wound healing, 183

Z

Zomepirac sodium, 193, 194